Women and Exercise:
Physiology and Sports Medicine
2nd Edition

MONA M. SHANGOLD, M.D.
Professor of Obstetrics and Gynecology
Director, Division of Reproductive Endocrinology
Director of the Sports Gynecology and Women's Life Cycle Center
Hahnemann University
Philadelphia, Pennsylvania

GABE MIRKIN, M.D.
Associate Clinical Professor
Georgetown University School of Medicine
Washington, D.C.

 F. A. DAVIS COMPANY • Philadelphia

F. A. Davis Company
1915 Arch Street
Philadelphia, PA 19103

ICOS2I079f

Printed in the United States of America

Last digit indicates print number: 10 9 8 7 6 5 4 3 2 1

Acquisitions Editor: Robert H. Craven
Medical Developmental Editor: Bernice M. Wissler
Production Editor: Gail Shapiro
Cover Design By: Donald B. Freggens, Jr.

As new scientific information becomes available through basic and clinical research, recommended treatments and drug therapies undergo changes. The author(s) and publisher have done everything possible to make this book accurate, up to date, and in accord with accepted standards at the time of publication. The authors, editors, and publisher are not responsible for errors or omissions or for consequences from application of the book, and make no warranty, expressed or implied, in regard to the contents of the book. Any practice described in this book should be applied by the reader in accordance with professional standards of care used in regard to the unique circumstances that may apply in each situation. The reader is advised always to check product information (package inserts) for changes and new information regarding dose and contraindications before administering any drug. Caution is especially urged when using new or infrequently ordered drugs.

Library of Congress Cataloging-in-Publication Data

Women and exercise : physiology and sports medicine / [edited by] Mona
    M. Shangold, Gabe Mirkin.—Ed. 2.
        p.   cm.
    Includes bibliographical references and index.
    ISBN 0-8036-7817-7
    1. Women athletes—Physiology.   2. Exercise for women-
-Physiological aspects.   3. Sports for women—Physiological aspects.
    4. Sports medicine.   I. Shangold, Mona M.   II. Mirkin, Gabe.
    [DNLM: 1. Physical Fitness.   2. Sports.   3. Sports Medicine.
    4. Women.   5. Exercise.   QT 260 W8715 1993]
    RC1218.W65W65 1993
    613.7′11′082—dc20
    DNLM/DLC   93-17937
    for Library of Congress   CIP

To Kenneth,
Our greatest treasure
and
Our greatest joy

Preface to the Second Edition

The success and warm reception of the first edition and the many advances in this field have led to the development of this second edition, in which all material has been updated and expanded. Much has happened since the publication of the first edition: Women athletes have set many new records; researchers have devoted increased attention to the consequences of exercise for women; clinicians have devoted greater attention to the needs and concerns of exercising women; and increasing numbers of female couch potatoes have acknowledged that exercise is beneficial and desirable.

The contributors remain accepted authorities and leaders in their fields. The same blend of basic and clinical science is presented, providing comprehensive coverage for both researchers and clinicians. Those caring for athletic women have shared their vast experience in a valuable composite of science and art. We believe this edition is even better than the first, and we hope it will surpass the first edition in providing satisfaction and inspiration.

Mona Shangold, M.D.
Gabe Mirkin, M.D.

Preface to the First Edition

We have prepared this book to assist physicians and other health care professionals in caring for women who exercise. Included are chapters covering the many fields necessary to provide comprehensive care to women who range from novice exercisers to elite athletes and who may require information about training, health maintenance, treatment of disease or injury, and rehabilitation. Chapters have been written by leading authorities in each of these fields to supply the necessary depth of scientific background and clinical experience. In each case, relevant basic science is explained, and pertinent literature is reviewed and interpreted. When sufficient data are present, most authors have outlined and justified their personal recommendations, based on these data. Because clinical medicine often requires action even when sufficient data are lacking or inconclusive, many contributors have outlined their advice for these situations, based on their own expertise and clinical experience. We believe readers will find these recommendations invaluable.

Contributors to this volume include both basic scientists and practicing physicians. We purposely have encouraged some basic scientists and clinicians to cover the same topics from their different perspectives. We feel that this approach adds greatly to the value of this book.

Although elementary textbooks must oversimplify in order to teach students, this book is aimed at scientists and educators, who appreciate that research may, at times, lead to conflicting conclusions and different recommendations based upon these conclusions. We are confident that the sophisticated reader will find the controversy generated by these different perspectives refreshing, stimulating, and representative of the state of the art in this field.

No other book to date has covered so many relevant topics dealing with exercise and sports medicine for women in the depth that is provided in this volume. We hope this volume meets the needs of generalists caring for women athletes and specialists wanting information outside of their own specialty. Above all, we hope it will enable exercising women to receive the best care possible.

Mona Shangold, M.D.
Gabe Mirkin, M.D.

Contributors

Oded Bar-Or, M.D.
Professor of Pediatrics
Director, Children's Exercise and Nutrition
  Centre
McMaster University
Hamilton, Ontario, Canada

Kelly D. Brownell, Ph.D.
Professor of Psychology
Professor of Epidemiology and Public
  Health
Co-Director, Yale Center for Eating and
  Weight Disorders
Yale University
New Haven, Connecticut

Marshall W. Carpenter, M.D.
Associate Professor, Obstetrics and
  Gynecology
Brown University
Director of Maternal-Fetal Medicine
Department of Obstetrics and Gynecology
Women and Infants Hospital of Rhode
  Island
Providence, Rhode Island

David H. Clarke, Ph.D.
Chair, Department of Kinesiology
University of Maryland
College Park, Maryland

Pamela S. Douglas, M.D.
Director of NonInvasive Cardiology
Beth Israel Hospital

Associate Professor of Medicine
Harvard Medical School
Boston, Massachusetts

Thomas D. Fahey, Ed.D.
Professor of Physical Education
California State University
Chico, California

Catherine Gilligan, B.A.
Associate Researcher
Biogerontology Laboratory
University of Wisconsin
Madison, Wisconsin

Letha Y. Griffin, M.D., Ph.D.
Staff Physician,
Peachtree Orthopaedic Clinic
Team Physician,
Georgie State University
Atlanta, Georgia

Carlos M. Grilo, Ph.D.
Director of Psychology
Yale Psychiatric Institute
Assistant Professor in
  Psychiatry
Yale University School of Medicine
New Haven, Connecticut

Christine Haycock, M.D.
Professor Emeritus
UMDNJ, New Jersey Medical School
Newark, New Jersey

Jack L. Katz, M.D.
Professor of Clinical Psychiatry
Cornell University Medical College
New York, New York
Chairman, Department of Psychiatry
North Shore University Hospital
Manhasset, New York

Robert M. Malina, Ph.D.
Professor
Departments of Kinesiology and Health
  Education and of Anthropology
University of Texas
Austin, Texas

Gabe Mirkin, M.D.
Associate Clinical Professor
Georgetown University School of Medicine
Washington, D.C.

Morris Notelovitz, M.D., Ph.D.
President and Medical Director
Women's Medical and Diagnostic Center
The Climacteric Clinic, Inc. and
  Midlife Centers of America, Inc.
Gainesville, Florida

Mary L. O'Toole, Ph.D.
Associate Professor
Director, Human Performance Laboratory
University of Tennessee-Campbell Clinic

Department of Orthopaedic Surgery
Memphis, Tennessee

Mona M. Shangold, M.D.
Professor of Obstetrics and Gynecology
Director, Division of Reproductive
  Endocrinology
Director of the Sports Gynecology and
  Women's Life Cycle Center
Hahnemann University
Philadelphia, Pennsylvania

Arthur J. Siegel, M.D.
Assistant Professor of Medicine
Harvard Medical School
Chief, Internal Medicine Department
McLean Hospital
Belmont, Massachusetts

Everett L. Smith, Ph.D.
Director, Biogerontology Laboratory
Department of Preventive Medicine
University of Wisconsin
Madison, Wisconsin

Denise E. Wilfley, Ph.D.
Research Scientist and Lecturer
Clinical Director Department of Psychology
Yale Center for Eating and Weight
  Disorders
Yale University
New Haven, Connecticut

Contents

I

Basic Concepts of Exercise Physiology

CHAPTER 1

Fitness: Definition and Development

MARY L. O'TOOLE, Ph.D., and PAMELA S. DOUGLAS, M.D.

COMPONENTS OF FITNESS
Muscular Strength and Endurance
Body Composition
Flexibility
Cardiovascular-Respiratory Capacity

BENEFITS OF FITNESS
For Healthy Individuals
Medical Implications

FITNESS EVALUATION
Muscular Strength and Endurance
Body Composition

Flexibility
Functional Capacity

FITNESS DEVELOPMENT AND
 MAINTENANCE
Fitness Development
Fitness Maintenance
Factors Affecting Fitness
 Development and Maintenance

TRAINING FOR COMPETITION
Interval Training
Cross Training

T he term "physical fitness" connotes a state of optimal physical well-being. However, a universally accepted definition of physical fitness is difficult to find. Cureton,[1] a pioneer in the fitness movement, defined it as "the ability to handle the body well and the capacity to work hard over a long period of time without diminished efficiency." Others have used physical fitness to describe a quality of life rather than a precise set of conditions. For example, in monographs published by the President's Council on Physical Fitness[2,3] to offer guidance to those interested in improving their physical fitness, a physically fit individual is described as one able to perform vigorous work without undue fatigue and still have enough energy left for enjoying hobbies and recreational activities, as well as for meeting emergencies. Exercise physiology texts[4-8] have similar descriptive rather than quantitative definitions of physical fitness. For example, Lamb[6] defines it as "the capacity to meet successfully the present and potential physical challenges of life." So, despite all the interest generated by physical fitness, a need remains for a clear definition of fitness to allow accurate assessment of an individual's level of fitness.

The most successful definitions used to quantify "fitness" have been based on its measurable components. Muscular strength and endurance, body com-

3

position, flexibility, and cardiovascular-respiratory capacity are generally agreed upon as the major components of physical fitness.[9] Therefore, for the purposes of this text, an operational measure of fitness based on combined capabilities in these four components will be assumed to quantify an individual's level of physical fitness.

A further problem in evaluating fitness is the wide variation in individual need for physical work capacity. For example, an adult who wishes to enjoy optimal health must maintain a certain degree of physical fitness, while a competitive ultraendurance athlete needs to maintain a greater capacity for physical work. Therefore, the adequacy of one's physical fitness cannot be judged simply by the attainment of some magic number. However, normative values for the parameters of muscular strength and endurance, body composition, flexibility, and cardiovascular-respiratory capacity have been developed based on age, gender, and habitual activity level.[10–12] An interested individual can compare her own values to the appropriate (based on desired activity level) normative values to assess the adequacy of her "fitness level."

COMPONENTS OF FITNESS

Muscular Strength and Endurance

Muscular strength refers to the force or tension that can be generated by a muscle or muscle group during one maximal effort.[5,6,9] Muscular endurance is the ability to perform many repetitions at submaximal loads.[5,6,13] For example, it takes a certain amount of strength to lift and swing a tennis racquet, but it takes muscular endurance to repeat that swing hundreds of times during the course of a 2-hour match. An individual may have a great deal of strength but little endurance, or may have extraordinary strength in one muscle group but not in others. Although women usually have a smaller muscle fiber area and, therefore, lower absolute strength levels than men, the trainability of

their muscles for strength and endurance performance is similar to that of men. The topics of muscular strength and endurance are covered in detail in Chapters 3 and 4.

Body Composition

Body composition makes an important contribution to an individual's level of physical fitness. Performance, particularly in activities that require one to carry one's body weight over distance, will be facilitated by a large proportion of active tissue (muscle) in relation to a small proportion of inactive tissue (fat).[14] In general, women have a greater percentage of fat than do men, whether trained or untrained. Therefore, when performing a weight-bearing activity such as distance running, women tend to be at a disadvantage compared with their male counterparts. The role of exercise in reaching and maintaining a desirable weight and percentage of body fat is discussed at length in Chapter 2.

Flexibility

Flexibility is the degree to which body segments can move or be moved around a joint.[5,6] The flexibility, or range of motion around a particular joint, is determined by the configuration of bony structures and the length and elasticity of ligaments, tendons, and muscles surrounding the joint.[5,6] Although there are no research data to support the concept that flexibility aids in coordinated movements, it certainly makes sense that by allowing free movement without unnecessary restriction, the body's efficiency and grace would be increased and the potential for injury reduced.[15]

Cardiovascular-Respiratory Capacity

The cardiovascular-respiratory component of fitness reflects the integrity of the heart and lungs as well as the ability of the muscle cells to use oxygen as fuel. It therefore reflects the degree to which an individual can increase metabolism above resting levels.[4-6,8,9] Incremental tests up to maximal oxygen uptake ($\dot{V}O_2$ max) are used to measure this component and to define the limits of physical work capacity. This measurement is considered to be the best single measure of an individual's overall functional capacity.[16] This and other measures of fitness will be discussed below.

BENEFITS OF FITNESS

Regular physical activity, resulting in fitness, has benefits to disease-free individuals as well as implications for the medical care of individuals with certain diseases.[4,17,18,20-23,25-28] There is general agreement that exercise performed by healthy individuals has both physical and psychologic benefits, including improved physical performance and enhanced quality of life. In contrast, although exercise clearly does not change the course of most diseases, there are certain medical implications that are important.

For Healthy Individuals

Physical Benefits

In reviewing the physiologic aspects of exercise in women, Drinkwater[17] cites numerous studies that support the hypothesis that women of all ages benefit from programs of physical conditioning. The observed changes in the women are similar to those in men and include increases in maximal aerobic capacity, maximal minute ventilation, O_2 pulse, and increases in submaximal work performance.[18,19] With training, one can perform the same amount of work with lower heart and respiratory rates and with a lower systolic blood pressure. Some studies show that beneficial effects occur after as little as 4 weeks of training.[17] Improvements reported by Getchell and Moore[27] are typical of the expected responses; that is, middle-

aged women and men responded to the exercise training program in a similar fashion, with a 21% increase in aerobic capacity and a 6% decrease in submaximal heart rates during posttraining exercise tests.

There have also been suggestions that exercise may affect longevity, or that a "reversal of aging" may occur. A number of epidemiologic studies have attempted to examine the long-term effects of exercise upon longevity. Although no study has yet demonstrated a negative effect, in general such studies may have limited applicability because of the many methodologic problems inherent in choosing subject populations for this type of study. From the viewpoint of this text, of primary importance is the fact that few have examined female populations. Other limitations include the inclusion of ex-athletes who may have had intense exercise training for short periods of time; classification of activity level based on workplace activity; and the interaction of a number of covariables such as obesity, smoking, environment, other life habits, and importantly, concomitant medical diseases.

Exercise training, however, has been well documented to modify or retard aspects of the aging process.[20,21] Exercise training slows the normal age-related declines in peak performance and maximal aerobic capacity, and it retards the loss of muscle and bone mass and the increase in body fat. The exercising older woman has an aerobic capacity and body composition similar to those of much younger, sedentary women.[22,23] It has been suggested that the rate of decline in many physiologic parameters may be reduced by approximately 50% in physically fit as compared with sedentary women.[24]

Psychologic Benefits

Although subjective parameters are extraordinarily difficult to measure, and a small number of participants may note a negative effect of exercise, it is generally thought that fitness leads to an improved quality of life. In several studies, the majority of participants in an exercise program noted an enhancement of mood, self-confidence, and feelings of satisfaction, achievement, and self-sufficiency.[25-28] Interestingly, in one study, those with the greatest improvement in endurance also had a more marked improvement on psychologic testing.[25] In general, women who exercise regularly are more likely to be more comfortable with day-to-day physical exertion and to have reduced anxiety and an improved body image.[26-28]

Medical Implications

Women with medical illnesses may have a lower level of fitness than their counterparts in a comparable but healthy, sedentary population. Although this may be due to limitations imposed by either the primary or an associated illness, it may also be related to the adoption of a less active lifestyle. In the latter case, increased fitness through participation in regular exercise programs encourages the patient to increase her level of activity in daily life and in recreation, thus yielding at least a subjective improvement in health.

Fitness or exercise training may have salutary effects upon specific medical disease in three ways: (1) as primary prevention (e.g., in modifying factors known to increase the risk of acquiring heart disease); (2) as secondary prevention or modification of the natural history of a disorder (e.g., decreases in both systolic and diastolic resting blood pressures); and (3) for rehabilitation or palliation of a specific disorder. The last is more closely related to task-specific exercise and is beyond our consideration of the benefits of overall fitness.

Cardiovascular Disease

Coronary Artery Disease. Although coronary artery disease is more common in men, it is the leading cause of death in women as well. Studies examining the effects of fitness upon the risk of developing coronary artery disease find either a re-

duced or, less often, an unchanged risk associated with higher levels of physical activity.[29,31-36] Unfortunately, methodologic problems similar to those inherent in studies of longevity also limit the applicability of many of these studies to women. One prospective study that did include 3120 women reported a decrease in both all-cause and cardiovascular disease mortality rates in physically fit versus inactive women.[30]

The amount of activity necessary to reduce cardiovascular risk is similarly unclear. It appears that no amount of exercise will lower the incidence of cardiovascular disease in those at especially high risk. However, in women at "usual" risk, it is likely that, as with men, moderate amounts of exercise are protective, with benefit accruing to those expending 200 to 500 kcal/d or 2000 kcal/wk pursuing vigorous activity. No studies have yet been performed to document this effect in women.[37-39] Although most studies have examined the effects of aerobic exercise, studies have shown that cardiovascular endurance may be increased by resistive exercise as well.[40]

The mechanisms by which exercise may improve cardiovascular health are unclear. Certainly, training enhances cardiac efficiency, allowing a given work rate to be achieved at a lower heart rate and blood pressure level. This is equally true in the healthy individual and in a patient with known coronary disease. Table 1-1 groups these and other physiologic changes occurring in the cardiovascular system with exercise according to the method by which they might prevent coronary heart disease, additionally noting the likelihood of each adaptation of being an important factor in prevention.[41] The beneficial effects of exercise are likely multifactorial, and the mechanisms are still unclear.

Exercise may also affect cardiovascular disease by altering risk factors for its development. In healthy women, higher levels of fitness, as determined by exercise duration on treadmill testing, have been associated with lower body weight, a lower percentage of body fat, lower incidence of cigarette

Table 1-1. BIOLOGIC MECHANISMS BY WHICH EXERCISE MAY CONTRIBUTE TO THE PRIMARY OR SECONDARY PREVENTION OF CORONARY HEART DISEASE*

Maintain or increase myocardial oxygen supply
  Delay progression of coronary atherosclerosis (possible).
    Improve lipoprotein profile (increase HDL-C/LDL-C ratio) (probable).
    Improve carbohydrate metabolism (increase insulin sensitivity) (probable).
    Decrease platelet aggregation and increase fibrinolysis (probable).
    Decrease adiposity (usually).
  Increase coronary collateral vascularization (unlikely).
  Increase coronary blood flow (myocardial perfusion) or distribution (unlikely).
Decrease myocardial work and oxygen demand
  Decrease heart rate at rest and submaximal exercise (usually).
  Decrease systolic and mean systemic arterial pressure during submaximal exercise (usually) and at rest (possible).
  Decrease cardiac output during submaximal exercise (probable).
  Decrease circulating plasma catecholamine levels (decrease sympathetic tone) at rest (probable) and at submaximal exercise (usually).
Increase myocardial function
  Increase stroke volume at rest and in submaximal and maximal exercise (likely).
  Increase ejection fraction at rest and in exercise (possible).
  Increase intrinsic myocardial contractility (unlikely).
  Increase myocardial function resulting from decreased "afterload" (probable).
  Increase myocardial hypertrophy (probable); but this may not reduce CHD risk.
Increase electrical stability of myocardium
  Decrease regional ischemia at rest or at submaximal exercise (possible).
  Decrease catecholamines in myocardium at rest and at submaximal exercise (probable).
  Increase ventricular fibrillation threshold due to reduction in cyclic AMP (possible).

*Expression of likelihood that effect will occur for an individual participating in endurance-type training program for 16 wk or longer at 65–80% of functional capacity for 25 min or longer per session (300 kcal) for 3 or more sessions per week ranges from unlikely, possible, likely, probable, to usually.
Abbreviations: HDL-C = high-density lipoprotein cholesterol; LDL-C = low-density lipoprotein cholesterol; CHD = coronary heart disease; AMP = adenosine monophosphate.
Source: Haskell,[41] p. 65, with permission.

smoking, lower systolic and diastolic blood pressures, lower total cholesterol with a higher high-density lipoprotein (HDL) subfraction, lower triglycerides, and, most importantly, a lower incidence of cardiovascular disease and lower mortality rate.[42] Using multiple regression analysis, Gibbons and colleagues[42] demonstrated independent associations between fitness level and lipid profiles, blood pressure, and smoking, suggesting that risk factors for coronary heart disease may be modified by fitness level. Other studies have partly confirmed these results, finding more favorable lipid profiles in active women;[43] however, an exercise-related increase in HDL cholesterol has been demonstrated only in men, not in women.[44]

The benefits of exercise in the modification of preexisting coronary disease are much less clear. At least one well-controlled study in men with heart disease showed a modest decrease in deaths due to myocardial infarction, with a trend toward a reduction in deaths from all causes in individuals pursuing exercise programs.[45] Although cardiac patients are generally encouraged to avoid resistive exercise because of the resultant unfavorable cardiac-loading conditions, some successfully used forms of exercise (e.g., rowing, bicycling) have significant resistive as well as aerobic components. No study has demonstrated a harmful effect of carefully performed exercise in selected cardiac patients.

Hypertension. Appropriately tailored exercise programs have been shown to result in 5- to 10-mm decreases in both systolic and diastolic resting blood pressures.[46-48] Although the mechanisms of these changes are unknown, exercise may be a useful adjunct to more conventional therapy. Care must be taken in the exercise prescription, however, because the normal increases in systolic and diastolic blood pressure levels with exercise are enhanced in patients with hypertension. Further, exercise blood pressure has been correlated with left ventricular mass, an independent risk factor for cardiovascular mortality.[49] Thus, it is important for the hypertensive individual to pursue dynamic or aerobic types of exercise that have less marked increases in blood pressure than those requiring resistive activity.

Associated with hypertensive disease are cerebrovascular accidents. Exercise has been shown to enhance fibrinolysis and may therefore reduce the incidence of or morbidity from stroke.[50]

Obesity

The benefits of exercise with regard to obesity are discussed in detail in Chapter 2. Obesity is probably an independent risk factor for cardiovascular disease in both sexes; its reduction would therefore be expected to contribute to cardiac health.[51] Exercise clearly increases caloric expenditure through the effort necessary to maintain activity, favorably alters metabolic rate and heat production, and is useful in preserving muscle mass during dieting. In addition to the subjective enhancement of perceived health, the toning effects of exercise may have a positive effect on self-image and may therefore encourage the dieter to adhere to both exercise and dietary programs.

Osteoporosis

With aging, the mineral content of bone decreases much more rapidly in women than in men, such that, after menopause, up to 8% of bone mass may be lost per decade. Although this has been regarded as an inevitable effect of aging and hormonal changes, it is clearly accelerated by inactivity or disuse. Further, most studies of athletes engaged in weight-bearing exercise (e.g., not swimmers) have shown up to a 40% increase in bone mass over more sedentary control subjects.[52,53] Controlled trials, with or without calcium supplementation, have demonstrated that exercise may retard or even reverse the normal loss of bone mineral content.[54-56] Thus, stresses imposed by exercise may be beneficial in preventing osteoporosis. However, exercise is more effective when estrogen and calcium supplements are also given.

Selected Other Diseases

Exercise training has been found to be of benefit in a variety of other chronic diseases. In general, it improves cardiovascular function, muscle strength, endurance, flexibility, adjustment to disease, activity level, and overall well-being. Additional benefits may be specific to the underlying disease. For example, in patients with chronic obstructive airways disease, exercise is useful for ventilatory muscle training, increased tolerance of dyspnea, and reduction in associated anxiety.[57] In those with end-stage renal disease, exercise may lower blood pressure and otherwise modify cardiovascular risk.[58] Additionally, in patients with both insulin-dependent and insulin-independent diabetes mellitus, a regularly followed exercise regimen may decrease insulin resistance, requirements, and circulating levels and improve glucose tolerance, thereby decreasing all diabetic "complications," especially cardiovascular disease. In patients with depression, exercise seems to improve mood or at least provide a physical vigor important in counteracting affective illness.[59]

FITNESS EVALUATION

Muscular Strength and Endurance

The strength of a particular muscle group can be quantified in several ways. Maximal isometric strength is the force generated during a maximal contraction against immovable resistance. Strain gauge tensiometers have long been used to measure isometric strength. Maximal isotonic strength is the greatest amount of weight that can be moved through the full range of motion only once (one repetition maximum, or 1 RM). Free weights or various pulley devices can be used to measure isotonic strength. Isokinetic strength is a measure of the maximal force that can be generated throughout the range of motion at a constant speed. Sophisticated isokinetic dynamometers can measure both concentric and eccentric muscle performance at varying speeds. Muscular endurance can be assessed by multiple repetitions (e.g., 20 to 30 RM) either isotonically or isokinetically. As with the other components of physical fitness, individual needs or desire for muscular strength and endurance will vary. The choice of methods to evaluate muscle performance will depend, in part, on the importance that the exerciser places on this component of physical fitness. See Chapter 3 for a complete discussion of muscular strength and endurance.

Body Composition

Evaluation of body composition is based on the classification of body components as either lean body mass or body fat. Commonly used methods for assessing body composition are hydrostatic weighing, anthropometric and skinfold thickness measurements, and bioelectric impedance measurements. A further discussion of body weight and body composition can be found in Chapter 2.

Flexibility

Flexibility can be measured directly or assessed indirectly during movement tasks.[5] Direct measurement of resting or static range of motion around a specific joint can be obtained with a goniometer. Dynamic flexibility or movement around a particular joint during an activity can be measured by digitizing of video, high-speed film analysis, or electrogoniometers. For a complete assessment of movement during activity, range of motion must be measured simultaneously in several planes. A less precise assessment of flexibility can be obtained using field tests such as the sit-and-reach test of Wells and Dillon[60] or the trunk flexion/extension tests of Cureton.[1]

As with the other components of fitness, each individual's need for flexibility may differ. However, the prevailing clinical opinion is that a normal range of motion for each joint is necessary for pain-free movement. These normal values can be found in texts on athletic training[61] or physical therapy.[62] The need for any additional flexibility varies among individuals and with activity interests.[61]

Functional Capacity

Terminology

Oxygen uptake measurements or estimations used to quantify activity or exercise can be reported in several different ways. In absolute terms, it is simply liters of oxygen used per minute. Because 1 L of oxygen is roughly equivalent to 5 kcal,[9] the approximate energy cost for any particular activity level can be calculated. One disadvantage of using liters per minute is the discrepancy between energy costs for individuals of varying weights.[9] For example, a 200-lb man will consume more oxygen during activity (or even sitting at rest) than will a 100-lb woman. For this reason, oxygen uptake is more often reported as milliliters of oxygen consumed per kilogram of body weight per minute ($mL \cdot kg^{-1} \cdot min^{-1}$). This allows the energy cost of various tasks to be compared among individuals without the bias of body weight. It is in these terms that $\dot{V}O_2$ max is most often reported for athletes. Although a high $\dot{V}O_2$ max may be taken as a "badge of honor" by endurance athletes, it actually has poor predictive ability for sports performance.[4] Nonetheless, a high $\dot{V}O_2$ max is indicative of a large aerobic capacity. The highest $\dot{V}_{O_2}$ max reported in the literature for men is 14 $mL \cdot kg^{-1} \cdot min^{-1}$ higher than that reported for women.[63,64] (This apparent gender discrepancy will be discussed later.)

With the advent of large-scale exercise testing and prescription at hospitals, universities, and health clubs, energy expenditure has been classified in metabolic equivalents (METs). One MET is the equivalent of resting oxygen consumption taken in a sitting position. For an average man, that is approximately 250 mL/min, and for an average woman, 200 mL/min.[9] METs can also be expressed in terms of oxygen consumption per unit of body weight, in which case, 1 MET is equivalent to 3.5 mL/kg per minute ($mL \cdot kg^{-1} \cdot min^{-1}$). One MET is also equal to 1 kcal/kg per hour ($kcal \cdot kg^{-1} \cdot hr^{-1}$).[70] The MET cost of a particular exercise can be calculated by dividing the metabolic rate ($\dot{V}_{O_2}$) during exercise by the resting metabolic rate. The American College of Sports Medicine (ACSM) has constructed tables listing the energy cost in METs for walking, jogging, and running during a range of speeds and grades of the treadmill (Tables 1–2 and 1–3).[65] Similar tables have been constructed for MET levels during bicycle ergometry and bench-stepping (Tables 1–4 and 1–5).[65] These tables are equally applicable to men and women.

Measurement

Maximal oxygen uptake ($\dot{V}_{O_2}$ max) is the best single measure of the overall functional capacity of an individual. Since human metabolism depends on oxygen utilization, an indirect estimate of energy metabolism can be made by measuring the amount of oxygen required to perform a given task. Oxygen uptake is frequently used to quantify an individual's maximal exercise capacity.

$\dot{V}_{O_2}$ max can be calculated from the actual measurement of expired oxygen and carbon dioxide during any exercise task of sufficient intensity and duration to require maximal use of aerobic energy systems.[4,6,9] The most commonly used exercise tests make use of a treadmill, cycle ergometer, or rowing ergometer. Any other device, such as bench stepping or simulated stair-climbing machines, that can be calibrated to allow the quantification of the exercise work, can also be used.[66] The volume and concentration of respiratory gases is measured either breath by breath or averaged for a certain time period (e.g., 15 seconds), using some kind of volume-metering device such as a Tissot spirometer or volume transducer, along with oxygen and carbon dioxide analyzers. Commercial metabolic carts with these components are available.

Table 1–2. APPROXIMATE ENERGY REQUIREMENTS IN METS FOR HORIZONTAL AND GRADE WALKING

% Grade	mph / m/min	1.7 / 45.6	2.0 / 53.7	2.5 / 67.0	3.0 / 80.5	3.4 / 91.2	3.75 / 100.5
0		2.3	2.5	2.9	3.3	3.6	3.9
2.5		2.9	3.2	3.8	4.3	4.8	5.2
5.0		3.5	3.9	4.6	5.4	5.9	6.5
7.5		4.1	4.6	5.5	6.4	7.1	7.8
10.0		4.6	5.3	6.3	7.4	8.3	9.1
12.5		5.2	6.0	7.2	8.5	9.5	10.4
15.0		5.8	6.6	8.1	9.5	10.6	11.7
17.5		6.4	7.3	8.9	10.5	11.8	12.9
20.0		7.0	8.0	9.8	11.6	13.0	14.2
22.5		7.6	8.7	10.6	12.6	14.2	15.5
25.0		8.2	9.4	11.5	13.6	15.3	16.8

Source: American College of Sports Medicine,[65] with permission.

Table 1–3. ENERGY REQUIREMENTS IN METS FOR HORIZONTAL AND UPHILL JOGGING/ RUNNING*

a. Outdoors on Solid Surface

% Grade	mph m/min	5 134	6 161	7 188	7.5 201	8 215	9 241	10 268
0		8.6	10.2	11.7	12.5	13.3	14.8	16.3
2.5		10.3	12.3	14.1	15.1	16.1	17.9	19.7
5.0		12.0	14.3	16.5	17.7	18.8	21.0	23.2
7.5		13.8	16.4	18.9	20.2	21.6	24.1	26.6
10.0		15.5	18.5	21.4	22.8	24.3	27.2	
12.5		17.2	20.6	23.8	25.4	27.1		

b. On the Treadmill

% Grade	mph m/min	5 134	6 161	7 188	7.5 201	8 215	9 241	10 268
0		8.6	10.2	11.7	12.5	13.3	14.8	16.3
2.5		9.5	11.2	12.9	13.8	14.7	16.3	18.0
5.0		10.3	12.3	14.1	15.1	16.1	17.9	19.7
7.5		11.2	13.3	15.3	16.4	17.4	19.4	21.4
10.0		12.0	14.3	16.5	17.7	18.8	21.0	23.2
12.5		12.9	15.4	17.7	19.0	20.2	22.5	24.9
15.0		13.8	16.4	18.9	20.3	21.6	24.1	26.6

*Differences in energy expenditures are accounted for by the effects of wind resistance.
Source: American College of Sports Medicine,[65] with permission.

Most often the test is incremental, with the work rate increased at the beginning of each of several stages.[4,6,9] During an incremental test, oxygen uptake will increase in a linear relationship with the increasing work rate. The test protocol ideally should reflect the exercise capabilities of the subject population being tested. Healthy individuals can usually begin with a work rate that re-quires an oxygen uptake of approximately 24 $mL \cdot kg^{-1} \cdot min^{-1}$. Work increments should require 3 to 7 $mL \cdot kg^{-1} \cdot min^{-1}$ increases in oxygen uptake. Because of expected higher maximal capacities, endurance athletes can be started at work rates greater than 30 $mL \cdot kg^{-1} \cdot min^{-1}$ with increments of 3 to 7 $mL \cdot kg^{-1} \cdot min^{-1}$. Elderly women or those with known or suspected limitations should

Table 1–4. ENERGY EXPENDITURE IN METS DURING BICYCLE ERGOMETRY

Body Weight		Exercise Rate (kg/min and watts)							
kg	lb	300 50	450 75	600 100	750 125	900 150	1050 175	1200 200	(kg/min) (watts)
50	110	5.1	6.9	8.6	10.3	12.0	13.7	15.4	
60	132	4.3	5.7	7.1	8.6	10.0	11.4	12.9	
70	154	3.7	4.9	6.1	7.3	8.6	9.8	11.0	
80	176	3.2	4.3	5.4	6.4	7.5	8.6	9.6	
90	198	2.9	3.8	4.8	5.7	6.7	7.6	8.6	
100	220	2.6	3.4	4.3	5.1	6.0	6.9	7.7	

Note: $\dot{V}O_2$ for zero-load pedaling is approximately 550 mL/min for 70- to 80-kg subjects.
Source: American College of Sports Medicine,[65] with permission.

Table 1–5. ENERGY EXPENDITURE IN
METS DURING STEPPING AT DIFFERENT
RATES ON STEPS OF DIFFERENT HEIGHTS

Step Height		Steps/min			
cm	in	12	18	24	30
0	0	1.2	1.8	2.4	3.0
4	1.6	1.5	2.3	3.1	3.8
8	3.2	1.9	2.8	3.7	4.6
12	4.7	2.2	3.3	4.4	5.5
16	6.3	2.5	3.8	5.0	6.3
20	7.9	2.8	4.3	5.7	7.1
24	9.4	3.2	4.8	6.3	7.9
28	11.0	3.5	5.2	7.0	8.7
32	12.6	3.8	5.7	7.7	9.6
36	14.2	4.1	6.2	8.3	10.4
40	15.8	4.5	6.7	9.0	11.2

Source: American College of Sports Medicine,[65] with
permission.

begin much lower and increase the work
rate more gradually. Duration of the early
stages should be at least 2 minutes to ensure
gradual physiologic adjustments. The later
stages can be 1 minute in duration. When the
maximal capacity for aerobic energy transfer has been reached, a further increase in

work rate will not be accompanied by an increase in oxygen uptake.[6]

Because the direct measurement of maximal oxygen uptake depends on subject motivation and the use of rather elaborate laboratory equipment, various submaximal
laboratory tests and field tests have been de-
vised to estimate maximal aerobic capacity.
Many of the submaximal predictive tests are
based on a linear relationship between heart
rate and oxygen uptake.[4,6,9] The slope of this
line is unique to each individual and depends on state of training but not on gender
(Fig. 1–1). A widely used predictive test is
the Åstrand-Rhyming Nomogram.[4] This nomogram allows the prediction of $\dot{V}O_2$ max
from the heart rate attained during one 6-
minute work bout on a cycle ergometer, but
can also be used with a step-test protocol.
Alternately, if oxygen uptake and heart rate
are measured at two submaximal exercise
intensities, the line representing the relationship between heart rate and oxygen uptake can then be extrapolated to the age-pre-
dicted maximal heart rate (200 − age) and
$\dot{V}O_2$ max estimated (Fig. 1–2). McArdle and
associates[9] have also developed a set of

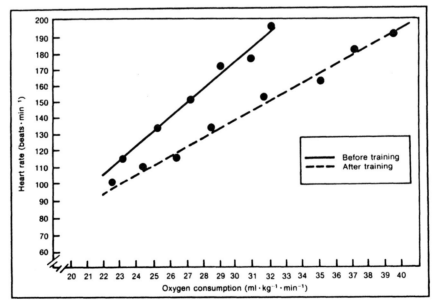

Figure 1–1. HR-$\dot{V}O_2$ line for a 20-year-old woman before and after a 10-week aerobic conditioning
program. (From McArdle, Katch, and Katch,[9] with permission.)

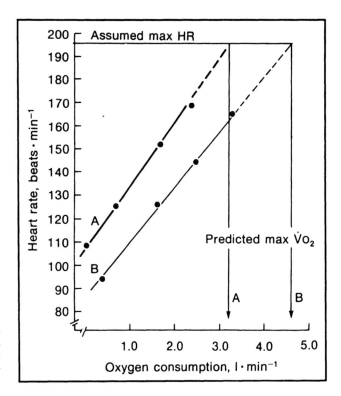

Figure 1–2. Application of the linear relationship between submaximal heart rate and oxygen consumption to predict $\dot{V}o_2$ max. (From McArdle, Katch, and Katch,[9] with permission.)

norms for the estimation of $\dot{V}o_2$ max from measurement of recovery heart rate following a bench-stepping protocol. Since one of the more practical uses of $\dot{V}o_2$ max test data is for monitoring an individual's progress in fitness programs over a period of time, it is unimportant which protocol is used as long as the same one is used in follow-up tests.

Several tests of distance covered in a given time period (walking, running, or a combination of the two) have also been used to predict aerobic capacity. The most widely known is the 12-minute walk/run test first suggested by Cooper in *Aerobics*.[67] Cooper[68] reported a correlation (based on tests of 47 male military personnel) of 0.90 between distance covered and maximal oxygen uptake actually measured in the laboratory. However, Maksud and colleagues,[69] repeating this correlation for women, reported a correlation of only 0.70 between actually measured oxygen uptake and distance covered, in a group of 26 female athletes. Katch and co-workers[70] noted a similarly low cor-

relation ($r = 0.67$) between these two measurements in 36 untrained female subjects. Because factors such as body weight, body fatness, and movement efficiency contribute to distance covered, these tests have error ranges of from 10% to 20% of actual maximal oxygen uptake.[9] They can be used only as a rough estimate of aerobic capacity.

Anaerobic Threshold

Traditionally, the term "anaerobic threshold" has been used to describe the level of exercise at which aerobic metabolism becomes insufficient to meet the required energy demands. This is assumed to be the point at which the resultant increase in anaerobic glycolysis causes lactate to accumulate in the muscles and blood.[6] Because this explanation is no doubt an oversimplification of the physiologic changes occurring, many investigators now avoid the term "anaerobic threshold" and prefer either "lactate breaking point" or "ventilation breaking point" to describe this alteration in metabolism.[71]

During light and moderate exercise, minute ventilation increases in a linear manner with increasing exercise intensity (oxygen uptake). However, at some point during the increasing exercise, the ventilation increases out of proportion to the increase in oxygen consumption. This point has been designated as the "ventilation breaking point." In an untrained individual, this point generally falls between 40% and 60% of $\dot{V}O_2$ max and is associated with a more rapid rise in blood lactate to a concentration of 2 millimoles (mmol) per liter (20 mg/dL blood). A second upswing in both ventilation and blood lactate can be seen at between 65% and 90% $\dot{V}O_2$ max and a lactate concentration of 4 mmol/L (36 mg/dL).[72] In highly trained athletes, these ventilation breaking points occur at higher percentages of $\dot{V}O_2$ max.

The mechanism of the ventilation breaking point has not been satisfactorily explained but is usually associated with the accumulation of lactic acid in the blood (hence, the appearance and rise of blood lactate).[6] The need to dispose of excess carbon dioxide produced from the buffering of excess hydrogen ions (from the lactic acid) drives the peripheral chemoreceptors that stimulate increased ventilation. Ventilation breaking points can be found during gas exchange measurements, whereas lactate breaking points can be found through frequent analysis of a small amount of blood, usually taken by a fingerstick. Most experiments with highly trained athletes use the 4-mmol value rather than the more reproducible 2-mmol value, since athletes can exercise for several hours with lactate values greater than 2 mmol but less than 4 mmol. As with the ventilation breaking point, there is no universally accepted explanation for the lactate breaking point. Among the explanations offered are increased production of lactate, decreased clearance of lactate, a combination of these two, and increased recruitment of fast-twitch (glycolytic) motor units.

FITNESS DEVELOPMENT AND MAINTENANCE

Fitness Development

Flexibility

Flexibility can best be improved through the use of sustained static stretches.[5,6,13] The muscles and connective tissue to be stretched should be slowly elongated to the point at which the exerciser feels a mild tension.[5,13] Usually, this position is then held for between 10 and 30 seconds.[13] During this time period, the exerciser should feel a gradual release of this feeling of tension as the stretch or myotatic reflex is overcome. As the tension is released, the exerciser should slowly move a fraction further, again to the point of tension, and continue to hold for approximately 30 seconds.[13] Stretching following an exercise session, when the muscle and connective tissues are warm, has been found to be the best time for improving flexibility.[6]

Cardiovascular Fitness

The ACSM has developed guidelines for building and maintaining fitness in healthy adults.[65,73] In recommending the quantity and quality of exercise, the ACSM cites five components that are applicable to the design of exercise programs for adults regardless of age, gender, or initial level of fitness: (1) type of activity, (2) intensity, (3) duration, (4) frequency, and (5) progression.

Type of Activity. The exercise program should include activities that use large muscle groups in a continuous rhythmic manner. Activities such as walking, hiking, jogging/running, swimming, bicycling, rowing, cross-country skiing, skating, dancing, and rope skipping are ideal. Because control of exercise intensity within rather precise limits is often desirable at the beginning of an exercise program, the most easily quantified activities, such as walking or stationary cycling, are particularly useful. Various endurance game activities such as field hockey, soccer, and lacrosse may also be suitable but may have high-intensity components, and therefore should not be used in the exercise prescription until participants are able to exercise comfortably at a minimum level of 5 METs.[65] If intensity, duration, and frequency are similar, the training result appears to be independent of the mode of aerobic activity. Therefore, a similar training effect on functional capacity can be expected, regardless of which endurance activity is used.

Intensity. The conditioning intensity of the aerobic portion of the exercise session is best expressed as a percentage of the individual's maximal or functional capacity. Effective training intensities are from 50% to 85% of $\dot{V}O_2$ max or 60% to 90% of the maximum heart rate achieved during a graded exercise test.[65,73,74] These intensities can be translated into MET levels. The intensity of training sessions comprised of most activities can be monitored through the use of target heart rates (Fig. 1–3) or through MET levels. The energy cost in METs of various activities can be found in the ACSM *Guidelines for Exercise Testing and Exercise Prescription* (see Tables 1–2 through 1–5).[65] Accurate quantification of some activities may be difficult. For example, target heart rates derived from treadmill exercise tests may not adequately quantify swimming or various other activities with a large upper-body component, such as aerobic dance.[75]

Duration. Each training session should last between 15 and 60 minutes, with an aerobic component of at least 15 minutes. Typically, an exercise session should include a 5- to 10-minute warm-up, 15 to 60 minutes of aerobic exercise at the appropriate training

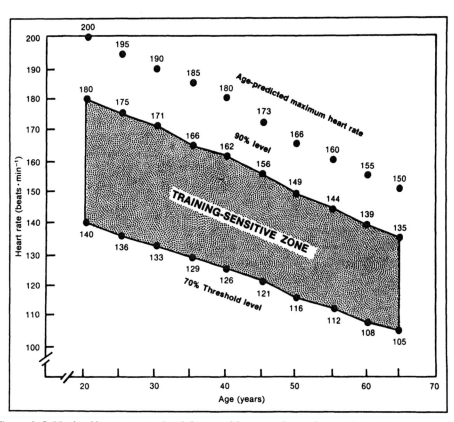

Figure 1–3. Maximal heart rates and training-sensitive zones for use in aerobic training programs for people of different ages. (From McArdle, Katch, and Katch,[9] with permission.)

level, and a cool-down of 5 to 10 minutes.[65,73,74] The function of the warm-up is gradually to increase the metabolic rate from the 1-MET level to the MET level required for conditioning. In planning the aerobic portion of the workout, one must consider that duration and intensity are inversely related. That is, the lower the exercise intensity, the longer the workout needs to be. Although significant cardiovascular improvements can be made with very intense (more than 90% $\dot{V}O_2$ max) exercise done for short periods of time (5 to 10 minutes), high-intensity, short-duration sessions are not appropriate for individuals starting a fitness program.[65] Because of potential hazards (including an unnecessary risk of injury) for untrained individuals embarking on a high-intensity program, low to moderate intensity for longer durations is recommended for those beginning a fitness program. Although the recommended duration of the aerobic or conditioning part of the workout is 15 to 60 minutes, an adequate training response can be elicited by maintaining the prescribed exercise intensity for a period of approximately 15 minutes.[65] With the warm-up and cool-down, a reasonable amount of total workout time for a person beginning an exercise program would be 30 minutes. The cool-down phase should include exercise of diminishing intensity to return the physiologic systems of the body to their resting states.

Frequency. The frequency of exercise sessions is somewhat dependent on the intensity and duration of the exercise. For example, exercise programs for individuals with very low functional capacities (less than 5 METs) may start out with several short (5-minute) sessions per day. For most individuals, exercise programs for improving one's fitness level should be done three to five times per week.[65]

Progression. The degree of improvement in $\dot{V}O_2$ max (the best measure of functional capacity) is directly related to the intensity, duration, and frequency of the training. Research has documented improvements in $\dot{V}O_2$ max ranging between 5% and 25%, with the largest changes usually seen in the individuals who have the lowest initial fitness levels.[76] Both men and women respond to aerobic training with similar increments in maximal oxygen uptake.[73] An individual starting a fitness program can expect a significant improvement in functional capacity to occur during the first 6 to 8 weeks.[4,6,9] The length of time necessary to reach one's true $\dot{V}O_2$ max depends on the initial fitness level and intensity of training. As conditioning takes place, the exercise intensity will need adjustment in order to keep the participant exercising in the training range. During the initial phases of a program, this is best done by changing the MET level to correspond to the desired exercise heart rate. Since with conditioning the heart rate will drop for any given submaximal work rate, intensity adjustments will result in more actual work being done during each exercise session.[65] Follow-up graded exercise tests should be done during the first year of the program to help in the intensity adjustment and in motivating the participant. The goals of the participant need to be taken into account to determine when the exercise program can be changed from one with a goal of increasing fitness level to one with the goal of maintaining the newly acquired level. Sample exercise programs for sedentary, active, and competing women are shown in Appendix 1–1. It must be stressed that no program should be undertaken lightly and that, for many women, the ideal program may be a highly individualized "exercise prescription" developed in conjunction with a physician and exercise physiologist.

Fitness Maintenance

Activity Level

Exercise must be continued on a regular basis in order to maintain a given fitness level. Hickson and colleagues[28,77,78] have shown that the duration and frequency of exercise may be reduced by as much as two thirds without affecting the training-induced $\dot{V}O_2$ max, but intensity plays a critical role in maintaining the training-induced changes.

When the duration of exercise sessions following 10 weeks of training was reduced from 40 minutes per day to 26 or 13 minutes per day for the next 5 weeks, no reduction in the exercise-induced $\dot{V}O_2$ max was seen.[77] Similarly, when sessions were reduced from 6 days/wk to 4 or 2 days/wk, there again was no reduction in $\dot{V}O_2$ max.[78] However, data suggest that in order to maintain training-induced gains, an individual must continue to exercise at an intensity of at least 70% of the training intensity.[28] Therefore, after achieving a desired level of fitness, an individual can theoretically be expected to maintain this level by exercising at least twice a week at 70% or more of her training intensity for a minimum of 13 minutes per session.

Caution is advised, however, in the interpretation of these data, since the subjects from whom these conclusions were reached were highly conditioned men and women, and the results may not be applicable to individuals training at lower intensities. It should also be kept in mind that body composition is one of the components of "physical fitness." Thus, if the participant is using the exercise program to maintain caloric balance and to keep body fat at a reasonable level, a maintenance program of 4 to 5 days/wk would be a better choice.

When an individual stops training, a significant detraining effect occurs within 2 weeks, as measured by a decrease in physical work capacity.[9] A 50% reduction of the newly acquired gain in fitness has been shown to occur by 4 to 12 weeks after cessation of training, while a return to pretraining fitness level can be expected after cessation of training between 4 weeks and 8 months.[73] Although much of this research is based on information from male subjects, the deconditioning pattern and time-course are expected to be similar in women.[76]

Role of Recreational Sports

Recreational sports that require an energy expenditure of sufficient intensity and duration to fall within ACSM guidelines for developing and maintaining fitness can be used for training.[65,73] Many recreational activities, however, are intermittent in nature and their energy expenditure is difficult to quantify. Although there are tables listing average energy expenditures,[9,73] the amount of energy expended often depends on the skill of the participants. For example, it is difficult to imagine that the energy expended by a professional tennis player such as Monica Seles is in any way similar to that expended by some weekend players. Recreational activities, then, are best used to supplement a planned program for the development and maintenance of physical fitness.

Factors Affecting Fitness Development and Maintenance

Age

Increased age alone is not a contraindication to participation in a fitness program. Regular training will result in positive physiologic adaptations, regardless of age.[6,73,79] Some studies have shown that older individuals may require longer to adjust to physical training programs and may not make as large an absolute improvement in fitness level as a younger person.[73] However, a comparison of improvements is often difficult because younger individuals tend to train at higher intensities than do older individuals. As an individual ages, there will be some decrease in $\dot{V}O_2$ max regardless of training, since there is an age-related drop in maximal heart rate, which, in turn, reduces maximal cardiac output.[4] An age-related decrease in $\dot{V}O_2$ max does not imply that an older individual cannot or should not participate in activities requiring a great deal of fitness. For example, each year there are several contestants and finishers over age 70 years in the Hawaiian Ironman Triathlon, a contest that takes 9 to 17 hours to complete.

Gender

Although most of the research supporting the quantity and quality of exercise necessary to develop and maintain fitness was initially derived from male subject data, it appears to be equally applicable to women. Numerous recent studies have documented similar training responses for men and women.[73] Before puberty, there is no difference in maximal aerobic power between boys and girls.[4] After that, however, the potential for absolute magnitude of aerobic capacity is higher for men. There seem to be at least three basic physiologic differences between men and women that affect the capacity for aerobic power.[17,19] Women usually have a higher percentage of body fat, a smaller oxygen-carrying capacity, and a smaller muscle-fiber area than do men. When the effects of body weight and percentage of body fat are corrected mathematically, the differences in $\dot{V}O_2$ max are lessened. Studies have averaged these differences to be approximately 50%, 20%, and 9% when $\dot{V}O_2$ max is expressed as liters per minute, milliliters per kilogram per minute, and milliliters per kilogram fat-free mass, respectively. The remaining difference (approximately 9%) is either still a difference in conditioning or more probably a gender-linked difference in the ability to transport and utilize oxygen. Since women usually have a lower hemoglobin concentration than men (normal range equals 12 to 16 g/dL for women; 14 to 18 g/dL for men) and a smaller blood volume, they have a smaller maximal oxygen-carrying capacity than men. In addition, endurance-trained women have approximately 85% of the muscle-fiber areas of endurance-trained men. Although the fiber area is different, the muscle composition is much the same for male and female endurance athletes.[17]

Underlying Disease

For any woman with known or suspected medical illness, embarking upon a fitness program should be preceded by consultation with a physician with special training in the patient's disease and, when indicated, by continued close medical supervision. Although it is rare that an individual should be excluded from exercise, many patients will need special considerations in the design and implementation of appropriate exercise training. Any aspect of an exercise program may be changed to adapt to the individual's needs, as long as the core features of exercise mode, intensity, duration, and frequency are preserved. Although reductions in intensity are most common, exercise modality may be altered (e.g., using non-weight-bearing or low-impact activities for the patient with arthritis, extreme obesity, or musculoskeletal abnormalities). Regardless of initial fitness level or absolute level of achievement, the positive effects of enhanced well-being, muscular strength, and activity tolerance may be expected. Monitoring methods may also need to be adapted to the individual situation (e.g., use of respiratory rate rather than heart rate for exercise intensity in the patient with a pacemaker). Detailed discussion of exercise prescription is beyond the scope of this chapter.

Sudden Death

Sudden death during exercise has been well publicized, yet is extremely rare and most unlikely in an otherwise healthy individual without known cardiac disease.[80-85] Although sudden death may occur more often during activity than during rest, most occurrences are related to usual daily activities and not to exercise programs.

The causes of sudden death during exercise have been examined in male athletes.[83] In the young, nearly 65% have some form of hypertrophic cardiomyopathy, 14% have congenital coronary artery anomalies, 10% have coronary heart disease, and 7% have ruptured aorta or Marfan's syndrome. In contrast, of those dying suddenly after age 35, more than 80% have coronary heart disease. Other associated diseases include hypertrophic cardiomyopathy, mitral valve prolapse, and acquired valvular disease. For this reason, women with known or suspected cardiovascular disease and previously sedentary individuals over 50 years of age should seek the advice of an internist or cardiologist before pursuing a vigorous exercise program. While most cardiovascular illnesses do not preclude the achievement of fitness, the exercise program should be individually tailored to meet the needs and limitations of the participant. Further, there are a small number of illnesses in which any form of vigorous activity should be strictly limited.

Injury

Most of the injuries resulting from participation in fitness programs are musculoskeletal injuries. Although occasionally there are traumatic injuries, such as fractures and torn ligaments, more frequently the injuries are the result of chronic microtrauma or overuse. These injuries include muscle strains, tendinitis, synovitis, bursitis, and stress fractures. In most cases, these injuries are not serious enough to prevent training but often require alterations in training patterns. Overuse injuries have been attributed mainly to errors in training, such as progressing too fast and not allowing enough time for recovery and adaptation.[84]

Practical Considerations

Practical considerations are often critical to whether or not an individual participates in a fitness program. The most important of these considerations for most people is time. Everyone has certain constraints on her time, whether they be job-related or home-related. An individual wishing to participate in an exercise program to improve fitness must make a time commitment. A minimum of at least 1 hour three times per week is necessary. This could comprise a bare minimum of 30-minute exercise sessions plus time to change clothes, travel, and so forth. Cost is another factor to be considered. Most exercise test evaluations with an exercise prescription cost between $100 and $400. Following this initial financial outlay, each individual can spend as little as the cost of a good pair of shoes and comfortable exercise clothing, or much more. Costs for the use of facilities can be from less than $100 per year for a YMCA/YWCA or local university-based program to $500 or $600 per year for a health club membership. Individuals can join exercise classes, such as one in aerobic dance, or they may choose to carry out their prescription on their own. Equipment for walking or jogging programs is minimal, but that for a bicycling program is more.

TRAINING FOR COMPETITION

Training for competition differs from training for fitness in that its main objective is improvement of performance rather than improvement of health. Training for competition should begin by using the same ACSM guidelines for intensity, frequency, and duration. A period of approximately 8 weeks is necessary to lay the groundwork for a more intense training program.[6] Physiologic adaptations occurring in ligaments and muscles during that time make them less susceptible to overuse injuries, which otherwise might occur as a result of high-intensity training. Once the fitness base is laid, the competitive athlete must overload her system further to continue improving. The overload should be progressive and individualized to the specific goals of the athlete. At this point, training should be as specific to the competition as possible. That is, the exerciser needs to train the specific muscles to be involved in the desired performance in a manner specific to the competition.

Interval Training

Because most competition involves an element of speed, the exerciser may benefit from interval as well as continuous training.[6] Interval training is a means of accomplishing a great deal of work in a short period of time by interspersing work intervals with rest intervals. The work intervals may be of any desired length, from just a few seconds to several minutes. The length of the work interval is determined by the specific demands of the competition and by the energy system the athlete wishes to train. Intervals of less than 4 seconds can be used to develop strength and power for activities such as a high jump, shot put, golf swing, or tennis stroke. Intervals of up to 10 seconds are used to develop sustained power for activities such as sprints, fast breaks, and so on. The length of these intervals forces the body to use immediate, short-term energy systems. Intervals of up to 1½ minutes are used to develop the intermediate, glycolytic energy systems for activities such as 200- to 400-meter dashes or 100-meter swims. Intervals lasting longer than 1½ minutes tax the aerobic as well as the glycolytic systems. Training intervals should include all the energy systems expected to be taxed during competition. Recovery times or rest between intervals should be of a length that allows recovery of that particular energy system before the next work bout.

Cross Training

Recently, the term "cross training" has been used to describe training in one exercise mode and deriving benefits in a different exercise mode. For example, triathletes often attribute improved running performance to concurrent bicycling training. Research, however, does not provide much support for a cross-training effect.

Although there is some evidence that the functional capacity of the cardiovascular system improves with different exercise modes, peripheral adaptation occurs only in the muscles involved in training.[85] Thus, while oxygen delivery may be enhanced through cross training, oxygen extraction is not. Therefore, cross training is not likely to improve competitive performance.

SUMMARY

In conclusion, physical fitness for women is very similar to physical fitness for men. That is, a certain level of fitness is necessary for general well-being and protection against some disease states. A greater degree of fitness is beneficial for certain recreational and competitive sport activities. Cardiovascular fitness can be developed according to the guidelines of the ACSM. Rate and degree of improvement for women can be expected to be similar to that for men and depends on intensity, duration, and frequency of exercise sessions.

REFERENCES

1. Cureton TK: Physical Fitness Appraisal and Guidance. CV Mosby, St. Louis, 1947.
2. President's Council on Physical Fitness: Adult Physical Fitness—A Program for Men and Women. US Government Printing Office, 1979.
3. President's Council on Physical Fitness: The Fitness Challenge . . . in the Later Years. US Government Printing Office, 1977.
4. Åstrand PO, and Rodahl K: Textbook of Work Physiology. Physiological Bases of Exercise, ed 3. McGraw-Hill, New York, 1986.
5. deVries HA: Physiology of Exercise for Physical Education and Athletics, ed 4. Wm. C. Brown, Dubuque, IA, 1986.
6. Lamb DR: Physiology of Exercise: Responses and Adaptations, ed 2. Macmillan, New York, 1984.
7. Mathews DK: Measurement in Physical Education, ed 2. WB Saunders, Philadelphia, 1963.
8. Mathews DK, and Fox EL: The Physiological Basis of Physical Education and Athletics, ed 2. WB Saunders, Philadelphia, 1976.
9. McArdle WD, Katch FL, and Katch VL: Exercise Physiology: Energy, Nutrition, and Human Performance. Lea and Febiger, Philadelphia, 1986.
10. Berg A, and Keul J: Physiological and metabolic responses of female athletes during laboratory and field exercise. Med Sport 14:77, 1981.
11. Drinkwater BL, Horvath SM, and Wells CL: Aerobic power of females, ages 10 to 68. J Gerontol 30:385, 1975.
12. Shvartz E, and Reibold RC: Aerobic fitness norm for males and females aged 6 to 75 years. Aviat Space Environ Med 61:3, 1990.
13. Gutin B: A model of physical fitness and dynamic health. Journal of Health, Physical Education, and Recreation 51:48, 1980.
14. Gutin B, Trinidad A, Norton C, et al: Morphological and physiological factors related to

endurance performance of 11- to 12-year-old girls. Res Q 49:44, 1978.

15. Anderson B: Stretching. Shelter Publications, Bolinas, CA, 1980.

16. Palgi Y, Gutin B, Young J, et al: Physiologic and anthropometric factors underlying endurance performance in children. Int J Sports Med 5:67, 1984.

17. Drinkwater BL: Women and exercise: Physiological aspects. Exerc Sport Sci Rev 12:21, 1984.

18. Flint MM, Drinkwater BL, and Horvath SM: Effects of training on women's response to submaximal exercise. Med Sci Sports 6:89, 1974.

19. Lewis DA, Kamon E, and Hodgson JL: Physiological differences between genders. Implications for sports conditioning. Sports Medicine 3:357, 1986.

20. Pollock ML, Miller HS, Jr, and Ribisl PM: Effect of fitness on aging. Phys Sportsmed 6:45, 1978.

21. Shepard RJ, and Kavanagh T: The effects of training on the aging process. Phys Sportsmed 6:33, 1978.

22. Vaccaro P, Dummer GM, and Clarke DH: Physiologic characteristics of female master swimmers. Phys Sportsmed 9:75, 1981.

23. Adams GM, and deVries HA: Physiological effects of an exercise training regimen upon women aged 52 to 79. J Gerontol 28:50, 1973.

24. Buskirk ER, and Hodgson JL: Age and aerobic power: The rate of change in men and women. Fed Proc 46:1824, 1987.

25. Prosser G, Carson P, Phillips R, et al: Morale in coronary patients following an exercise programme. J Psychosom Res 25:587, 1981.

26. Franklin B, Buskirk E, Hodgson J, et al: Effects of physical conditioning on cardiorespiratory function, body composition and serum lipids in relatively normal weight and obese middle-aged women. Int J Obes 3:97, 1979.

27. Getchell LH, and Moore JC: Physical training: Comparative responses of middle-aged adults. Arch Phys Med Rehabil 56:250, 1974.

28. Hickson R, Foster C, Pollock ML, et al: Reduced training intensities and loss of aerobic power, endurance, and cardiac growth. J Appl Physiol 58:492, 1985.

29. Morris JN, Heady JA, Raffle PAB, et al: Coronary heart-disease and physical activity. Lancet 2:1053, 1111, 1953.

30. Blair SN, Kohl HW, Paffenbarger RS, et al: Physical fitness and all-cause mortality: A prospective study of healthy men and women. JAMA 262:2395, 1989.

31. Paffenbarger RS, Wing AL, and Hyde RT: Physical activity as an index of heart attack in college alumni. Am J Epidemiol 108:161, 1978.

32. Morris JN, Pollard R, Everitt MG, et al: Vigorous exercise in leisure time: Protection against coronary heart disease. Lancet 2:1207, 1980.

33. Costas R, Garcia-Palmieri MR, Nazario E, et al: Relation of lipids, weight and physical activity to incidence of coronary heart disease: The Puerto Rico Heart Study. Am J Cardiol 42:653, 1978.

34. Salonen JT, Puska P, and Tuomilehto J: Physical activity and risk of myocardial infarction, cerebral stroke and death: A longitudinal study in Eastern Finland. Am J Epidemiol 115:526, 1982.

35. Chapman JM, and Massey FJ: The interrelationship of serum cholesterol, hypertension, body weight and risk of coronary disease. J Chronic Dis 17:933, 1964.

36. Paul O: Physical activity and coronary heart disease. Part II. Am J Cardiol 23:303, 1969.

37. Skinner JS, Benson H, McDonough JR, et al: Social status, physical activity and coronary proneness. J Chronic Dis 19:773, 1966.

38. Rose G: Physical activity and coronary heart disease. Proc R Soc Med 62:1183, 1969.

39. Paffenbarger RS Jr, Brand RJ, Sholtz RI, et al: Energy expenditure, cigarette smoking, and blood pressure level as related to death from specific diseases. Am J Epidemiol 108:12, 1978.

40. Stewart KJ, and Kelemen MH: Circuit weight training: A new approach to cardiac rehabilitation. Practical Cardiology 12:41, 1986.

41. Haskell WL: Cardiovascular benefits and risks of exercise: The scientific evidence. In Strauss RH: Sports Medicine. WB Saunders, Philadelphia, 1984, pp 57–76.

42. Gibbons LW, Blair SN, Cooper KH, et al: Association between coronary heart disease risk factors and physical fitness in healthy adult women. Circulation 67:977, 1983.

43. Haskell WL, Taylor HL, Wood PD, et al: Strenuous physical activity, treadmill exercise test performance and plasma high-density lipoprotein cholesterol. Circulation 62(Suppl IV):53, 1980.

44. Busby J, Notelovitz M, Putney K, et al: Exercise high density lipoprotein cholesterol and cardiorespiratory function in climacteric women. South Med J 78:769, 1985.

45. Shaw LW: Effects of a prescribed supervised exercise program on mortality and cardiovascular morbidity in patients after a myocardial infarction: The National Exercise and Heart Disease Project. Am J Cardiol 48:39, 1981.

46. Tipton CM, Matthes RD, Bedford TB, et al: Exercise, hypertension, and animal models. In Lowenthal DT, Bharadwaja K, and Oaks WW

(eds): Therapeutics Through Exercise. Grune and Stratton, New York, 1979, pp 115–132.

47. Choquette G, and Ferguson RJ: Blood pressure reduction in "borderline" hypertensives following physical training. Can Med Assoc J 108:699, 1973.

48. Hagberg JM, Goldring D, Ehsani AA, et al: Effect of exercise training on the blood pressure and hemodynamic features of hypertensive adolescents. Am J Cardiol 52:763, 1983.

49. Douglas PS, O'Toole ML, Hiller WDB, et al: Left ventricular structure and function by echocardiography in ultraendurance athletes. Am J Cardiol 58:805, 1986.

50. Williams RS, Logue EE, Lewis JL, et al: Physical conditioning augments the fibrinolytic response to venous occlusion in healthy adults. N Engl J Med 302:987, 1980.

51. Hubert HB, Feinleib M, McNamara PM, et al: Obesity as an independent risk factor for cardiovascular disease: A 26-year follow-up of participants in the Framingham Heart Study. Circulation 67:968, 1983.

52. Aloia JF, Cohn SH, Babu T, et al: Skeletal mass and body composition in marathon runners. Metabolism 27:1793, 1978.

53. Lane NE, Bloch DA, Jones HH, et al: Long-distance running, bone density, and osteoarthritis. JAMA 255:1147, 1986.

54. Krolner B, Toft B, Nielsen SP, et al: Physical exercise as prophylaxis against involutional vertebral bone loss: A controlled trial. Clin Sci 64:541, 1983.

55. Smith EL, Reddan W, and Smith PE: Physical activity and calcium modalities for bone mineral increase in aged women. Med Sci Sports Exerc 13:60, 1981.

56. Aloia JF, Cohn SH, Ostuni JA, et al: Prevention of involutional bone loss by exercise. Ann Intern Med 89:356, 1978.

57. Unger KM, Moser KM, and Hansen P: Selection of an exercise program for patients with chronic obstructive pulmonary disease. Heart Lung 9:68, 1980.

58. Richter EA, Ruderman NB, and Schneider SH: Diabetes and exercise. Am J Med 70:201, 1981.

59. Brown RS, Ramirez DE, and Taub JM: The prescription of exercise for depression. Phys Sportsmed 6:35, 1978.

60. Wells KF, and Dillon EK: Sit and reach: A test of back and leg flexibility. Res Q 23:115, 1952.

61. Klafs CE, and Arnheim DD: Modern Principles of Athletic Training. CV Mosby, St. Louis, 1973.

62. Rothstein JM: Measurement in Physical Therapy. Churchill Livingstone, New York, 1985, p 105.

63. Bergh U, Thorstensson A, Sjodin B, et al: Maximal oxygen uptake and muscle fiber types in trained and untrained humans. Med Sci Sports 10:151, 1978.

64. O'Toole ML, Hiller WDB, Crosby LO, et al: The ultraendurance triathlete: A physiological profile. Med Sci Sports Exerc 19:45, 1987.

65. American College of Sports Medicine: Guidelines for Graded Exercise Testing and Exercise Prescription, ed 3. Lea and Febiger, Philadelphia, 1986.

66. Olson MS, Williford HN, Blessing DL, et al: The cardiovascular and metabolic effects of bench stepping exercise in females. Med Sci Sports Exerc 23:1311, 1991.

67. Cooper KH: Aerobics. Bantam Books, New York, 1968.

68. Cooper K: Correlation between field and treadmill testing as a means for assessing maximal oxygen intake. JAMA 203:201, 1968.

69. Maksud MG, Cannistra C, and Dublinski D: Energy expenditure and VO_2max of female athletes during treadmill exercise. Res Q 47:692, 1976.

70. Katch FL, McArdle WD, Czula R, et al: Maximal oxygen intake, endurance running performance, and body composition in college women. Res Q 44:301, 1973.

71. Gutin B: Prescribing an exercise program. In Winick M (ed): Nutrition and Exercise. John Wiley & Sons, New York, 1986, pp 30–50.

72. Skinner JS, and McLellan TH: The transition from aerobic to anaerobic metabolism. Res Q Exerc Sport 51:234, 1980.

73. American College of Sports Medicine: Position statement on the recommended quantity and quality of exercise for developing and maintaining fitness in healthy adults. Med Sci Sports 19:vii, 1978.

74. Wilmore JH: Individual exercise prescription. Am J Cardiol 33:757, 1974.

75. Parker SB, Hurley BF, Hanlon DP, et al: Failure of target heart rate to accurately monitor intensity during aerobic dance. Med Sci Sports Exerc 21:230, 1989.

76. Pollock ML: The quantification of endurance training programs. Exerc Sports Sci Rev 1:155, 1973.

77. Hickson RC, Kanakis C Jr, Davis JR, et al: Reduced training duration effects on aerobic power, endurance, and cardiac growth. J Appl Physiol 53:225, 1982.

78. Hickson R, and Rosenkoetter MA: Reduced training frequencies and maintenance of aerobic power. Med Sci Sports Exerc 13:13, 1981.

79. Hagberg JM, Graves JE, and Limacher M: Cardiovascular responses of 70–79 year old men and women to exercise training. J Appl Physiol 66:2589, 1989.

80. Gibbons LW, Cooper KH, Meyer B, et al: The acute cardiac risk of strenuous exercise. JAMA 244:1799, 1980.
81. Thompson P, Stern M, Williams P, et al: Death during jogging or running: A study of 18 cases. JAMA 242:1265, 1979.
82. Thompson P, Funk E, Carleton R, et al: Incidence of death during jogging in Rhode Island from 1975 through 1980. JAMA 247:2535, 1982.
83. Maron BJ, Epstein SE, and Roberts WC: Causes of sudden death in competitive athletes. J Am Coll Cardiol 7:204, 1986.
84. Clancy WG: Runners' injuries. Am J Sports Med 8:137, 1980.
85. Clausen JP: Effect of physical training on cardiovascular adjustments to exercise in man. Physiol Rev 57:779, 1977.

APPENDIX 1-1

Sample Training Programs

The following are sample training schedules for women starting a fitness program. They are, however, only examples of types of activities that would be appropriate for women in these categories and should not be undertaken without proper medical and fitness evaluation. Also included are general guidelines to be followed by an athlete training for competition. Since a competitive athlete must train specifically for the requirements of her sport, a program appropriate for one athlete may be of little benefit to someone in another sport.

SAMPLE 8-WEEK PROGRAM FOR A SEDENTARY 30-YEAR-OLD WOMAN

Weeks 1-4. (Initial Stage—The energy cost of the exercise in this stage should be approximately 200 kcal per session. Exercise sessions should be three times per week or every other day.)

Warm-up. 5 min walking (heart rate [HR] = 110 beats per minute [bpm]; 5 min stretching (areas to stretch: Achilles tendon, hamstrings, lower back, and shoulders).

Aerobic Phase. 15 min vigorous walking, jogging, stationary cycling, or any combination of these (HR = 135–145 bpm). After the second week, the time for this phase should be gradually increased (by 1 min every other day) to 20 min.

Cool-down. 5 min walking (HR = 100–110 bpm); 5 min stretching (same as in warm-up).

Weeks 4-8. (Improvement Stage—The energy cost of exercise in this stage should be approximately 300 kcal per session. Exercise sessions should be three to five times per week.)

Warm-up. 5 min walking (HR = 115 bpm); 5 min stretching, as previously.

Aerobic Phase. 20 min initially; gradually increase to 25 min, as above. Aerobic activities can include walking, jogging, cycling, or any other continuous, rhythmic exercise. (HR = 140–150 bpm.)

Cool-down. 5 min walking (HR = 100–110 bpm); 5 min stretching, as previously.

Week 8 and Afterward. (Maintenance Stage—The energy cost should still be approximately 300 kcal per session.)

Warm-up. Same as above.

Aerobic Phase. Intensity and duration of sessions should be the same as in Improvement Stage. Exercise should be done at least 3 times per week. Recreational sport activities of approximately the same intensity may be substituted 1 day per week.

Cool-down. Same as above.

SAMPLE 8-WEEK PROGRAM FOR SEDENTARY 60-YEAR-OLD WOMAN

Weeks 1–4. (Initial Stage—200 kcal per session; three times per week.)

Warm-up. 5 min walking (HR = 100 bpm); 5 min stretching (areas to stretch: Achilles tendon, hamstrings, lower back, and shoulders).

Aerobic Phase. 12–15 min vigorous walking or stationary cycling (HR = 110–120 bpm).

Cool-down. 5 min walking (HR = 95–105 bpm); 5 min stretching, as previously.

Weeks 4–8. (Improvement Stage—300 kcal per session, three to five times per week.)

Warm-up. 5 min walking (HR = 110 bpm); 5 min stretching, as previously.

Aerobic Phase. 15 min initially; gradually increase to 25 min of walking, jogging, stationary cycling, or any combination of these (HR = 120–130 bpm).

Cool-down. 5 min walking (HR = 100–105 bpm); 5 min stretching, as previously.

Week 8 and Afterward. (Maintenance Stage—The energy cost per session should remain at 300 kcal. Exercise should be done at least three times per week.) Exercise program can remain the same as in the Improvement Stage with recreational sport activities substituted once a week if desired.

SAMPLE 8-WEEK PROGRAM FOR A MODERATELY ACTIVE 45-YEAR-OLD WOMAN

Weeks 1–2. (Initial Stage—Energy cost approximately 300 kcal per session. The purpose of this stage in a moderately active woman is to allow adaptation [particularly musculoskeletal] to occur in response to specific aerobic activity, such as jogging.)

Warm-up. 5 min walking or slow jogging (HR = 120–125 bpm); 5 min stretching (Achilles tendon, hamstrings, lower back, shoulders).

Aerobic Phase. 25 min of vigorous walking, jogging, stationary cycling, rowing, or any other continuous, rhythmic activity of choice. (HR = 135–140 bpm.)

Cool-down. 5 min slow jogging and/or walking (HR = 110 bpm); 5 min of stretching, as previously.

Weeks 3–8. (Improvement Stage—300–500 kcal per session.)

Warm-up. 10 min (same as previously).

Aerobic Phase. 25 min initially; gradually increase to 45 min per session. Any activity that will keep the heart rate 140–145 bpm for this length of time may be used.

Cool-down. 10 min (same as previously).

Week 8 and Afterward. (Maintenance Stage—Exercise sessions should be similar to those in the Improvement Stage and should be done at least three times per week with an energy cost of 500 kcal per session.)

GUIDELINES FOR THE COMPETITIVE ATHLETE

1 Training should be in three stages, comparable to those shown earlier but on a higher level—laying a base, increasing intensity, and fine tuning.
2 When adding sport-specific activities, training should be under conditions as similar to competitive conditions as possible.
3 Set reasonable goals in a reasonable time frame.
4 Keep a training diary to discover your own personal pattern of optimal training and to discover practices that lead to injury for you.
5 Use an overload/adaptation/progression system. That is, allow enough time for adaptation to occur after a hard workout, by following the hard workout with several easy or moderate ones. For example, after a race, some running coaches suggest waiting one day for each mile that was run before beginning the next hard workout.
6 Balance the high energy output of training with a high caloric intake.

SAMPLE PROGRAM FOR A USTS DISTANCE TRIATHLETE

(0.9-mile swim, 25-mile bike, 6.2-mile run)

Weeks 1–4. (Initial Stage—Goals are gradually to increase weekly mileage to 3 miles of swimming, 45 miles of bicycling, and 20 miles of running.)

Each workout should follow the format given previously (that is, warm-up, aerobic phase, and cool-down). The warm-up and cool-down phases should include gradual transition from rest to swimming, cycling, or running, as well as stretching of the muscles specific to that activity.

Each activity should be done three times per week, or nine total workouts for the week. Since there are a variety of muscle groups being used, each with its own stresses, the triathlete can safely exercise every day. In order to complete the nine workouts, single workouts can be done on 5 days, and double workouts on 2 other days. Workouts in the same sport should not be done on 2 consecutive days.

Training mileages per workout should be up to 1500 meters swimming, 25 miles cycling, and 6 miles running. No interval training should be done. All training mileages should be accomplished aerobically; that is, at the end of the workout, the triathlete should feel that she could repeat the workout immediately.

Weeks 4–12. (Improvement Stage—The time to increase the intensity of the workouts.)

Mileages should be increased to 5 miles of swimming, 75 miles of bicycling, and 25 miles of running per week.

During this stage, the emphasis should be on increasing the mileages so that some workouts are done slower than race pace at distances longer than race distances. Other workouts should be done using interval training. One interval training workout per week per sport is sufficient, and interval training should probably not be done on consecutive days. Time trials at race distances can be added during this phase.

Each activity should be done four or five times per week for a total of no more than 15 workouts per week. Hard workouts should be followed by easy workouts in each activity so that hard workouts are not done on two consecutive days. Occasionally, a swim workout should be immediately followed by a bike workout and a bike workout immediately followed by a run.

Weeks 12 Through the Competitive Season. The emphasis during this time should be on race performance. The total amount of training should be cut down, particularly on weeks when the triathlete is competing. The emphasis in workouts should be on quality rather than quantity. Short intervals concentrating on speed rather than endurance should be done once a week for each activity. Other days can either be at race pace for distances shorter than the race, or slower for longer distances. One day a week can be complete rest or a very easy workout.

CHAPTER 2

Exercise and Regulation
of Body Weight*

DENISE E. WILFLEY, Ph.D., CARLOS M. GRILO, Ph.D., and
KELLY D. BROWNELL, Ph.D.

People are searching frantically for the ideal body. In 1989, U.S. consumers spent an estimated $32 billion on weight control programs and products.[1] This drive for thinness has created a burgeoning marketplace for physical fitness equipment, attire, and health clubs. This stems from a clear belief that exercise aids in weight maintenance in persons at normal weight and in weight loss in overweight individuals. In fact, women often state that exercise is one of their primary methods of weight control.

The concern for thinness and dieting behavior is especially prevalent among

*Preparation of this chapter was supported in part by a MacArthur Foundation Fellowship to Carlos M. Grilo and in part by a grant from the Jenny Craig Foundation for the Fellowship Program of the Yale Center for Eating and Weight Disorders.

women. The eating disorders of anorexia and bulimia, both of which involve preoccupation with weight, are seen almost exclusively in women. Obesity occurs equally in women and men, yet women are more frequently the consumers of weight control products and are more likely to attend clinical programs.

In our culture, the search for the perfect body begins at a young age and is especially pronounced among women. A recent survey, the Youth Risk Behavior Surveillance System (YRBSS), revealed interesting findings regarding weight control practices among adolescents. Using self-administered questionnaires in comparable national, state, and local surveys, the YRBSS measures the prevalence of health-risk behaviors of adolescents.[2,3,4] The 1990 YRBSS included 11,631 students from grades 9 through 12.

Substantial differences were found in the weight perceptions of boys and girls. Female students were twice as likely as male students to consider themselves "too fat" (34% versus 15%, respectively). Moreover, many more female students were engaging in weight control strategies. Among female students, 44% reported that they were currently trying to lose weight, 26% were trying to keep from gaining weight, 7% were trying to gain weight, and only 23% were not trying to do anything about their weight. Among male students, 15% reported that they were trying to lose weight, 15% were trying to keep from gaining weight, 26% were trying to gain weight, and 44% were not trying to do anything about their weight. Female students reported using exercise (51%) and skipping meals (49%) as the two most common means of weight control.

In sum, weight control is widely sought after by both female adolescents and adults in the United States.[4] Among high school girls in 1990, 70% of girls versus 30% of boys reported that they were either trying to lose weight or maintain their current weight. Data collected on adults looks very similar. Among 60,912 adults in the 1989 Behavior Survey and Behavioral Risk Factor Surveillance System (BRFSS), about 70% of women

and 50% of men reported they were currently either trying to lose weight or to maintain their current weight.[4]

There are countless variations among women in the combinations of diet and exercise programs they follow. It is important, therefore, to understand the physiologic and psychologic effects of such programs and to identify approaches that are safe and effective. Exercise physiology and sports medicine are central to this endeavor. In spite of the fitness boom, many women and men are too inactive to attain the psychologic and health benefits of exercise, and many of those who begin exercise programs do not continue exercising long enough to achieve their health and fitness goals.[5]

In this chapter, we discuss the prevalence, severity, and refractory nature of weight problems. The effects of exercise on food intake, metabolism, and regulation of body weight are outlined, with specific focus on the effects of exercise on women. We discuss mechanisms by which exercise facilitates long-term weight loss, because there appear to be multiple pathways linking exercise to weight change. We then discuss ways to increase adherence, with particular focus on the importance of tailoring exercise interventions to the special physical and psychosocial needs of overweight persons. We also examine special issues such as how our culture's preoccupation with shape and weight may perpetuate unhealthy attitudes toward dieting and exercise, how to establish criteria for a "reasonable weight" for an individual, and when exercise can be psychologically and/or physically harmful. We end by describing the role exercise can play in weight regulation and by outlining an approach to exercise that accounts for metabolic variables, cultural factors, psychologic issues, and the challenge of long-term adherence.

THE NATURE AND SEVERITY OF WEIGHT DISORDERS

Overweight is a prevalent problem with serious adverse effects on health and longevity. Approximately 27% of women and 24% of men are overweight, using a criterion of 20% or more above desirable weight.[6] Overweight is associated with elevated serum cholesterol, elevated blood pressure, cardiovascular disease, and noninsulin-dependent diabetes.[7,8] It also increases the risk for gallbladder disease and some types of cancer, and it has been implicated in the development of osteoarthritis of the weight-bearing joints.[9]

Overweight clearly affects a large proportion of the U.S. population. The burdens of overweight are shouldered disproportionately by the poor and members of certain ethnic groups. Overweight is multidetermined in nature, reflecting biologic, envi-

ronmental, cultural, socioeconomic, and psychologic factors.

Careful measurement of height and weight is currently the first step in the clinical assessment of the overweight.[10] The body mass index (BMI), the weight in kilograms divided by the square of the height in meters, a measure of relative weight, is a more useful measurement of degree of overweight than weight tables, since it correlates highly (0.8) with more precise laboratory assessments of body composition and is adjusted for height in order to compare body weight across individuals or groups.[7] For persons of average weight, one BMI unit is equivalent to approximately 6.8 lb in men and 5.8 lb in women (Fig. 2–1). Since risk is approxi-

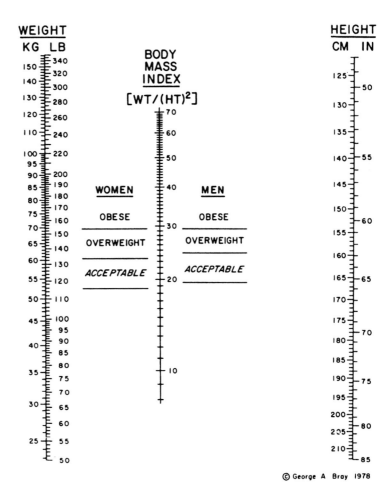

Figure 2–1. Nomogram for body mass index (BMI). To determine BMI, place a ruler or other straightedge between the body weight column on the left and the height column on the right and read the BMI from the point where it crosses the center. (©George A. Bray, M.D., 1978, reprinted with permission.)

© George A Bray 1978

RISK CLASSIFICATION ALGORITHM

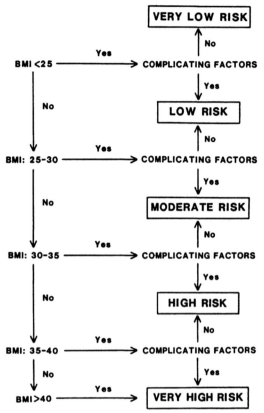

Figure 2–2. Risk classification algorithm. After measuring the BMI, the individual risk is increased or decreased based on the presence of complicating factors. (George A. Bray, M.D., 1988, reprinted with permission.)

mately proportional to degree of overweight, Bray[10] classifies the degree of risk on a scale from Class 0, *very* low risk, to Class IV, *very* high risk (Fig. 2–2).

Weight loss programs have shown dramatically improved short-term results over the past two decades, but long-term results are still discouraging. This resistance to treatment, combined with the high prevalence and striking severity noted earlier, make obesity a public health problem of considerable magnitude.[11]

At the other end of the continuum of weight concerns lies anorexia nervosa (see Chapter 17). This involves a morbid and persistent dread of fat, with pathologic diet-ing and physical activity to the point where body weight drops low enough to be life-threatening. It occurs primarily in adolescents and young adults in their early 20s, and with few exceptions is confined to females. It is not the "flip side" of obesity. Anorexics have characteristic family backgrounds and patterns that are not common among the overweight. There are also few overweight persons who develop anorexia nervosa.

Another eating disorder characterized by excessive weight preoccupation and concerns is bulimia nervosa. It involves fluctuations between extreme dietary restriction and out-of-control eating (binge eating). Most women with bulimia nervosa report the onset of binge eating following a severe diet.[12] The binge eating is followed by some compensatory behavior such as self-induced vomiting, use of diuretics or laxatives, strict dieting or fasting, or vigorous exercise in order to prevent weight gain. As with anorexia nervosa, bulimia nervosa is most common among females. Among the contributing factors are cultural pressures to be thin, mothers' criticism of daughters' weight and appearance, dysfunctional family patterns, low self-esteem, social self-consciousness, and dieting itself.[13–15]

Both anorexia nervosa and bulimia nervosa are most common in the populations who are most invested in dieting and weight loss—predominately white, middle to upper class females.[16] In contrast, obesity is negatively correlated with socioeconomic status.[17] There is an overall correlation between the cultural pressure to be thin and prevalence of eating disorders, both across and within ethnic groups.[18] It is also well documented that eating disorders are more prevalent in occupations (e.g., modeling) and other life activities (e.g., gymnastics) that place pressure on females to be thin.[19]

In each of these disorders, complex interactions exist among food intake, physical activity, metabolism, psychology, and culture. The remainder of this chapter will discuss the interplay of these factors in the lives and health of women.

THE ASSOCIATION BETWEEN PHYSICAL ACTIVITY AND WEIGHT

During the last century, overweight has become increasingly common despite an overall *decrease* in the average daily caloric intake of the population.[11,20,21] Several important changes have occurred during this period of time that may help explain this phenomenon. Daily energy expenditure has decreased as society has progressed from an agricultural, to an industrial, to an information-based economy, with fewer and fewer jobs requiring physical exertion. Our culture has also adopted a technology-oriented philosophy of saving energy and increasing comfort. As a result, daily energy expenditure has dropped dramatically during this century.

In 1984, the U.S. Department of Agriculture estimated that between the years of 1965 and 1977 the average daily energy expenditure dropped by 200 calories per day (the equivalent of almost 21 lb/y).[22] A report issued by the Centers for Disease Control (CDC) in 1992, based on the national school-based Youth Risk Behavior Survey, estimated that only 37% of students in grades 9 to 12 were vigorously active three or more times per week. A comparison of these 1992 CDC findings with the 1984 report issued by the National Children and Youth Fitness Study, suggests that participation in vigorous activity in adolescents is decreasing.[2,23,24] Another report issued by the CDC in 1987 revealed that fewer than 20% of U.S. adults engage in regular vigorous activity, while approximately 50% lead sedentary lives.[24,25] These declines in physical activity among adolescents and adults are unquestionably related to the increased prevalence of obesity in the United States.

During this century, more has changed than physical activity. Despite lower caloric intake, changes in dietary habits may play a role in increased weight. These changes include increased fat consumption and meal irregularity (fewer meals are consumed). These changes must be considered in concert with the significant decline in physical activity. Given the effects of changes in dietary composition and exercise on metabolism and body composition, it is not difficult to posit a relationship between these factors and increased obesity.

Research generally shows that overweight individuals are less active than their average-weight peers.[26] Physical activity is inversely related to body weight, body composition,[27,28] and waist-to-hip ratio, although its relation to different degrees of obesity is less clear. There are factors, however, that must be considered when interpreting these results. First, many studies with both children and adults have failed to find meaningful differences in activity levels between overweight and average-weight persons.[26] Studies with those who are *extremely* overweight, however, have found significantly lower activity levels than for average-weight persons. A second factor is that lower levels of activity may not necessarily represent a lower energy expenditure. For example, an overweight person will require more energy to perform the same activity than a normal-weight person because of additional energy required to carry the excess weight. Therefore, an overweight person may actually expend more calories than a lighter-weight person who exercises more. A third factor may be the most important. Although overweight individuals may be less active than average-weight persons, it is possible that physical inactivity is a *consequence*—not a cause—of being overweight. We speculate that since physical activity becomes increasingly difficult with increased weight, this may lead to marked declines in exercise.

We have addressed the underuse of activity and its association with increased weight. Later we will address the overuse (abuse) of activity. Discussing both the underuse and overuse of exercise is important for understanding the relationship between exercise and weight regulation. We will now discuss the role that exercise plays in weight loss and maintenance and outline possible links between them.

EXERCISE AND WEIGHT CONTROL

Data reveal a pattern of weight regain when dietary interventions are used alone to control weight, whereas diet combined with exercise leads to better maintenance.[29] The importance of exercise for weight control is clear: regular exercise is a central component of losing weight and is the single best predictor of long-term weight maintenance.[11,29–37]

Correlational studies reveal consistently that exercise is associated with successful weight loss and maintenance.[35,38–41] Kayman and associates[35] studied formerly obese women who lost weight and kept it off and compared them with obese women who had lost weight and regained. Of the maintainers, 90% were exercising regularly (minimum of three times a week for >30 minutes), compared to only 34% of the regainers (Fig. 2–3).

Experimental weight loss treatment studies with random assignment and control groups comparing exercise to no exercise provide the strongest scientific support for the role of exercise in weight control. Many of these studies,[29,34,37,42–46] but not all,[47–49]

have found that combining exercise and dietary change produces greater weight loss than diet change alone.

It appears, however, that exercise exerts a special impact on weight maintenance. Behavior modification dietary programs, exercise, and combinations of diet and exercise have about the same short-term effect on weight loss.[26] Thus, physical activity has a modest effect on initial weight loss, perhaps because dietary compliance is good early in a program and there is little room for additional weight loss. However, long-term effects are clear: exercise is critical for weight maintenance. When the participants in experimental studies are followed for 1 or 2 years, striking effects of exercise emerge. A study by Pavlou and colleagues[29] provides persuasive evidence for the benefit of exercise in weight maintenance—regardless of the type of dietary intervention. In this study, 160 male members of the Boston Police Department and the Metropolitan District Commission were randomly assigned to one of four 12-week programs (balanced caloric-deficit diet [BCDD] of 100 kcal; a ketogenic protein-sparing modified fast [PSMF]; and two liquid forms of these balanced and ketogenic diets [DPC-70 and DPC-

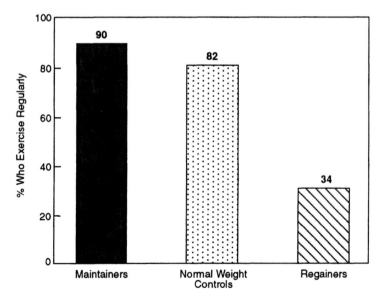

Figure 2–3. Maintenance and relapse after weight loss in women. (Adapted from Kayman et al,[35] p 803, with permission.)

800]) and to either an exercise or nonexercise group. Figure 2–4 displays 8- and 18-month follow-up data,[29] showing no difference between the initial and the 18-month follow-up weight for those who did not exercise, regardless of the four types of diets used for weight loss. In sharp contrast, the exercise group maintained weight loss. Furthermore, whether one added or stopped exercise following treatment predicted weight maintenance. As shown in Fig. 2–5, participants who ceased exercise at the end of treatment regained weight, whereas those who started exercise at the end of treatment maintained their weight loss at an 18-month follow-up. In sum, exercisers were much less likely to regain their weight during follow-up. No comparable studies have been performed using women, but we may tentatively assume that the findings would be similar.

Exercise facilitates maintenance with both balanced diets[29,50] and very low calorie diets.[29,37] Furthermore, even minimal increases in lifestyle activities (e.g., walking instead of riding, doing errands by walking),

which bolster energy expenditure by as little as 200 to 400 calories per day, result in enhanced maintenance in children.[51,52] We would like to underscore the connection between exercise and weight maintenance, because for many people, keeping the weight off is a greater challenge than losing weight initially.

LIKELY MECHANISMS LINKING EXERCISE AND WEIGHT CONTROL

Conventional wisdom suggests that overweight persons should exercise more, presumably because "it burns calories." It is unlikely, however, that exercise exerts its powerful effects on weight control simply because it burns calories. Exercise can alter body weight, body composition, appetite, and basal metabolism, and can affect health, independent of weight loss. Moreover, exercise can enhance psychologic well-being, improve self-esteem, and increase motiva-

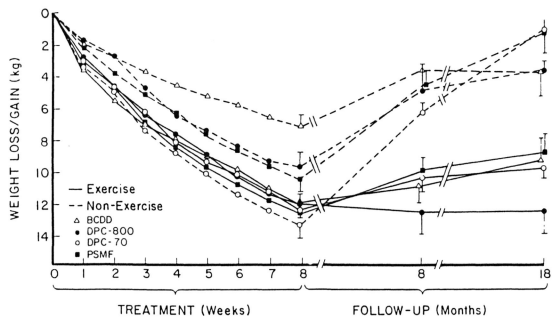

Figure 2–4. Exercise as an adjunct to weight-loss maintenance in moderately obese subjects. Follow-up data after 18 months confirm the long-term effectiveness of exercise intervention for as short a period as 8 weeks. There is no difference between initial and 18-month follow-up weight for those who did not exercise, regardless of the diet used for weight loss. In contrast, the exercise group maintained weight loss. (From Pavlou et al,[29] p 1121, with permission.)

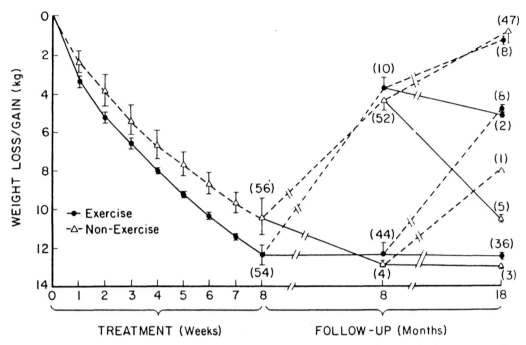

Figure 2–5. The addition or removal of learned exercise would appear to be a major contributing factor relative to weight maintenance. Subjects who ceased exercise regained or demonstrated a strong tendency to return to pre-study weights. Poststudy introduction of exercise (learned but nonsupervised) creates a positive effect. (Number of subjects given in parentheses.) (From Pavlou et al,[29] p 1122, with permission.)

tion. Although the exact links are not fully understood, there are multiple pathways by which exercise may aid in weight control (Table 2–1).

Understanding the potential mechanisms is crucial for prescribing exercise programs

Table 2–1. POSSIBLE LINKS BETWEEN EXERCISE AND WEIGHT CONTROL

1. Exercise expends energy.
2. Exercise may decrease appetite.
3. Exercise may enhance metabolic rate.
4. Exercise may preserve lean body tissue.
5. Exercise may limit preference for dietary fat.
6. Exercise enhances health.
7. Exercise improves risk factors associated with overweight.
8. Exercise has positive psychologic effects:
    Improves self-esteem and psychologic well-being,
    Decreases mild stress and anxiety,
    Increases confidence,
    May enhance dietary adherence.

Source: Adapted from Grilo et al.,[26] p 257, with permission.

for individuals. For example, if metabolic variables emerge as important, the types and amount of exercise needed to boost metabolic rate should be prescribed. If psychologic mechanisms are important, consistency, rather than type or amount, may be the central feature of a program. As a result, different programs might be prescribed depending on the nature of the links between exercise and weight control.

Energy Expenditure

Exercise Expends Energy

Any activity uses energy, so any increase in activity can aid in weight control. Table 2–2 provides values for caloric expenditure of various physical activities. Several important points are highlighted by this chart. First, routine activities like using stairs and walking are useful ways of expending energy. For example, walking up and down two

Table 2–2. CALORIC VALUES FOR 10
MINUTES OF ACTIVITY

	Body Weight					Body Weight		
	125	175	250			125	175	250
Personal Necessities					*Light Work*			
Sleeping	10	14	20		Assembly line	20	28	40
Sitting (watching TV)	10	14	18		Auto repair	35	48	69
Sitting (talking)	15	21	30		Carpentry	32	44	64
Dressing or washing	26	37	53		Bricklaying	28	40	57
Standing	12	16	24		Farming chores	32	44	64
					House painting	29	40	58
Locomotion					*Heavy Work*			
Walking downstairs	56	78	111					
Walking upstairs	146	202	288		Pick and shovel work	56	78	110
Walking at 2 mph	29	40	58		Chopping wood	60	84	121
Walking at 4 mph	52	72	102		Dragging logs	158	220	315
Running at 5.5 mph	90	125	178		Drilling coal	79	111	159
Running at 7 mph	118	164	232					
Running at 12 mph	164	228	326		*Recreation*			
Cycling at 5.5 mph	42	58	83		Badminton	43	65	94
Cycling at 13 mph	89	124	178		Baseball	39	54	78
					Basketball	58	82	117
Housework					Bowling (nonstop)	56	78	111
Making beds	32	46	65		Canoeing (4 mph)	90	128	182
Washing floors	38	53	75		Dancing (moderate)	35	48	69
Washing windows	35	48	69		Dancing (vigorous)	48	66	94
Dusting	22	31	44		Football	69	96	137
Preparing a meal	32	46	65		Golfing	33	48	68
Shoveling snow	65	89	130		Horseback riding	56	78	112
Light gardening	30	42	59		Ping-pong	32	45	64
Weeding garden	49	68	98		Racquetball	75	104	144
Mowing grass (power)	34	47	67		Skiing (alpine)	80	112	160
Mowing grass (manual)	38	52	74		Skiing (water)	60	88	130
					Skiing (cross-country)	98	138	194
Sedentary Occupation					Squash	75	104	144
Sitting writing	15	21	30		Swimming (backstroke)	32	45	64
Light office work	25	34	50		Swimming (crawl)	40	56	80
Standing, light activity	20	28	40		Tennis	56	80	115
Typing (electric)	19	27	39		Volleyball	43	65	94

Source: From Brownell,[135] pp 66–67, with permission.

flights of stairs per day, in place of using an elevator, would account for approximately 6 lb of weight loss per year for an average-weight man.[53] Second, heavier people burn more calories than normal-weight people while doing the same activity, because more energy is required to move the extra mass.

Despite these facts, many people are disappointed when they learn that even very rigorous physical activities produce relatively small energy deficits.[54] For example, a typical fast-food meal consisting of a quarter-pound cheeseburger, a small order of french fries, and a chocolate shake contains about 1100 calories. To expend 1100 calories through exercise would require running 11 miles or playing tennis for 3 hours.

However, Bray[55] and others have observed that weight loss in people who exercise tends to be greater than would be expected through the direct expenditure of energy. Consequently, other physiologic or psychologic mechanisms are likely to be important.

Exercise May Enhance Metabolic Rate

Resting metabolic rate (RMR) accounts for approximately 60% to 75% of a person's total daily energy needs.[55-57] Thus, small changes that either decrease or increase RMR can have a dramatic effect on a person's total daily energy expenditure. For instance, dieting can lead to a rapid and significant reduction in RMR.[55,57-62] Since dieting and weight loss often lower RMR, it is important to find ways to help offset this metabolic slowdown.[57,63]

Exercise may prevent or at least reduce the decline in the body's metabolic rate produced by dieting.[57,60,64,65] Tremblay and colleagues[65] found a significant increase in RMR (8% of pretraining value) in obese individuals who engaged in an 11-week training program, despite significant reductions in body weight and body fat mass. Broeder and colleagues[66] observed that 12 weeks of either high-intensity endurance or resistance training helped to prevent an attenuation in RMR normally observed during extended periods of negative energy balance, by either preserving the person's fat-free mass via endurance training, or increasing it via resistance training. In contrast, Phinney and colleagues[49] found that when physical activity was added while on a very low calorie diet, it further depressed the metabolic rate rather than raised it. These conflicting findings underscore the need for more research to define the amount and types of exercise that have the most beneficial metabolic effects.

Another dilemma confronting dieters is the potential metabolic consequences of successive episodes of weight loss followed by regain (i.e., weight cycling or yo-yo dieting). There is inconclusive evidence about whether weight cycling produces greater drops in RMR with repeated dieting efforts.[26] To the extent that this does occur, it may be particularly important to use exercise interventions with weight-cyclers, as they may bolster RMR.[46]

Appetite and Hunger

Exercise May Decrease Appetite

A number of studies with both humans and animals have examined the association between exercise and appetite.[26] A frequent misconception is that increased activity will be met with increased food intake, so there is no net benefit of the exercise. Although the effects of exercise on appetite are complex, this regulatory mechanism tends to be in effect for only certain levels of activity.[26]

Studies with humans suggest that exercise can be effective in regulating appetite. Increasing physical activity moderately tends to decrease appetite, food intake, and body weight, whereas increasing exercise to vigorous levels leads to increased appetite but stable body weight.[67-70] However, women may benefit less from the suppression effects of exercise on appetite than do men.[67] Some studies have found that increased physical activity does not decrease appetite in lean women, and that they may in fact eat more,[67,70,71] although their appetite does not appear to increase beyond the level needed to maintain weight.

In sum, exercise is unlikely to increase appetite beyond the level to keep body weight stable, and often may lead to decreased food intake. However, a potential problem exists, since people may "believe" they will be hungrier after they exercise. Monitoring one's feelings of hunger before and after exercise may help dispel this myth. In fact, some individuals find it useful to exercise at times when they are tempted to overeat.

Exercise May Limit Preference for Dietary Fat

Another potential benefit of exercise may be its influence on the intake of fat in the diet. Several animal studies have found that weight cycling (repeated cycles of weight loss and regain) results in a higher consumption of dietary fat,[72,73] accompanied by larger adipose tissue depots.[72] Exercise, however, seems to limit this increased dietary fat selection in weight-cycled female rats, and reduces the amount of body fat regained during refeeding periods.[73] These findings may have important implications for the treatment of overweight in humans, since weight cycling is common.

Body Composition

Exercise May Preserve Lean (Muscle) Tissue

Unfortunately, weight loss is not due solely to the loss of body fat. Weight loss is accounted for by several changes, including the loss of both lean and fat body tissue. As much as 25% of the weight lost by dieting alone can be lean body mass (LBM).[57] In fact, the often observed slowing of weight loss despite continued dieting (reaching a plateau) may be due partly to the loss of lean tissue, since lean tissue requires more energy to sustain itself.

The loss of LBM decreases when exercise (even low to moderate) is combined with diet.[74] Several studies have found that regular aerobic exercise, even in the absence of dietary restriction, can produce significant body fat loss with minimal loss of lean tissue.[75–77] More recently, resistance training has been used to improve the ratio of lean to fat tissue, which may have the added benefit of increasing energy expenditure.[78] Since increasing LBM and decreasing body fat may increase metabolic rate (because muscle requires more calories than does fat), exercise prescriptions with this goal in mind may be especially useful.

Physical Activity and Health

Prospective studies reveal an inverse relationship between exercise or fitness level and morbidity and mortality in overweight men and women.[79–82] Substantial evidence

exists that regular physical activity is associated with good health.[82–84] Moreover, even modest levels of exercise are sufficient for significant health benefits.[79,85,86] Lee[87] reviewed the literature pertaining to women and aerobic exercise and concluded that middle-aged and older women incur the same physiologic and health benefits from exercise as do men (see Appendices 2–1 and 2–2).

One study provides convincing evidence that even low levels of activity can have a substantial health impact. Blair and colleagues[79] calculated the age-adjusted all-cause death rates over an 8-year period in 10,224 men and 3120 women who were apparently healthy at baseline. Each person was assigned to a fitness category (based on entry maximal treadmill testing), ranging from the very unfit (Fitness Level 1) to the very fit (Fitness Level 5). In all BMI strata, the low-fit men and women had higher death rates than moderate- and high-fit subjects. Therefore, physically fit individuals had much lower mortality rates (Fig. 2–6). The largest reductions in risk, however, came from moving from very low to moderate levels of fitness, not from being extremely active. This study and others have helped counter the notion that one must exercise vigorously to obtain the health benefits of exercise,[83,85] and is *critically important* for overweight persons, in whom adherence is

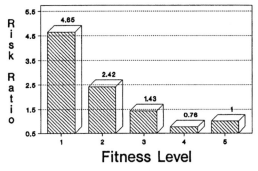

Figure 2–6. The relationship between fitness level and death rate in women. (From Brownell,[135] p 178, with permission, based on findings of Blair et al.[79])

greatest in the low to moderate intensity range.[5,33,51]

Exercise Improves Medical Conditions Often Associated with Overweight

Exercise helps offset medical conditions prevalent in the overweight. Conditions such as high blood pressure, elevated cholesterol, and diabetes improve with exercise.[83] Exercise can provide these benefits independent of weight loss.[53,54,83,88,89] Several studies have now shown an association between distribution of body fat (abdominal fat) and increased health risk (e.g., higher incidence of myocardial infarctions and strokes).[90] Recent population-based studies show that physically active men and women have lower (more favorable) waist-to-hip ratios.[91-94] Therefore, in the absence of clinical intervention data, it seems reasonable to recommend exercise for overweight persons with a high waist-to-hip ratio, although research is needed to document whether exercise reduces abdominal fat.

Psychologic Changes

Exercise has important psychologic effects and is associated with positive psychologic health. Physical activity improves mood, psychologic well-being (especially immediately following exercise), and self-concept, and also decreases mild anxiety, depression, and stress.[95,96] In persons attempting to lose or maintain weight, exercise may relieve stress or other negative feelings that precede dietary lapses.[97]

Surprisingly low levels of exercise seem to complement dieting by increasing dietary adherence.[51,96] Rodin and Plante[96] reported that findings from their weight control studies suggest that people who engage in modest exercise (i.e., jumping jacks for 10 minutes a day, three times a week) are substantially more successful at weight control than nonexercisers. Similarly, Epstein and colleagues[51] found that adherence to

diet was related to adherence to exercise, and that adherence was better in programs with lower rather than higher caloric expenditure.

In these studies,[51,96] *low* calorie expenditure was related to increased dietary adherence and weight loss. Physiologic factors (e.g., increased metabolic rate) alone cannot account for the weight loss when the amount of exercise is so minimal. These findings raise the important issue of whether perceived or actual fitness is the key factor in linking exercise to weight control. Since adherence is better for low- to moderate-intensity exercise, low levels may evoke feelings of mastery. Improved self-concept due to exercising may then generalize to other aspects of functioning, thereby increasing confidence for controlling dietary practices. One's perception of being physically fit thus may be more important than physical fitness per se.[95] Developing the self-image of an exerciser should enhance self-efficacy, which could lead to increased self-determination.

Collectively, these studies show that exercise of low to moderate intensity is associated with improved dietary patterns and weight loss. These results parallel others that suggest that exercise may not need to be aerobic or of high intensity to engender positive psychologic correlates.[98-101] Indeed, high-intensity exercise can increase negative mood states such as tension, anxiety, and fatigue.[102] Such negative consequences are important to avoid, since they represent potential barriers to exercise adherence.

In sum, exercise is an important predictor of success at weight reduction and maintenance and has numerous health and psychologic benefits. The link between exercise, weight control, and positive psychologic functioning dictates the importance of finding strategies to help individuals become more active. In the next section, we will discuss the challenge of adherence and suggest ways to maximize an overweight person's ability to comply with exercise regimens.

THE CHALLENGE OF ADHERENCE

Poor adherence has long been considered a challenge in exercise programs. Although there have been over 200 studies conducted in the past 20 years on various determinants of exercise behavior,[103] little systematic investigation has been conducted on overweight persons. We will draw from the existing studies on adherence relevant for overweight persons and suggest ways to develop a program. The reader is referred to prior reviews for a more general overview of exercise adherence, since they provide a framework from which a program for the overweight individual can be established.[5,26,83,103]

Adherence and the Demographics of Obesity

Although most people who are overweight know that increased exercise may help them lose weight, many are unable to establish and maintain a personal exercise program. Professionals are confronted with the challenge of helping these individuals increase their level of physical activity.

One reason that exercise adherence is a special challenge in overweight persons is that groups most likely to be overweight are also least likely to exercise. Overweight occurs with especially high prevalence in minority populations[104,105] and in persons with lower socioeconomic status (SES).[21,106] In addition, the incidence of obesity increases with age, particularly in women.[21,107] For African-American women ages 45 to 75 years, obesity rates are as high as 60%.[21] Exercise rates for obese persons, the elderly, minority groups, and those with low SES, however, are very low.[103,108]

Obstacles to Exercise for the Overweight Individual

Several obstacles can impede the transition from the desire to exercise to the act of exercising. Careful attention to potential

Table 2-3. POTENTIAL PHYSICAL AND PSYCHOLOGIC BARRIERS TO EXERCISE IN OVERWEIGHT PERSONS

Physical Barriers
Poor fitness
Excess weight
Psychologic Barriers
Negative experiences
Teased by peers
Picked last for teams
Social Anxiety
Shame of being observed
Body image dissatisfaction
Lack of confidence
Lack of knowledge or experience

Source: Adapted from Grilo et al,[26] p 264, with permission.

physical and psychologic barriers to exercise among overweight individuals is critical. Table 2-3 summarizes potential barriers to exercise.

Physical Burden

For many overweight persons, exercise is unpleasant due to poor physical conditioning and excess weight. Weight becomes a burden that must be overcome. Increasing physical activity may be difficult, painful, and fatiguing. Starting a program too quickly or vigorously may lead to excess fatigue, physical discomfort, and injuries, each of which can deter a person from future efforts. Starting overweight people with a low- to moderate-paced program is crucial for preventing injuries, enhancing exercise self-efficacy, and sustaining adherence.

Negative Associations

Psychologic barriers are sometimes formidable obstacles for overweight people to overcome in order to exercise regularly. For people who have been overweight since childhood, early memories such as being teased, being picked last for teams, and suffering from poor athletic performance leave many obese persons ashamed and self-conscious about their bodies.[109,110] Overweight is often associated with social rejection.[111,112] Consequently, many overweight persons manifest disturbances in areas of life affected by weight, such as body image, social interactions, and self-esteem.[112]

It is not surprising that thoughts of exercise may evoke unpleasant memories, feelings of inadequacy, and shame at the prospect of being observed. Not only does the excess weight add a physical burden, but a persistent negative body image may discourage a person from exercising with others, and the lack of self-confidence may prevent a person from starting an exercise program. It is important to be sensitive to such experiences and to create a supportive atmosphere so that overweight persons can identify and initiate activities they enjoy in a positive way. Helping overweight persons identify clothing that they feel comfortable wearing, from shoes to workout apparel, and explaining where to obtain exercise clothing in large sizes is useful and appreciated. It is essential to encourage patients to experiment with different activities until they experience pleasure and satisfaction. This may include exploring community options that provide opportunities to exercise with other overweight individuals.

Developmental and Gender Issues

Exercise initiation and maintenance may be enhanced by tailoring interventions to specific developmental milestones.[113] An executive woman with an ill mother will have different developmental and practical issues than a teenager with minimal responsibilities. Table 2–4 presents features and examples of physical activity programs for several important periods. It is also important to tailor interventions specifically for women. For example, many women have not been involved in physical activity programs. The fact that inactivity is considered a problem for women reflects a substantial shift in attitudes in the past 25 years.[114] Many women over 30 were never encouraged to participate in team sports or recreational physical activity; instead, many learned to

diet for weight control. It will be important to keep this inexperience in mind when developing exercise programs for these individuals.

Adherence Studies

Exercise adherence has been understudied with overweight persons. This is unfortunate, since overweight persons have low exercise participation rates and are at a high risk for health problems that can be improved with exercise.[103] For instance, Gwinup[115] found that only 32% of overweight women enrolled in a walking exercise program remained in the program for 1 year. In a prospective study with a large community sample, Sallis and co-workers[116] found that overweight subjects were less likely to adopt exercise than were normal-weight subjects.

Intensity

Less intense, "lifestyle" activity or moderate-intensity activities (those that require less than 60% of maximal capacity, such as walking) generally have superior initiation and adherence rates and lower drop-out rates than do vigorous activities.[51,83,87,116,117] This seems to hold true among widely diverse groups of people. A large community study in California[116] found that both men and women were more likely to adopt moderate activity than a vigorous fitness regimen. Moderate activity programs showed a dropout rate (25% to 35%) roughly one half of that seen for vigorous exercise (50%). Additionally, moderate activity appears to be more readily maintained over the life span, whereas participation in vigorous activity declines dramatically with age.[118] This is especially important to consider with overweight persons, since overweight increases with age. In fact, low-intensity exercise (30% to 45% MHR) has produced significant increases in fitness for women in their 60s and 70s.[119] Overweight children also do better when low-intensity, lifestyle exercise regimens are prescribed, versus high-intensity activities; Epstein and colleagues[52,120] found

Table 2-4. PHYSICAL ACTIVITY PROGRAMS FOR SEVERAL MAJOR DEVELOPMENTAL MILESTONES

Milestone (Critical Period)	Specific Features	Goals/Strategies
Adolescence	Rapid physical and emotional changes Increased concern with appearance and weight Need for independence Short-term perspective Increased peer influence	Exercise as part of a program of healthy weight regulation (both sexes) Noncompetitive activities that are fun, varied Emphasis on independence, choice Focus on proximal outcomes (e.g., body image, stress management) Peer involvement, support
Initial work entry	Increased time and scheduling constraints Short-term perspective Employer demands	Choice of activities that are convenient, enjoyable Focus on proximal outcomes Involvement of worksite (environmental prompts, incentives) Realistic goal setting, injury prevention Coeducational, noncompetitive activities
Parenting	Increased family demands and time constraints Family-directed focus Postpartum effects on weight, mood	Emphasis on benefits to self and family (e.g., stress management, weight control, well-being) Activities appropriate with children (e.g., walking) Flexible, convenient, personalized regimen Inclusion of activities of daily living Neighborhood involvement, focus Family-based public monitoring, goal-setting Availability of child-related services (child care)
Retirement age	Increased time availability and flexibility Longer-term perspective on health; increased health concerns, "readiness" Caregiving duties, responsibilities (parents, spouse, children, or grandchildren)	Identification of current and previous enjoyable activities Matching of activities to current health status Emphasis on mild- and moderate-intensity activities, including activities of daily living Use of "life path point" information and prompts Emphasis on activities engendering independence Garnering support of family members, peers Availability of necessary services (e.g., caretaking services for significant other)

Source: From King,[113] p 250, with permission.

that lifestyle exercise was superior to programmed aerobic exercise for long-term weight maintenance (Fig. 2-7). It may be that since lifestyle programs are more flexible and easily incorporated into one's daily routine, fewer barriers emerge to preclude continued participation.[51,121]

In sum, prescription of lifestyle activity over vigorous, programmed exercise may represent one key to adherence for overweight persons. Beginning individuals with modest activity goals that are readily incorporated into their daily life is preferable to approaches that promote sweat, pain, and extreme effort. Adherence is increased when the activity can be readily incorporated into daily life; this, in turn, may enhance one's confidence in the ability to perform physical activity (self-efficacy), which may improve adherence. Moderate-intensity activity has many of the health benefits of vigorous exercise,[79,116,122] with the added benefit of easier maintenance.[83]

Relapse Prevention Strategies

Cognitive behavioral therapy (CBT) programs for exercise adherence that have in-

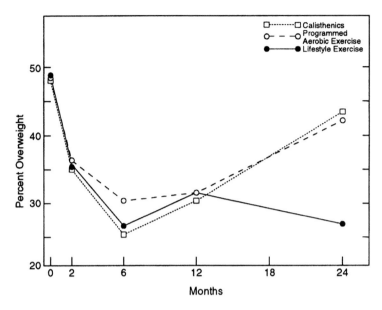

Figure 2-7. Percent overweight for children in three groups (calisthenics, programmed aerobic exercise, and lifestyle exercise) at 0, 2, 6, 12, and 24 months. (From Epstein et al,[120] p 351, with permission.)

corporated components of Marlatt and Gordon's[123] relapse prevention model result in better physical activity rates at followup.[124–128] Although originally developed for other areas such as smoking and alcohol, this model offers several important suggestions to persons trying to maintain any behavior change. Three elements are particularly useful for increasing adherence: (1) flexible rather than rigid exercise goals,[128] (2) training individuals in specific techniques to cope with missed exercise sessions,[126] and (3) identifying potential situations that might interfere with exercise or lifestyle changes and developing plans for coping with those high-risk situations and setbacks.[124] Moreover, relapse training, in comparison to a treatment with no relapse training, results in significantly greater weight maintenance.[124] Even minimal intervention strategies such as telephone contacts or mailings, however, may enhance adherence and maintenance of weight loss.[31,36]

Stages of Change in Exercise Adoption and Maintenance

Recently, several researchers have suggested that individuals proceed through specific stages in the initiation and mainte-

nance of exercise and proposed that individuals in the different stages may require different cognitive and behavioral approaches.[5,129,130] This model proposes that people proceed through five stages: precontemplation, contemplation, preparation, action, and maintenance, as follows:[131]

Precontemplation. Precontemplators do not intend to change their behavior in the foreseeable future. These individuals are unaware of the benefits of exercise or are uncertain about whether the benefits are greater than the negative aspects. Movement to the next stage would require acknowledging and becoming more aware of the negative aspects of their lack of exercise.

Contemplation. Contemplators are aware of the negative aspects of their lack of exercise and are seriously considering taking action. Both the positive and negative aspects are considered. Contemplators have not, however, committed themselves to the necessary steps for change. Exercisers will progress to the next stage only after a decision to change their lack of exercise.

Preparation. Exercisers in the preparation stage are characterized by a readiness and intention to begin exercise or change their behavior in the foreseeable future. These individuals have evaluated past successes and failures and are on the verge of taking action. Movement to the next stage requires setting attainable goals and steps for action.

Action. Persons in the action stage begin to make changes in their behavior. A central focus is setting appropriate goals and taking action to implement them. They are aware of the cognitive, behavioral, and/or environmental factors that may interfere with continued progress.

Maintenance. Persons in the maintenance stage focus their attention on preventing relapse to former behaviors as well as continuing the exercise patterns begun in the action stage. Exercisers in the maintenance stage are concentrating on identifying potential situations that may interfere with their continued success.

A potential major contribution of this model for increasing and maintaining exercise lies in its consideration of the readiness of individuals for change.[5] Awareness of variables such as readiness can facilitate patient-treatment matching, thus improving outcome.[132] In fact, a recent study[129] found that exercise programs must accommodate the large percentage of individuals who are not ready to change their exercise habits. Research is needed on how to best match exercise interventions to patient's stages of change. The concepts of readiness and patient-treatment matching apply not only to exercise in overweight persons, but also to dieting itself.[11]

Social Support

All health behaviors, including exercise, are influenced by social context. Attempts to improve weight loss by involving significant others have met with mixed results,[133] perhaps because of a failure to assess the needs and characteristics of the target groups. One

study[134] found a significant interaction between weight loss treatment and gender: women did better when treated with their spouses, whereas men did better when treated alone. This study is an example of the potential need to match particular support interventions to the individual's needs and characteristics.

Equivalent studies looking at social support and exercise adherence in overweight persons have not been done. Our clinical experience suggests, however, that there tend to be "solo" versus "social" exercisers. The "solo" type individual typically does not desire the company of others and tends to select activities such as walking or jogging alone. A "social" exerciser may prefer an aerobics class or jogging with a partner. Our experience is that a better match between personality type and type of exercise results in a better fit.[135]

Further research is needed to identify the factors that predict success with spouse, family, or peer interventions for exercise and dietary adherence with obese persons. Brownell[135] and Brownell and Rodin[136] provide specific strategies and techniques to aid overweight individuals in identifying and pursuing the type of social support they need.

PROGRAM RECOMMENDATIONS

Three basic issues confront the clinician: (1) the type of exercise to prescribe, (2) ways to maximize adherence, and (3) relapse prevention. Table 2–5 outlines our recommendations for exercise programs for overweight persons. Important elements are discussed below.

Avoid a Threshold Mentality

Any activity, even those not normally labeled as exercise, can provide substantial benefit. It is important to avoid the trap of defining physical activity in traditional terms (70% of maximal heart rate, three

Table 2–5. RECOMMENDATIONS FOR MAXIMIZING EXERCISE ADHERENCE IN OBESE PERSONS

General Principles

1. Be sensitive to psychologic barriers.
2. Be sensitive to physical barriers.
3. Decrease focus on exercise threshold.
4. Increase focus on enhanced self-efficacy.
5. Emphasize consistency and enjoyment, not amount and type.
6. Begin at a person's level of fitness.
7. Encourage people to define routine activities as "exercise."
8. Focus on compliance and avoid emphasis on minor metabolic issues (e.g., whether to exercise before or after a meal).
9. Consider life-span developmental context.
10. Consider sociocultural issues and gender influences.
11. Evaluate social support network.
12. Evaluate stage of change and intervene accordingly.

Specific Interventions

1. Prescription
   a. Provide clear information about importance of activity, including the psychologic benefits.
   b. Maximize routine activity. Define daily activities as exercise.
   c. Maximize walking (e.g., walk while doing errands).
   d. Increase use of stairs in lieu of escalators and elevators.
   e. Incorporate a programmed activity that is enjoyable, fits with lifestyle, and is feasible as client's fitness improves.
2. Behavioral
   a. Introduce self-monitoring, feedback, and goal-setting techniques.
   b. Identify important targets other than weight loss, including physical changes, increased mobility (flexibility, endurance, ease), and lowered heart rate.
   c. Suggest that exercise may help soothe emotional distress when risk for overeating is high.
   d. Stimulus control: increase exercise cues (e.g., reminders for increasing activity) and decrease competing cues (e.g., do not schedule exercise when it might conflict with work or social obligations).
3. Maintenance and relapse prevention
   a. Use flexible guidelines and goal-setting, but avoid rigid rules.
   b. Identify potential high-risk situations for skipping exercise (e.g., stressful times, busy schedule).
   c. Develop plans to cope with high-risk situations.

d. Use exercise following dietary lapses to psychologically regain a sense of control, mastery, and commitment.
e. Convey philosophy that a lapse can be used as a signal to re-initiate small amounts of physical activity (e.g., a 2-minute walk). Encourage notion that all exercise has a cumulative effect on a number of domains (health, mood, sense of mastery).
f. Use of minimal intervention strategies, including phone contacts, may foster exercise maintenance.

Source: Adapted from Grilo et al,[26] p 266, with permission.

times per week, for at least 15 minutes). This three-part equation (frequency, intensity, and duration) has been defined as essential for cardiorespiratory conditioning,[57] but it implies an exercise "threshold"—that is, that exercise must occur in a specific amount to be beneficial. This threshold may motivate physically active or athletic persons, but it may deter others, including the overweight. Since any exercise is worthwhile, the threshold mentality may hinder more than help. As a professional working with overweight people, it is important for you to stress that low to moderate levels of exercise provide many health,[79] psychologic,[96] and weight-loss benefits.[52,120] Showing overweight persons data such as Figure 2–6 can help make this point.

Consistency May Be More Important than the Type or Amount of Exercise

We believe the most important question to ask about exercise is, "Will I be doing this a year from now?" It is important to help patients choose activities that will be enjoyable in the long run. Developing a consistent form of activity, or a consistent set of activities, is the primary focus. It is preferable to have a person regularly play tennis twice a week and walk for one additional day than to run 4 miles/d for a week and then stop entirely. Lifestyle change, consistency, and moderation are the key goals.

Provide Thorough Education

It is important to emphasize that even low-intensity exercise leads to enhanced dietary adherence and weight control. Otherwise, people will feel they are always exercising "less than they should." Education regarding the physical and psychologic benefits of exercise can expand the patient's understanding of the potential benefits. Dispelling erroneous notions such as "no pain, no gain" is an essential component. Poor health behaviors can result from inadequate information as well as nonadherence.

Be Sensitive to the Special Needs of Overweight Persons

Since obese persons have special psychologic and physical barriers to exercise, helping them feel comfortable with exercise and helping them define even low levels of activity as exercise is an important step toward adherence. Simply conveying understanding and sensitivity can be helpful.

SPECIAL ISSUES

It is important to develop "reasonable" weight-loss goals and healthy attitudes regarding exercise and diet. Our culture's preoccupation with shape and weight may foster unhealthy attitudes. Health care professionals should be aware of methods to encourage the pursuit of "reasonable" weight-loss goals.

The Role of Exercise in the Search for the Perfect Body

Today's aesthetic ideal is becoming increasingly lean, coupled with an added pressure to be physically fit.[137-140] The symbolic connotations of having the ideal body (success, self-control, acceptance), current standards about ideal body weight and shape, and the overstated health benefits of slenderness are important factors responsible for the increase in dieting and exercise behavior.[137] Consumers are frantically searching for information to achieve the perfect body. One need only look at the multibillion dollar industry to help people look more attractive—diets, exercise paraphernalia, cosmetics, fashions, and various forms of cosmetic surgery—to realize the extent to which there is societal pressure to "look good."[141]

Two beliefs fuel this search for the "ideal" body. The first belief is that the body is infinitely malleable, and that with the right diet, exercise program, and personal effort, an individual can achieve the aesthetic ideal. The second belief is that once the ideal is achieved, there will be considerable rewards, such as career advancement, wealth, interpersonal attraction, and happiness.[137]

Ideal Versus Healthy Versus Reasonable Weight

The body cannot be shaped at will. Genetic factors play a substantial role in limiting our ability to change body weight[142,143] and body shape.[144] Certain individuals may be prone to gain weight or to have specific body shapes and these factors may resist attempts to lose weight.[11] This creates a mismatch between cultural pressures and biologic realities.[137]

This collision between cultural pressures and biologic realities leads to the critical question of how much control a person has over weight and shape.[145] Scientists have estimated that current aesthetic ideals (popular models and actresses) have 10% to 15% body fat, compared with 22% to 26% for healthy, normal-weight women.[137,140,146] For instance, a study by Wiseman and colleagues[140] found that the majority of Playboy centerfolds and Miss America contestants were 15% or more below their expected weight, one of the criteria for anorexia nervosa. One may speculate that many of our "ideals" have eating disorders. Miss America contestants work out an average of 14 hours per week, with some approaching 35 hours.[147] Although the current societal ideal is unattainable and/or unrealistic for most people, those who do not meet the ideal are often judged to be lazy, indulgent, and lacking willpower. The exercise and weight loss needed to pursue the aesthetic ideal, however, is far in excess of what is necessary (or recommended) for healthy living.[146]

Weight-loss programs typically identify some "goal weight" or "ideal weight" as the desired outcome. Moreover, whether or not there are formal goals developed by program staff, patients often have self-imposed goals influenced by visualizations of an aesthetic ideal. The notion of ideal weight may be useful for people who are only mildly overweight (because the ideal is potentially attainable), or for prevention efforts in which excess weight beyond the standard signals the need for intervention. For many people, however, the ideal generates a search for an elusive goal, which often leads to poor long-term results.

Brownell and Wadden[11] suggest that it is important to think not only of an ideal

weight, but a reasonable weight. Table 2-6 lists questions to formulate a reasonable weight for an individual patient. The calculation of reasonable weight would take into account the individual's weight history, developmental stage, social circumstances, metabolic profile, and other factors. For instance, specific milestones, transitions, and life periods affect how women feel toward their bodies. Females begin life with more body fat than males, and this difference continues to increase during specific developmental stages over the life span (at puberty, pregnancy, and menopause). These physiologic changes promote weight gain.[148] Discussing these developmental transitions can help women develop an acceptance and understanding of the physiologic changes while also using this information to formulate a reasonable weight goal.

In some cases, reasonable weight and health ideals may be the same (e.g., the individual can sustain the effort, calorie restriction, and exercise necessary to maintain that weight). On the other hand, the reasonable weight might exceed the ideal weight if biologic, psychologic, developmental, or cultural variables interfere.

Nonetheless, any weight loss is likely to be beneficial, particularly if it can be maintained. For some individuals, a small weight loss can lead to significant improvements in medical conditions[149,150] and may have a number of positive outcomes, such as feeling more energetic, improved mobility, or less dependence on others for basic needs. Thus, patients should be encouraged to set goals according to several parameters, since this may help to prevent the common trap of viewing anything but goal weight as failure. Tracking changes in physiologic factors that are likely to change with increased physical activity and weight loss (e.g., blood sugar, blood pressure, serum cholesterol); anthropometric measures (e.g., skinfold thickness and circumferences); and psychologic changes may provide clear evidence of accomplishment to both patients and health professionals. Maintaining these benefits

Table 2-6. QUESTIONS USED AS CLINICAL CRITERIA TO HELP ESTABLISH A "REASONABLE WEIGHT" FOR AN INDIVIDUAL*

1. Is there a history of excess weight in your parents or grandparents?
2. What is the lowest weight you have maintained as an adult for at least one year?
3. What is the largest size of clothes that you feel comfortable in, at the point you say "I look pretty good considering where I have been"? At what weight would you wear these clothes?
4. Think of a friend or family member (with your age and body frame) who looks "normal" to you. What does the person weigh?
5. At what weight do you believe you can live with the required changes in eating and/or exercise?

*These questions are based in part on criteria proposed by Brownell and Rodin[136] and represent clinical impression. Research-based criteria have not been established.
Source: Reprinted from Brownell and Wadden,[11] p 509, with permission.

can be one central goal of treatment, even if more weight is to be lost.

Exercise Overuse (Abuse)

As we have noted, exercise is an important aspect of weight control and is generally viewed as a healthy and positive endeavor. Unfortunately, exercise can become compulsive when done in pursuit of excessive thinness. An enduring fear of being fat is a hallmark of anorexia nervosa and bulimia nervosa.[14,151–153] Vigorous exercise can be a means of weight loss or one of several tactics used by the individual to counteract the ingestion of excess calories or deal with body image concerns. Intense fears of becoming fat may exist in people across all weight groups and body shapes.

Even exceptionally lean persons may have body image disparagement. In fact, a growing body of research with athletes suggests that a disproportionately high rate of fear of fatness and extreme dieting measures may exist in these lean and fit individuals.[19] One group of researchers investigated the functional role of exercise in a group of 112 women who were regular exercise participants.[154] While only a handful were overweight, 77% of these relatively slender and active women wanted to lose weight, and most of them were dieting (57%). Another study revealed that 19% of a group of female runners met diagnostic criteria for bulimia nervosa,[155] which is a much higher prevalence than expected in this group.[156] Of the bulimic women, most cited exercise as their most common compensation tactic for binge-eating episodes. Results did not indicate a particular weight or running profile (that is, the bulimics were not significantly different on mileage per week or fastest time for a 10-K race than nonbulimics), but did reveal associated psychologic factors (dietary restraint and depression). A survey conducted in *Runner's World* magazine[157] revealed that among the 4000 runners who responded, 48% of the females and 21% of the

males said that they were often, usually, or always "terrified of being fat."

This "terror of being fat" can cause some individuals to fall into the trap of excessively exercising while still falling short of the "perfect body." Many studies evaluate whether people diet or exercise, but minimal attention has been paid to *why* they do so. A substantial subset of runners may be motivated by the fear of being fat and may be running away from a vision of being fat. Because both diet and exercise are excessive in some individuals, knowing the motivation may be helpful in detecting unhealthy exercise and dietary behaviors. Table 2–7 presents questions that might aid health professionals in determining whether exercise is excessive or potentially problematic.[158] These questions are based on our clinical experience and may not predict exercise abuse. Rather, affirmative responses suggest the need for further evaluation and understanding of that individual's use (or potential abuse) of exercise. It is critically

Table 2–7. ASSESSMENT QUESTIONS TO SCREEN FOR POTENTIAL EXERCISE ABUSE

1. Are there times during the day when you feel unable to stop thinking about exercise, even if you want to?
2. Do you feel anxious, irritable, or uncomfortable when you miss an exercise session?
3. If you miss an exercise session, do you feel that you need to make up for it (e.g., by staying up later or getting up earlier to do it, by increasing the amount of exercise you do the next day)?
4. Have you sometimes exercised despite being advised against it (i.e., by a doctor, friend, family member)? What advice was given? Why did you exercise?
5. Do you try to increase your exercise session (or add an additional exercise) when you feel you have overeaten or when you eat "junk foods"?
6. Do you worry about putting on weight or becoming fat if you miss an exercise session?
7. When you exercise, do you think about the calories or the amount of fat you are burning off?

Source: From Grilo and Wilfley,[158] p 163, with permission.

important for health professionals to recognize possible signs and symptoms of exercise abuse.

SUMMARY

Weight control is widely sought after by women in the United States. This pervasive desire for thinness leads women to seek out many different combinations of diet and exercise programs. It is critical, therefore, to understand the physiologic and psychologic effects of such programs and to identify programs that are safe and effective.

Physical activity is central to this endeavor. It is the most powerful predictor of long-term weight maintenance. Exercise programs of low to moderate intensity have superior adherence to those of high intensity and have many health, psychologic, and weight-loss benefits. We feel it is critical to encourage overweight and inactive women to view any activity as beneficial and that consistency is the key variable.

Conversely, it is important to recognize possible signs of exercise abuse. Sadly, many women are in pursuit of the current societal ideal, which is often unattainable and/or unrealistic. Women should be encouraged to develop reasonable expectations for weight control and exercise. Focus on lifestyle change, consistency, and moderation may be the best treatment philosophy.

REFERENCES

1. Begley CE: Government should strengthen regulation in the weight loss industry. J Am Diet Assoc 91:1255, 1991.
2. Centers for Disease Control: Body-weight perceptions and selected weight-management goals and practices of high school students—United States, 1990. MMWR 40:741, 1991.
3. Kolbe LJ: An epidemiological surveillance system to monitor the prevalence of youth behaviors that most affect health. Health Educ 21:44, 1990.
4. Serdula M: Weight control practices in U.S.

adolescents and adults: Youth risk behavior survey and behavioral risk factor surveillance system. In Methods for Voluntary Weight Loss and Control. NIH Technology Assessment Conference, 1992, p 46.
5. Dishman RK: Increasing and maintaining exercise and physical activity. Behav Ther 22:345, 1991.
6. Kuczmarski RJ: Prevalence of overweight and weight gain in the United States. Am J Clin Nutr 55:495S–502S, 1992.
7. Bray GA: Effects of obesity on health and happiness. In Brownell KD, and Foreyt JP (eds): Handbook of Eating Disorders: Physiology, Psychology, and Treatment of Obesity, Anorexia, and Bulimia. New York, Basic Books 3, 1986.
8. Pi-Sunyer FX: Health implications of obesity. Am J Clin Nutr 53:1595S, 1991.
9. National Institutes of Health Consensus Development Panel on the Health Implications of Obesity: Health implications of obesity. National Institutes of Health consensus development conference statement. Ann Intern Med 103:1073, 1985.
10. Bray GA: Pathophysiology of obesity. Am J Clin Nutr 55:488S, 1992.
11. Brownell KD, and Wadden, TA: Etiology and treatment of obesity: Toward understanding a serious, prevalent, and refractory disorder. J Consult Clin Psychol 60:505, 1992.
12. Pyle RL, Mitchell JE, Eckert ED, et al: Maintenance treatment and 6-month outcome for bulimic patients who respond to initial treatment. Am J Psychiatry 147:871, 1990.
13. Pike KM, and Rodin J: Mothers, daughters, and disordered eating. J Abnorm Psychol 100:198, 1991.
14. Striegel-Moore RH, Silberstein LR, and Rodin J: Toward an understanding of risk factors for bulimia. Am Psychol 41:246, 1986.
15. Striegel-Moore RH, Silberstein LR, and Rodin J: The social self in bulimia nervosa: Public self-consciousness, social anxiety, and perceived fraudulence. J Abnorm Psychol (in press).
16. Wilson, GT: Short-term psychological benefits and adverse effects of weight loss. In Methods for Voluntary Weight Loss and Control NIH Technology Assessment Conference, 1992, p 134.
17. Rand CSW, and Kuldau, JM: The epidemiology of obesity and self-defined weight problem in the general population. Int J Eat Dis 9:329, 1990.
18. Hsu G: Eating Disorders. Guilford Press, New York, 1990.
19. Brownell KD, Rodin J, and Wilmore JH: Eat-

ing, Body Weight and Performance in Athletes. Lea and Febiger, Philadelphia, 1992.

20. Brownell KD, and Wadden, TA: The heterogeneity of obesity: Fitting treatments to individuals. Behav Ther 22:153, 1991.

21. Van Itallie TB: Health implications of overweight and obesity in the United States. Ann Intern Med 103:983, 1985.

22. U.S. Department of Agriculture: Nationwide food consumption survey. Nutrient intakes, individuals in 48 years, year 1977–1978, Report No. I-2, Consumer Nutrition Division, Human Nutrition Information Service. 1984. Hyattsville, MD.

23. McGinnis JM: The public health burden of a sedentary lifestyle. Med Sci Sports Exerc 24:S196, 1992.

24. Centers for Disease Control: Sex-, age-, and region-specific prevalance for sedentary lifestyle in selected states in 1985—The Behavioral Risk Factor Surveillance System. MMWR 36:195, 1987.

25. Centers for Disease Control: CDC surveillance summaries. MMWR 39(No. SS-2):8, 1990.

26. Grilo CM, Brownell KD, and Stunkard AJ: The metabolic and psychological importance of exercise in weight control. In Stunkard AJ, and Wadden T (eds): Obesity: Theory and Therapy, ed 2. Raven Press, New York, 1993, pp 253–273.

27. Klesges RC, Eck LH, Isbell TR, et al: Physical activity, body composition, and blood pressure: A multimethod approach. Med Sci Sports Exerc 23:759, 1991.

28. Strazzulo P, Cappuccio M, Trevisan M, et al: Leisure time physical activity and blood pressure in schoolchildren. Am J Epidemiol 127:726, 1988.

29. Pavlou KN, Krey S, and Steffee WP: Exercise as an adjunct to weight loss and maintenance in moderately obese subjects. Am J Clin Nutr 49:1115, 1989.

30. King AC, Taylor CB, and Haskell WL: Expanding methods for achieving sustained participation in community-based physical activity. The First International Congress of Behavioral Medicine, Upsala, Sweden. International Society of Behavioral Medicine, 1990.

31. Perri MG, McAdoo WG, McAllister DA, et al: Enhancing the efficacy of behavior therapy for obesity: Effects of aerobic exercise and a multicomponent maintenance program. J Consult Clin Psychol 54:670, 1986.

32. Craighead LW, and Blum MD: Supervised exercise in behavioral treatment for moderate obesity. Behav Ther 20:49, 1989.

33. Epstein LH, McCurley J, Wing RR, and Valoski A: Five-year follow-up of family-based behavioral treatments for childhood obesity. J Consult Clin Psychol 58:661, 1990.

34. Hill JO, Schlundt DG, Sbrocco T, et al: Evaluation of an alternating-calorie diet with and without exercise in the treatment of obesity. Am J Clin Nutr 50:248, 1989.

35. Kayman S, Bruvold W, and Stern JS: Maintenance and relapse after weight loss in women. Behavioral aspects. Am J Clin Nutr 52:800, 1990.

36. King, AC, Frey-Hewitt B, Dreon DM, and Wood PD: Diet versus exercise in weight maintenance: The effects of minimal intervention strategies on long-term outcomes in men. Arch Intern Med 149:2741, 1989.

37. Sikand G, Kondo A, Foreyt JP, Jones PH, and Gotto AM: Two-year follow-up of patients treated with a very-low-calorie-diet and exercise training. Am Diet Assoc 88:487, 1988.

38. Colvin RH, and Olson SB: A descriptive analysis of men and women who have lost significant weight and are highly successful at maintaining the loss. Addict Behav 8:287, 1983.

39. Gormally J, Rardin D, and Black S: Correlates of successful response to a behavioral weight control clinic. J Counsel Psychol 27:179, 1980.

40. Gormally J, and Rardin D: Weight loss and maintenance changes in diet and exercise for behavioral counseling and nutrition education. J Consult Clin Psychol 28:295, 1981.

41. Marston AR, and Criss J: Maintenance of successful weight loss: Incidence and prediction. Int J Obes 8:435, 1984.

42. Dahlkoetter J, Callahan EJ, and Linton J: Obesity and the unbalanced energy equation: Exercise vs. eating habit change. J Consult Clin Psychol 47:898, 1979.

43. Duddleston AK, and Bennion M: Effect of diet and/or exercise on obese college women: Weight loss and serum lipids. J Am Diet Assoc 56:126, 1970.

44. Harris MB, and Hallbauer ES: Self-directed weight control through eating and exercise. Behav Res Ther 11:523, 1973.

45. Stalonas PM, Johnson WG, and Christ M: Behavior modification for obesity: The evaluation of exercise, contingency management, and program adherence. J Consult Clin Psychol 46:463, 1978.

46. Van Dale D, and Saris WHM: Repetitive weight loss and weight regain: Effects on weight reduction, resting metabolic rate, and lipolytic activity before and after exercise and/or diet treatment. Am J Clin Nutr 49:409, 1989.

47. Belko AZ, Van Loan M, Barbieri TF, and

Maclin P: Diet, exercise, weight loss, and energy expenditure in moderately overweight men. Int J Obes 11:93, 1987.

48. Lennon D, Nagle F, Stratman F, Shrago E, and Dennis S: Diet and exercise training effects on resting metabolic rate: Int J Obes 9:39, 1985.

49. Phinney SD, La Grange BM, O'Connell M, and Danforth E: Effects of aerobic exercise on energy expenditure and nitrogen balance during very low calorie dieting. Metabolism 37:758, 1988.

50. Hill JO, Newby FD, Thacker SV, Sykes MN, and Di Girolamo M: Influence of food restriction coupled with weight cycling on carcass energy restoration during ad libitum refeeding. Int J Obes 12:547, 1988.

51. Epstein LH, Koeske R, and Wing RR: Adherence to exercise in obese children. J Cardiac Rehab 4:185, 1984.

52. Epstein LH, Wing RR, Koeske R, Ossip DJ, and Beck S: A comparison of lifestyle change and programmed aerobic exercise on weight and fitness changes in obese children. Behav Ther 13:651, 1982.

53. Brownell KD, Stunkard AJ, and Albaum JM: Evaluation and modification of exercise patterns in the natural environment. Am J Psychiatry 137:1540, 1980.

54. Bjorntorp P: Exercise and obesity. Psychiatr Clin North Am 1:691, 1978.

55. Bray G: The obese patient. WB Saunders, Philadelphia, 1976.

56. Danforth E, and Landsberg L: Energy expenditure and its regulation. In Greenwood MRC (ed): Obesity. New York, Churchill Livingstone, 1983, p 103.

57. McArdle WD, Katch FI, and Katch VL: Exercise Physiology: Energy, Nutrition, and Human Performance. Lea and Febiger, Philadelphia, 1991.

58. Barrows K, and Snook JT: Effect of a high-protein, very-low-calorie diet on resting metabolism, thyroid hormones, and energy expenditure of obese middle-aged women. Am J Clin Nutr 45:391, 1987.

59. Elliot DL, Goldberg L, Kuehl KS, and Bennett WM: Sustained depression of resting metabolic rate after massive weight loss. Am J Clin Nutr 49:93, 1989.

60. Mole PA, Stern JS, Schultz CL, Bernaver EM, and Holcomb, BJ: Exercise reverses depressed metabolic rate produced by severe caloric restriction. Med Sci Sports Exerc 21:29, 1989.

61. Ravussin E, Burnand B, Schutz Y, and Jequier E: Energy expenditure before and during energy restriction in obese patients. Am J Clin Nutr 41:753, 1985.

62. Welle SL, Amatruda JM, Forbes GB, and Lockwood DH: Resting metabolic rates of obese women after rapid weight loss. J Clin Endocrinol Metab 59:41, 1984.

63. Brownell KD, and Grilo CM: Weight management. In Durstine JL and Robertson M (eds): Resource Manual for Guidelines for Exercise Testing and Prescription, 1993, p 455.

64. Tremblay A, Despres JP, and Bouchard C: The effects of exercise-training on energy balance and adipose tissue morphology and metabolism. Sports Med 2:223, 1985.

65. Tremblay A, Fontaine E, Poehlman ET, et al: The effect of exercise-training on resting metabolic rate in lean and moderately obese individuals. Int J Obes 10:511, 1986.

66. Broeder CE, Burrhus KA, Svanevik LS, and Wilmore JH: The effects of either high-intensity resistance or endurance training on resting metabolic rate. Am J Clin Nutr 55:802, 1992.

67. Anderson B, Xu X, Rebuffe-Scrive M, et al: The effects of exercise training on body composition and metabolism in men and women. Int J Obes 15:75, 1991.

68. Epstein LH, Wing RR, and Thompson JK: The relationship between exercise intensity, caloric intake, and weight. Addict Behav 3:185, 1978.

69. Holm G, Bjorntorp P, and Jagenberg R: Carbohydrate, lipid, and amino acid metabolism following physical exercise in man. J Appl Physiol 45:128, 1978.

70. Woo R, Garrow JS, and Sunyer FXP: Effect of exercise on spontaneous calorie intake in obesity. Am J Clin Nutr 36:470, 1982.

71. Woo R, and Pi-Sunyer FX: Effect of increased physical activity on voluntary intake in lean women. Metabolism 34:836, 1985.

72. Reed DR, Contreras RJ, Maggio C, Greenwood MRC, and Rodin J: Weight cycling in female rats increases dietary fat selection and adiposity. Physiol Behav 42:389, 1988.

73. Gerardo-Gettens T, Miller GD, Horwitz BA, et al: Exercise decreases fat selection in female rats during weight cycling. Am J Physiol 260:R518, 1991.

74. Ballor DL, McCarthy JP, and Wilterdink EJ: Exercise intensity does not affect the composition of diet- and exercise-induced body mass loss. Am J Clin Nutr 51:142, 1990.

75. Bouchard C, Tremblay A, Després J-P, et al: The response to long-term overfeeding in identical twins. N Engl J Med 322:1477, 1990.

76. Després J-P, Bouchard C, Tremblay A, Savard R, and Marcotte M: Effects of aerobic training on fat distribution in male subjects. Med Sci Sports Exerc 17:113, 1985.

77. Segal KR, and Pi-Sunyer FX: Exercise, resting metabolic rate, and thermogenesis. Diabet Metabol Rev 2:19, 1986.
78. Donnelly JE, Pronk NP, Jacobsen DJ, Pronk SJ, Jakicic JM: Effects of a very-low-calorie diet and physical-training regimens on body composition and resting metabolic rate in obese females. Am J Clin Nutr 54:56, 1991.
79. Blair SN, Kohl HW, Paffenbarger RS, Clark DG, Cooper KH, and Gibbons LW: Physical fitness and all-cause mortality. J Am Med Assoc 262:2395, 1989.
80. Helmrich SP, et al: Physical activity and reduced occurrence of noninsulin-dependent diabetes mellitus. N Engl J Med 325:147, 1991.
81. Manson JE, Colditz GA, Stampfer MJ, et al: Physical activity and incidence of non-insulin-dependent-diabetes mellitus in women. Lancet 338:774, 1991.
82. Paffenbarger RS, Hyde RT, Wing AL, and Hsieh CC: Physical activity, all-cause mortality, and longevity of college alumni. N Engl J Med 314:605, 1986.
83. Dubbert PM: Exercise in behavioral medicine. J Consult Clin Psychol 60:613, 1992.
84. Hanson DF, and Nedde WH: Long-term physical training effect in sedentary females. J Appl Physiol 37:112, 1978.
85. DeBusk RF, Stenestrand U, Sheehan M, and Haskell HL: Training effects of long versus short bouts of exercise in healthy subjects. Am J Cardiol 65:1010, 1990.
86. Leon AS, Connett J, Jacobs DR, Rauramaa R: Leisure-time physical activity levels and risk of coronary heart disease and death. JAMA 258:2388, 1987.
87. Lee C: Women and aerobic exercise: Directions for research development. Ann Behav Med 13:133, 1991.
88. Powell, Caspersen CJ, Koplan JP, and Ford ES: Physical activity and chronic disease. Am J Clin Nutr 49:999, 1989.
89. Wood PD, Stefanick ML, Dreon DM, et al: Changes in plasma lipids and lipoproteins in overweight men during weight loss through dieting as compared with exercise. N Engl J Med 319:1173, 1988.
90. Lapidus L, Bengtsson C, Larsson B, Pennert K, Rybo E, and Sjostrom L: Distribution of adipose tissue and risk of cardiovascular disease and death: 12 year follow-up of participants in the population study of women in Gothenburg, Sweden. Br Med J 289:1261, 1984.
91. Seidell JC, Cigolini M, Després J-P, Charzewski J, et al: Body fat distribution in relation to physical activity and smoking habits in 38-year-old European men: The European Fat Distribution Study. Am J Epidemiol 133:257, 1991.
92. Tremblay A, Després J-P, Leblanc C, et al: Effect of intensity of physical activity on body fatness and fat distribution. Am J Clin Nutr 51:153, 1990.
93. Troisi RJ, Heinold JW, Vokonas PS, and Weiss ST: Cigarette smoking, dietary intake, and physical activity: Effects on body fat distribution—the Normative Aging Study. Am J Clin Nutr 53:1104, 1991.
94. Wing RR, Matthews KA, Kuller LH, Meilahn EN, and Plantinga A: Waist to hip ratio in middle-aged women: Associations with behavioral and psychosocial factors and with changes in cardiovascular risk factors. Arteriosclerosis Thrombosis 11:1250, 1991.
95. Plante TG, and Rodin J: Physical fitness and enhanced psychological health. Curr Psychol: Res Rev 9:3, 1990.
96. Rodin J, and Plante TG: The psychological effects of exercise. In Williams RS, and Wallace A (eds): Biological Effects of Physical Activity. Human Kinetics Books. Champaign, IL, 1989, p 127.
97. Grilo CM, Shiffman S, and Wing RR: Relapse crises and coping among dieters. J Consult Clin Psychol 57:488, 1989.
98. Doyne EJ, Ossip-Klein DJ, Bowman ED, Osborn KM et al: Running versus weight lifting in the treatment of depression. J Consult Clin Psychol 55:748, 1987.
99. King AC, Taylor CB, Haskell WL, and De Busk RF: Influence of regular aerobic exercise on psychological health: A randomized, controlled trial of healthy middle-aged adults. Health Psychol 8:305, 1989.
100. Martinsen EW, Medhus A, and Sandvik L: Effects of aerobic exercise on depression: A controlled study. Br Med J 291:109, 1985.
101. Martinsen EW, Strand J, Paulsson G, and Kaggestad J: Physical fitness level in patients with anxiety and depressive disorders. Int J Sports Med 10:58, 1989.
102. Steptoe A, and Cox S: Acute effect of aerobic exercise on mood. Health Psychol 7:329, 1988.
103. Sallis JF, and Hovell MF: Determinants of exercise behavior. In Pandolf KB, and Holloszy JO (eds): Exercise and Sport Sciences Reviews, vol 18. Williams & Wilkins, Baltimore, 1990, p 307.
104. Ernst ND, and Harlan, WR: Obesity and cardiovascular disease in minority populations: Executive summary. Conference highlights, conclusions, and recommendations. Am J Clin Nutr 53:1507S, 1991.
105. Pawson IG, Martorell R, and Mendoza F:

Prevalence of overweight and obesity in U.S. Hispanic populations. Am J Clin Nutr 53:1522S, 1991.

106. Sobal J, and Stunkard AJ: Socioeconomic status and obesity: A review of the literature. Psychol Bull 105:260, 1989.

107. Williamson DF, Kahn HS, Remington PL, and Anda RF: The 10-year incidence of overweight and major weight gain in U.S. adults. Arch Intern Med 150:665, 1990.

108. Caspersen CJ, Christenson GM, and Pollard RA: Status of the 1990 physical fitness and exercise objectives-evidence from NHIS. Public Health Rep 101:587, 1986.

109. Thompson JK: Body image disturbance: Assessment and treatment. Pergamon, Elmsford, NY, 1990.

110. Thompson JK, Fabian LJ, Moulton DO, Dunn ME, and Altabe MN: Development and validation of the physical appearance related teasing scale. J Pers Assess 56:513, 1991.

111. Allon N: The stigma of overweight in everyday life. In Wolman B (ed): Psychological Aspects of Obesity: A Handbook. Van Nostrand Reinhold, New York, 1982, p 130.

112. Wadden TA, and Stunkard AJ: Social and psychological consequences of obesity. Ann Int Med 103:1062, 1985.

113. King A: Community intervention for promotion of physical activity and fitness. In Pandolf KB, and Holloszy JO (eds): Exercise and Sport Sciences Reviews, vol 19. Williams & Wilkins, Baltimore, 1991, p 211.

114. Dubbert PM, and Martin JM: Exercise. In Blechman EA, and Brownell KD (eds): Handbook of Behavioral Medicine for Women. Pergamon, New York, 1988, p 291.

115. Gwinup G: Effect of exercise alone on the weight of obese women. Arch Int Med 135:676, 1975.

116. Sallis JF, Haskell WL, Fortmann SP, Vranizun KM, Taylor CB, and Solomon DS: Predictors of adoption and maintenance of physical activity in a community sample. Prev Med 15:331, 1986.

117. Dishman RK, Sallis JF, and Orenstein DR: The determinants of physical activity and exercise. Public Health Rep 100:158, 1985.

118. Sallis JF, Haskell WL, Wood PD, et al: Physical activity assessment methodology in the Five-City Project. Am J Epidemiol 121:91, 1985.

119. Foster VL, Hume GJ, Byrnes WC, et al: Endurance training for elderly women: Moderate vs low intensity. J Gerontol 44:M184, 1989.

120. Epstein LH, Wing RR, Koeske R, and Valoski A: A comparison of lifestyle exercise, aerobic exercise, and calisthenics on weight loss in obese children. Behav Ther 16:345, 1985.

121. Brownell KD, and Stunkard AJ: Physical activity in the development and control in obesity. In Stunkard AJ (ed): Obesity. WB Saunders, Philadelphia, 1980, p 300.

122. King AC, Haskell WL, Taylor CB, et al: Group- vs home-based exercise training in healthy older men and women: A community-based clinical trial. JAMA 266:1535, 1991.

123. Marlatt GA, and Gordon J (eds): Relapse Prevention: Maintenance Strategies in the Treatment of Addictive Behaviors. New York, Guilford Press, 1985.

124. Baum JG, Clark HB, and Sandler J: Preventing relapse in obesity through posttreatment maintenance systems: Comparing the relative efficacy of two levels of therapist support. J Behav Med 14:287, 1991.

125. Belisle M, Roskies E, and Levesque MM: Improving adherence to physical activity. Health Psychol 6:159, 1987.

126. King AC, and Frederiksen LW: Low-cost strategies for increasing exercise behavior: Relapse preparation training and social support. Behav Modif 8:3, 1984.

127. King AC, Taylor CB, Haskell WL, and DeBusk RF: Strategies for increasing early adherence to and long-term maintenance of home-based exercise training in healthy middle-aged men and women. Am J Cardiol 61:628, 1988.

128. Martin JE, Dubbert P, Katell AD, et al: Behavioral control of exercise in sedentary adults: Studies 1 through 6. J Consult Clin Psychol 52:795, 1984.

129. Marcus BH, Rossi JS, Selby VC, et al: The stages and process of exercise adoption and maintenance in a worksite sample. Health Psychol, in press.

130. Prochaska JO, Harlow LL, Redding CA, et al: Stages of change, self-efficacy, and decisional balance of condom use in a high HIV-risk sample. Am J Commun Psychol, in press.

131. DiClemente CC, Prochaska JO, Fairhurst SK, et al: The process of smoking cessation: An analysis of precontemplation, contemplation and preparation stages of change. J Consult Clin Psychol 59:295, 1991.

132. Fowler JL, Follick MT, Abrams DB, and Rickard-Figueroa K: Participant characteristics as predictors of attrition in worksite weight loss. Addict Behav 10:445, 1985.

133. Black DR, Gleser LJ, and Kooyers KJ: A meta-analytic evaluation of couples' weight-loss program. Health Psychol 9:330, 1990.

134. Wing RR, Marcus MD, Epstein LH, and Jawad A: A "family-based" approach to the treatment of obese type II diabetic patients. J Consult Clin Psychol 59:156, 1991.

135. Brownell KD: The LEARN program for weight control. American Health Publishing Company, Dallas, 1991.

136. Brownell KD, and Rodin J: The weight maintenance survival guide. American Health Publishing Company, Dallas, 1990.

137. Brownell KD: Dieting and the search for the perfect body: Where physiology and culture collide. Behav Ther 22:1, 1991.

138. Freedman R: Beauty Bound. Lexington Books, Lexington, MA, 1986.

139. Rodin J: Body Traps, Morrow, New York, 1992.

140. Wiseman CV, Gray JJ, Mosimann JE, and Ahrens AH: Cultural expectations of thinness in women: An update. Int J Eat Dis 11:85, 1992.

141. Rodin J: Cultural and psychosocial determinants of weight concerns. In Methods for Voluntary Weight Loss and Control. NIH Technology Assessment Conference 1992, p 17.

142. Stunkard AJ, Foch TT, and Hrubec Z: A twin study of human obesity. JAMA 256:51, 1986.

143. Stunkard AJ, Harris JR, Pedersen NL, McClearn GE: The body mass index of twins who have been reared apart. N Engl J Med 322:1483, 1990.

144. Bouchard C, and Johnson FE (eds): Fat distribution during growth and later health outcomes. Alan Liss, New York, 1988.

145. Brownell KD: Personal responsibility and control over our health: When expectation exceeds reality. Health Psychol 10:303, 1991.

146. Katch FI, and McArdle WD: Nutrition, Weight Control and Exercise, ed 3. Lea and Febiger, Philadelphia, 1988.

147. Trebbe A: Ideal is body beautiful and clean cut. USA Today, September 15, 1979, p 1.

148. Rodin J, and Larson L: Social factors and the ideal body shape. In Brownell KD, Rodin J, and Wilmore JH (eds): Eating, Body Weight and Performance in Athletes. Lea and Febiger, Philadelphia, 1992, p 146.

149. Blackburn GL, and Kanders BS: Medical evaluation and treatment of the obese patient with cardiovascular disease. Am J Cardiol 60:55g, 1987.

150. Wassertheil-Smoller SW, Blaufox MD, Oberman A, Langford HG, and Davis BR: TAIM Study: Adequate weight loss as effective as drug therapy for mild hypertension. Paper presented at American Heart Association Conference on Cardiovascular Disease Epidemiology, San Diego, 1990.

151. Fairburn CG, and Cooper, PJ: The clinical features of bulimia nervosa. Br J Psychiatry 144:238, 1984.

152. Garfinkel PE, and Garner DM: Anorexia nervosa: A multidimensional perspective. Brunner/Mazel, New York, 1982.

153. Wilson GT: Bulimia nervosa: Models, assessment, and treatment. Curr Opinion Psychiatry 2:790, 1989.

154. Davis C, Fox J, Cowles M, Hastings P, and Schwass K: The functional role of exercise in the development of weight and diet concerns in women. J Psychosom Res 34:563, 1990.

155. Prussin RA, and Harvey PD: Depression, dietary restraint, and binge eating in female runners. Addict Behav 16:295, 1991.

156. Pope HG, Jr, Hudson JI, and Yurgelen-Todd D: Anorexia nervosa and bulimia among 300 women shoppers. Am J Psychiatry 141:292, 1984.

157. Brownell KD, Rodin J, and Wilmore JH: Eat, drink, and be worried? Runner's World 28, August 1988, p 28–34.

158. Grilo CM, and Wilfley DE: Weight control: Exercise adherence and abuse. Weight Control Digest 2:161, 1992.

159. Adams GM, and DeVries HA: Physiological effects of an exercise training regimen upon women aged 52 to 79. J Gerontol 28:50, 1973.

160. Badenhop DT, Cleary PA, et al: Physiological adjustments to higher- or lower-intensity exercise in elders. Med Sci Sports Exerc 15:496, 1983.

161. Bassey EJ, Patrick JM, Irving JM, Blecher A, and Fenten PH: An unsupervised "aerobics" physical training programme in middle-aged factory workers: Feasibility, validation and responses. Eur J Appl Physiol 52:120, 1983.

162. Blumenthal JA, Schocker DD, Needels TL, and Hindle P: Psychological and physiological effects of physical conditioning on the elderly. J Psychosom Res 26:505, 1982.

163. Blumenthal JA, Emery CF, Madden DJ, et al: Cardiovascular and behavioral effects of aerobic exercise training in healthy older men and women. J Gerontol 44:M147, 1989.

164. Cavanaugh DJ, and Cann CE: Brisk walking does not stop bone loss in postmenopausal women. Bone 9:201, 1988.

165. Cowan MM, and Gregory LW: Responses of pre- and post-menopausal females to aerobic conditioning. Med Sci Sports Exerc 17:138, 1985.

166. Franklin B, Buskirk E, Hodgson J, et al: Effects of physical conditioning on cardiorespiratory function, body composition and serum lipids in relatively normal-weight and obese middle-aged women. Int J Obes 3:97, 1979.

167. Getchell LH, and Moore JC: Physical training: Comparative response of middle-aged

adults. Arch Physical Med Rehab 56:250, 1975.

168. Haber P, Honiger B, Kilicpera M, and Niederberger M: Effects on elderly people 67–76 years of age of three-month endurance training on bicycle ergometer. Eur Heart J 5:37, 1984.

169. Jarvie GJ, and Thompson, JK: Appropriate use of stationary exercycles in the natural environment: The failure of instructions and goal setting to appreciably modify exercise patterns. Behav Ther 8:187, 1985.

170. Jette M, Sidney K, and Campbell J: Effects of a twelve-week program on maximal and submaximal work output indices in sedentary middle-aged men and women. J Sports Med Physical Fitness 28:59, 1988.

171. Juneau M, Rogers F, DeSantos V, et al: Effectiveness of self-monitored, home-based, moderate-intensity exercise training in middle-aged men and women. Am J Cardiol 60:66, 1987.

172. Kukkonen K, Rauramaa R, Siitonen U, and Hanninen O: Physical training of obese middle-aged persons. Ann Clin Res 14:80, 1982.

173. Lewis S, Haskell WL, Wood PD, et al: Effects of physical activity on weight reduction in obese middle-aged women. Am J Clin Nutr 29:151, 1976.

174. Morrison DA, Boyden TW, Pamenter RW, et al: Effects of aerobic training on exercise tolerance and echocardiographic dimensions in untrained postmenopausal women. Am Heart J 112:561, 1986.

175. Netz Y, Tenenbaum G, and Sagir M: Patterns of psychological fitness as related to patterns of physical fitness among older adults. Percept Motor Skills 67:647, 1988.

176. Seals DR, Hagberg JM, Hurley BF, Ehsani AA, and Holloszy JO: Endurance training in older men and women I. Cardiovascular response to exercise. J Appl Physiol 57:1024, 1984.

177. White MK, Yeater RA, Martin RB, et al: Effects of aerobic dancing and walking on cardiovascular function and muscular strength in post-menopausal women. J Sports Med 24:159, 1984.

178. MacKeen PC, Franklin BA, Nicholas C, and Buskirk ER: Body composition, physical work capacity and physical activity habits at 18-months follow-up of middle-aged women participating in an exercise intervention program. Int J Obes 7:61, 1983.

179. Blumenthal JA, Emery CF, Madden DJ, et al: Long-term effects of exercise on psychological functioning in older men and women. J Gerontol, in press.

ACKNOWLEDGMENTS

We are grateful to Adele Jones for her assistance with the preparation of this manuscript.

APPENDIX 2–1

Research Examining Physiologic Effects of Exercise in Adult Women: Subject and Program Characteristics

Authors	Subjects			Program			Weeks' Duration	Control Group
	N	Age	Notes	Session Time (min)	Freq/Week	Intensity		
Adams and DeVries[159]	23	52–79	17 ex 6 control	40	3	60% MHR	13	Last six to volunteer
Badenhop et al.[160]	32	>60	26 F, 8 M 14 mod ex 14 low ex 4 control	50	3	60%–75% MHR 30%–45% MHR	9	Those unable to commit time
Bassey et al.[161]	108	55–60	53 F 55 M	20–40	5	?	12	Randomly assigned to successive programs
Blumenthal et al.[162]	24	65–85	18 F 6 M	30	3	70%–85% MHR	11	None
Blumenthal et al.[163]	101	60–83	51 F, 50 M 33 aerobic 34 yoga control 34 wait list control	60	3	70% MHR	16	Random
Cavanaugh and Cann[164]	17	m = 56	8 ex 9 control	25–50	3	60% MHR	52	Those unable to commit time
Cowan and Gregory[165]	38	35–66	20 pre-menopause 18 post-menopause	50	4	80% MHR	9	Randomly assigned to ex or control
Franklin et al.[166]	36	29–47	23 obese 13 normal	45	4	75% $\dot{V}o_2$max	12	None
Foster et al.[119]	16	67–89	9 mod ex 9 low ex	17–42	5	60% MHR 40% MHR	10	None
Getchell and Moore[167]	23	28–57	11 F 12 M	30	3–4	75%–85% MHR	10	None

APPENDIX 2-1

Research Examining Physiologic Effects of Exercise in Adult Women: Subject and Program Characteristics (*Continued*)

Authors	Subjects			Program				
	N	Age	Notes	Session Time (min)	Freq/ Week	Intensity	Weeks' Duration	Control Group
Haber et al.[168]	12	67–76	8 F 4 M	20–40	3	60% MHR	12	None
Jarvie and Thompson[169]	16	26–52	12 F 4 M	25	7	pulse?	17	Wait list
Jette et al.[170]	26	35–53	12 F 14 M	30	3	60% $\dot{V}o_2max$	12	Random 50% in no-ex gp
Juneau et al.[171]	120	40–60	60 F 60 M	50	5	65%–77% MHR	24	Random 50% in no-ex gp
Kukkonen et al.[172]	169	35–50	97 F 72 M	30–60	3–6	60%–70% MHR	68	None
Lewis et al.[173]	22	30–52		25 and 60	2 and 2	80% MHR and low	17	None
Morrison et al.[174]	32	m = 51	22 ex 10 control	40	3	65%–75% MHR	32	Random
Netz et al.[175]	24	50–64	13 F 11 M	60	3	70% MHR	12	None
Seals et al.[176]	24	60–69	14 ex 10 control	30 and 60	3	40% MHR and 85% MHR	48*	Assignment method not specified
White et al.[177]	72	50–63	36 walk 36 dance	33	4	70% MHR	24	None

*Subjects spent 24 weeks in low-intensity activity and then 24 weeks in higher-intensity.

MHR = age-adjusted maximal heart rate; $\dot{V}o_2max$ = maximal oxygen capacity.

Source: Adapted from Lee,[87] p 134, with permission.

Outcomes of Studies Listed in Appendix 2-1

Authors	Program Type	% Drop Out	Physical Outcomes		Follow-up
			Improved	No Change	
Adams and DeVries[159]	Supervised	0	PWC V̇O₂max O₂ pulse RHR Weight	RSBP RDBP Skinfolds	None
Badenhop et al.[160]	Supervised	0	PWC, EHR V̇O₂max		None
Bassey et al.[161]	Home-based	53	EHR phys. activity		12-week follow-up of 29 Ss—some maintenance
Blumenthal et al.[162]	Supervised	8	PWC Endurance	RSBP, RDBP RHR, EHR Weight	None
Blumenthal et al.[163]	Supervised	4	V̇O₂max RHR Endurance Anaerobic threshold Total cholesterol, LDL	Bone density Grip strength	Blumenthal et al.[179]
Cavanaugh and Cann[164]	Supervised	0	RHR Phys. activity	Bone density % fat	None
Cowan and Gregory[165]	Supervised? (not specifically stated)	0	% fat V̇O₂max Endurance	Weight Lean mass	None
Foster et al.[119]	Supervised	24	V̇O₂max PWC	Weight Blood lactate EHR Total cholesterol HDL	None

APPENDIX 2-2

Outcomes of Studies Listed in Appendix 2-1 (*Continued*)

Authors	Program Type	% Drop Out	Physical Outcomes Improved	Physical Outcomes No Change	Follow-up
Franklin et al.[166]	Supervised	0	EHR Weight Skinfolds % fat ESBP RSBP, RDBP, EDBP (obese only)	Rate-pressure prod Lean mass	See MacKeen et al.[178]
Getchell and Moore[167]	Supervised? (not specifically stated)		EHR Skinfolds $\dot{V}O_2$max Lactic acid	Weight	None
Haber et al.[168]	Supervised	0	PWC Max work load $\dot{V}O_2$max	EHR	None
Jarvie and Thompson[169]	Home-based	75	$\dot{V}O_2$max	$\dot{V}O_2$max Skinfolds Weight	None
Jette et al. (1970)	Supervised	0	$\dot{V}O_2$max EHR	Blood lactate	None
Juneau et al.[171]	Home-based	6	$\dot{V}O_2$max Weight (M only)	RHR EHR % fat Lean mass	None
Kukkonen et al.[172]	Home-based	44	Weight BMI $\dot{V}O_2$max RSBP, RDBP (M only) Serum triglyceride (F only)	Total cholesterol	Program continued for 17 months; tested at 2, 5, 11, and 17

Lewis et al.[173]	Supervised	9	% fat Weight RHR, EHR ESBP HDL:LDL ratio Endurance	Serum triglyceride Total cholesterol	None
MacKeen et al.[178]	18-month follow-up of Franklin et al.[166]	64		Physical activity $\dot{V}O_2$max % fat	Yes
Morrison et al.[174]	Supervised	22	$\dot{V}O_2$max Endurance Cardiac efficiency		None
Netz et al.[175]	Supervised	?high	EHR Weight		
Seals et al.[176]	Home-based then supervised	22	$\dot{V}O_2$max Weight RHR ESBP Blood lactate Cardiac efficiency	EHR Cardiac output Blood lactate	None
White et al.[177]	One class/wk supervised plus home-based	29	RHR Weight RSBP (down) RDBP (up) Muscle strength Endurance		

Endurance = time spent in standard exercise task; EDBP = exercising diastolic blood pressure; HDL = high-density lipoprotein level; RDBP = resting diastolic blood pressure; RHR = resting heart rate; $\dot{V}O_2$max = maximal oxygen capacity; EHR = exercising heart rate; ESBP = exercising systolic blood pressure; LDL = low-density lipoprotein level; RSBP = resting systolic blood pressure; PWC = physical work capacity.

Source: Adapted from Lee,[87] pp 136–137, with permission.

CHAPTER 3

Training for Strength

DAVID H. CLARKE, Ph.D.

With proper training, women can become very strong. However, even with the same strength-training program, their muscles will not enlarge as much as those of men. The data-based studies regarding the adaptations resulting from strength training have come predominantly from research conducted on male subjects, but, aside from questions raised concerning muscle hypertrophy, it seems tenable to conclude that principles that apply to men also apply to women.

DEFINITION OF STRENGTH

The first concept that needs to be defined is that of strength. A dictionary definition is unacceptable, as the terms "tough," "powerful," and "muscular" do very little to describe what is actually a functional concept. Attempts at obtaining a true measure of muscle force show that maximum tension varies from 1.5 to 2.5 $kg \cdot cm^{-2}$ in vertebrate nonhuman muscles and perhaps slightly higher in the normal human.[1] Thus, if one assumes a value of 3 $kg \cdot cm^{-2}$ and that large muscles of the thigh may have 100 cm^2 of cross section, the resulting internal force that could be developed would be 300 kg. Obviously, the amount of useful torque that can be marshaled during normal activities must be expressed somewhat differently, since it is not feasible to determine true internal tensions. Thus, it is customary to employ the concept of the maximal voluntary contraction (MVC), which implies that the effort is not submaximal or created by some external stimulus, such as a tetanic shock. Yet one does not know whether the contraction resulted in any movement, whether it caused any muscle shortening or lengthening, and, if movement did occur, whether it was at a fixed speed or whether the tension on the muscle was constant or variable.

Mastering the terminology helps one not only to understand the literature on strength training but also to comprehend the difficulty faced by investigators in quantifying the results of various training regimens. There are few absolute standards available for the assessment of strength, so a wide variety of procedures has been employed. Thus, there has been great difficulty in making clear comparisons among various studies. In the present context, *isotonic strength* (or dynamic strength) of a muscle is defined as the maximum force that can be exerted by that muscle during contraction as it moves through its full range of motion. This can be further delineated into concentric (i.e., shortening) and eccentric (i.e., lengthening) forms. *Isometric strength* (or static strength) is a single MVC performed by a muscle group in a static position, in which no shortening or lengthening of the muscle occurs; *isokinetic strength* resembles the isotonic contraction, since the joint moves through a range of motion, but the speed of movement is held constant. This latter system requires specialized equipment to control for a variety of movement speeds.

ISOTONIC TRAINING

The usual method of training has been to follow a routine of isotonic exercises. A system described by DeLorme and Watkins[2] during the period immediately following World War II became known as progressive resistance exercise (PRE) and was based on a set of 10 repetitions maximum (10 RM), which is the heaviest weight that can be lifted and lowered 10 times in succession. The manner in which these exercises were to be employed was first to perform a set of 10 repetitions of one half of the weight of the 10 RM, then to perform a second set of 10 repetitions at three fourths of the weight of the 10 RM, and finally to perform as many repetitions as possible at the weight of the

10 RM. When an appropriate number of additional repetitions of the 10 RM could be performed, more weight was added and the process continued at this new 10-RM weight. It is generally thought that keeping the total number of repetitions for the three sets somewhere in the range of 30 to 35 enhances the development of muscular strength. Using a program with reduced resistance and increased repetitions is thought to emphasize muscular endurance. Houtz, Parrish, and Hellebrandt[3] applied the PRE principle to female subjects, exercising the quadriceps and forearm muscles, and found that strength more than doubled in 4 weeks. Thus, it seems probable that the principles of strength development can be successfully applied to women as well as men.

Interest in refining the procedures for PRE for effective strength gains has been the subject of fairly intense investigation in the subsequent years. Berger[4] has provided considerable insight into the strength development process, using various combinations of repetitions, sets (number of repeated sequences the exercise is performed during a given session), and number of training sessions per week. The criterion measure of muscular strength was the 1 RM, defined as the maximum amount of weight that could be successfully moved through a complete range of motion for one repetition. In one study,[4] Berger trained six groups for 12 weeks employing the bench press exercise. The groups used resistances of 2, 4, 6, 8, 10, and 12 RM as their training modalities and performed only one set of repetitions per training session. At the end of this time it was found that those training at four, six, and eight repetitions gained significantly greater amounts of strength than any of the other groups, suggesting that an optimum target for training would be to perform between three and nine repetitions. Using one, two, and three sets of repetitions and employing 2, 6, and 10 RM as the weights and numbers of repetitions in each set, he found that no advantage was gained by exercising with heavier loads for 2 RM than with lighter loads at 10 RM.[5] All combinations resulted in significant strength increases, but strength gains were maximal when the number of repetitions per set was 6 RM for three sets. To determine whether increasing the number of sets beyond three would lead to greater gains in strength, Berger[6] compared the strength achieved by performing 2 RM for six sets, 6 RM for three sets, and 10 RM for three sets. He found that all three groups gained significantly and similarly in strength. This suggests that there is a point beyond which gains in muscular strength should not be anticipated.

Berger and Hardage[7] studied an alternate, somewhat unique modification of the 10-RM training technique. One group performed 10 repetitions for one set, but each repetition was adjusted so that it required maximum effort, that is, a 1 RM. Subsequent repetitions were performed by gradually reducing the load, so that at the 10th repetition the subjects were still exerting maximum tension. When compared with the regular 10-RM group, it was found that both groups improved significantly in the 1-RM bench press after 8 weeks of training. However, the 1-RM group improved significantly more than the regular 10-RM group, indicating the relative importance of intensity of effort in training. It should be noted that almost all studies have shown the importance of attaining maximal tension of the muscles during the course of the exercise.

To compare the strength achieved by performing many repetitions using light weight with that gained by performing few repetitions using heavy weight, Anderson and Kearney[8] trained 43 male subjects using three sets of 6 to 8 RM for one group, 30 to 40 RM for a second group, and 100 to 150 RM for a third group, all subjects employing the bench press three times per week for 9 weeks. Strength was assessed with the 1-RM bench press, administered before and after the training. Gains in strength were achieved by all three groups, but only the high-resistance, low-repetition (6- to 8-RM) group was significantly stronger than the other two groups, which did not differ from

each other. Thus, it appears that strength gains are greatest when resistance is high. Since few repetitions can be done using high resistance, a smaller time expenditure is required for this training.

The question of whether an effective training response can be elicited for women may be answered in the affirmative, at least if the intensity of the training program is high enough, and if the program lasts long enough. Staron et al.[9] submitted adult women to such a program of high-intensity, heavy-resistance exercises of the lower extremity for 20 weeks. A significant increase in the 1 RM was found for each exercise, even though the subjects trained only twice a week.

A consideration for most individuals engaging in weight training exercise has to do with how long the results of training will persist if the training frequency is reduced. Graves et al.[10] recruited both male and female subjects who trained for either 10 or 18 weeks on knee extension, using a 7- to 10-RM regimen. Following this 10-week period, the subjects reduced their training fequency from a minimum of three times per week to less. Subjects who stopped training altogether lost 68% of the previously gained strength, but those who reduced to 2 and even 1 day per week did not change significantly in strength. Thus, a maintenance routine would seem to be possible when training only once per week.

It has generally been found that men have greater absolute amounts of strength than women under most conditions.[11-14] Even untrained men who have not been specifically weight training[15] exhibit greater upper and lower body strength than female athletes trained in such sports as basketball and volleyball but not weight training. The ratios comparing the strength of women to that of men are on the order of 0.46 to 0.73 when compared on maximal strength of elbow flexion, shoulder flexion, back extension, and hand grip.[16] Even though this is the case, the established principles of strength training are applicable to both men and women.

ISOMETRIC TRAINING

The systematic use of isometric training principles can probably be traced to the 1953 report of Hettinger and Muller,[17] who found an average strength increase of 5% per week when the muscle tension was held for 6 seconds at two thirds of maximum strength. Even when the tension was increased to 100%, or when the length of time was increased, very little additional improvement was noted. Isometric exercises are normally performed by establishing a given joint angle and exerting isometric tension at that point in the range of motion (e.g., pushing against a stationary wall). As with isotonic exercises, more than one set may be performed and the length of time for which the tension is exerted may vary. However, the amount of the strength gain suggested by Muller[18] has not been confirmed in subsequent experimentation. It seems more likely that the amount of strength gain would depend on the relative state of training of a given muscle group. Thus, the closer one is to a theoretic maximum, the more likely the gains are to be small.[19]

Isometric exercise does increase muscular strength. Josenhans[20] employed isometric exercises for the grip and the flexor and extensor muscles of the finger, the elbow, and the knee and found a 40% increase in muscular force at the end of the training period. When 5-second maximal isometric contractions of the quadriceps muscles were employed, it was found that strength increases vary between 80% and 400%.[21] Morehouse[22] separated some trained subjects into high- and low-strength groups and employed either 1, 3, 5, or 10 maximum isometric contractions each session. Subjects increased significantly in strength after 5 weeks, with similar improvements found regardless of level of initial strength. Apparently, most individuals can anticipate increases in strength regardless of how strong they are at the outset, unless they are already in an advanced state of muscular training.

These principles were applied to postpubescent young men who were trained in wrist flexion employing the Hettinger and Muller strategy[17] of two-thirds maximum tension for one 6-second period each day. This was compared with a technique in which 80% of maximum strength was employed in five 6-second periods.[23] Both groups of subjects improved significantly after 4 weeks of training, although no significant difference resulted between the two groups. This suggests that a single 6-second bout of isometric exercise on a daily basis is about as effective for developing muscular strength as bouts practiced more frequently and at higher tensions. Furthermore, high school boys and girls training for one contraction per day at 25%, 50%, 75%, and 100% of maximum isometric elbow flexion strength were compared after training.[24] With the exception of the 25% resistance group, all groups became stronger. Thus, the age of subjects seems to be of little consequence for achieving strength-training results.

Increasing the number of isometric contractions appears to increase the strength gain over a greater range of motion.[25] One group of subjects held three maximum isometric contractions at an elbow joint angle of 170 degrees' flexion, each for 6 seconds, in a program that was of 6 weeks' duration. Another group performed twenty 6-second maximum contractions at the same joint angle. Maximum strength was assessed before and after the experiment at angles of both 90 and 170 degrees. All tests used isometric maximum contractions. The subjects who performed more contractions gained strength significantly at both joint angles, while those who performed fewer contractions became stronger only at the angle of 170 degrees, the training angle. Thus, the longer duration of work seems to be more beneficial for strength development, but the difference is small compared with the amount of effort required. The evidence for joint-angle–specific effects of isometric training is fairly strong, especially when the muscles are placed at a relatively short length. This can be accomplished by manipulating the joint angle. This specificity of training response is difficult to justify if the training adaptation results in changes in muscle size. An alternate explanation would involve some sort of neural adaptation. Thus, Kitai and Sale[26] trained the ankle plantar flexor muscles of women at a joint angle of 90 degrees employing two sets of five maximal voluntary isometric contractions each held for 5 seconds. The training program was 6 weeks in duration and resulted in significant increases in voluntary strength at the training angle and the two adjacent angles at 5 and 10 degrees in either direction only. Examination of peak strength of maximum twitch of the involved muscles would point to a neural mechanism as being responsible for this joint specificity in isometric training. This point has been reinforced by the finding of an increase in maximal integrated electrical activity at the specific training angle.[27]

Whereas most investigations have employed either male subjects or a combination of male and female subjects, Hansen[28,29] used female subjects, employing sustained and repeated isometric contractions. The gains in isometric strength in this study ranged from approximately 4% to 11% over a 5-week training program.

A more recent development has been the incorporation of functional isometrics into an isotonic strength training program. In a given range of motion, it is common to locate a given point at which the muscle is most inefficient. Weight lifters refer to this as the "sticking point" of exercise. It represents the point at which the force available is equal to the resistance of the weight. To determine whether the incorporation of maximum isometric contractions at this point would permit the development of strength beyond that provided by the isotonic exercise alone, subjects[30] in a control group trained on the bench press exercise using an isotonic training procedure employing 6 to 8 RM, while the experimental group added to this routine an isometric program consist-

ing of six maximal voluntary contractions at a predetermined "sticking point" in the bench press. Analysis of the 1-RM bench press before and after the training program revealed significant improvements for both groups. However, the experimental group was significantly stronger than the control group, providing evidence that isometric training enhances the standard isotonic training routine in the achievement of maximum strength.

ISOTONIC VERSUS ISOMETRIC TRAINING

It has been difficult to compare the improvements in strength resulting from isotonic and isometric training methods, because the intensities of training in the two methods cannot be equated. The ideal method of comparison would employ two exercise regimens, both of equal workloads. However, this has been difficult to accomplish because isometric exercises involve no movement and, thus, are difficult to quantify in physical terms.

Despite the problems inherent in comparing isotonic and isometric training effects, Rasch and Morehouse,[31] in one of the earlier studies, compared these two methods by having one group (isotonic) perform a 5-RM procedure involving three sets of arm presses and curls, taking a total of 15 seconds to perform, and having the other group (isometric) employ a 15-second exercise period contracting the muscles isometrically at two-thirds maximum. Following 6 weeks of training, substantial increases were found for the isotonic exercise group in elbow flexion and arm elevation and for the isometric exercise group in arm elevation alone. No significant gain was made in elbow flexion for the isometric training group. Thus, subjects employing isotonic exercise gained a greater amount of strength than did those subjects employing isometric exercises. It was suggested by the investigators that some of the strength development may have come from the acquisition of skill, since subjects tended to do better when performing familiar procedures. This may help explain sudden early increases in strength; they may be attributable more to neuromuscular coordination than to true muscle hypertrophy.

Isometric and isotonic training procedures were applied to subjects engaging in exercise over a 12-week training period, exercising three times per week and employing the larger muscles of the back.[32] The isometric group trained with a back pull machine, contracting the muscles for 6 seconds maximally, three sets per exercise session, and the isotonic group employed back hyperextension exercises based on an 8- to 12-RM regimen. Both groups improved significantly in muscular strength, but the isometric group gained significantly more when an isometric test was employed, and the isotonic group performed better when a test of isotonic strength, such as the 1-RM procedure, was used. This finding suggests that training is specific, a concept that has received additional support from some studies.

This is in contrast, however, to the work of many other investigators who have reported similar gains in strength from these two different training methods. For example, Berger[33] trained subjects for 12 weeks both isometrically and isotonically and used the criterion of the 1-RM test. The final strength of the isometrically trained group was not significantly different from seven of the nine groups that trained isotonically. Coleman[34] employed the elbow flexor muscle in a program of 12 weeks' duration, using an isometric regimen consisting of two 10-second contractions and an isotonic training program consisting of a 5-RM regimen. In this instance, there was an attempt to equate the load, duration, and range of motion of the exercise. No significant difference was found between the two methods, although both produced significant strength gains.

Salter[35] investigated the effect on muscular strength of maximum isometric and isotonic contractions, performed at different repetition rates. The isometric group gradually increased force to maximum over approximately 4 seconds. The isotonic group lifted a load equivalent to 75% of maximum as far as possible, also over a duration of 4 seconds. The exercise involved supination of the left hand and included 12 male and 8 female subjects. All training procedures resulted in a significant improvement in strength. However, no significant differences were found between the different procedures. Chui[36] noted similar findings. Two groups trained with rapid and slow isotonic contractions and were compared with a group employing isometric contractions. The slow isotonic contractions required a cadence of 4 seconds for movement and recovery, and the isometric contractions were held for 6 seconds. All groups employed a weight equal to a 10-RM resistance. No advantage was found for either procedure over the other, although each group gained significantly in muscular strength. When isometric contractions were lengthened to 30 seconds,[37] the development of strength was found to be less than by isotonic methods by some 14%, even though both isotonic and isometric methods caused increases in muscular strength.

Thus, it would seem desirable to employ isotonic procedures whenever possible. Gains in strength with isometric exercise tend to be less consistent than those with isotonic exercise, when many training techniques and strength tests are employed.

ECCENTRIC TRAINING

As pointed out earlier, isotonic movement can be divided into a concentric (shortening) and an eccentric (lengthening) phase. It is generally concluded that in isotonic training the greatest force is exerted concentrically, and this usually means that the muscle is shortening and the load is being lifted against gravity. Thus, loads are adjusted so that the greatest tension is provided during this phase. The eccentric phase is ordinarily employed to complete the movement so that the muscle returns to its original length. The weight is simply lowered slowly with gravity assistance. It is generally accepted that the amount of weight that can be lowered maximally is about 20% greater than that which can be lifted against gravity. Logically, one would expect the added force that can be resisted with an eccentric contraction to be a greater stimulus to strength gain. However, scientific studies have failed to show any advantage of eccentric over concentric training.

Bonde Petersen[38] studied isometric, isotonic, and eccentric contractions in female and male subjects for a period lasting from 20 to 36 days. Training for each subject consisted of one of the following protocols: 1 maximum isometric contraction daily, 10 maximum isometric contractions daily, or 10 eccentric contractions daily. It was found that performance of one maximum isometric contraction daily had no effect on the isometric strength of the subjects; performance of 10 isometric contractions daily caused no change in the strength of the female subjects but led to a significant increase (13%) for the male subjects. Subjects who trained with the 10 daily eccentric contractions failed to demonstrate any significant increase in strength. This lack of significant strength gain may have been due to training every day rather than every other day. It is possible that insufficient time was allowed between training sessions to recover completely from the previous training session.

Singh and Karpovich[39] designed a study to determine the effect of eccentric training on a muscle group as well as on its antagonist (the opposing muscle complex). In this instance, the forearm extensors were given 20 maximum eccentric contractions four times per week for 8 weeks, and the extensors as well as the forearm flexors were tested for maximum strength before and after training. Concentric and isometric strength of the exercised muscles increased approximately 40%, but the eccentric strength increased only 23%. When the antagonistic muscles were examined, it was found that they also increased in strength, ranging from 17% to

31%. This suggests that during maximum contractions in eccentric movement, the antagonistic muscles are also contracted. By palpation and by examination of the electromyographic activity emanating from the antagonistic muscle, the investigators verified that this occurs. This finding illustrates the fact that it is very difficult to isolate muscle activity in the human body.

More recently, Johnson and co-workers[40] trained subjects with eccentric movements on one arm and leg and concentric movements on the opposite arm and leg, three times weekly for a period of 6 weeks. The specific exercises included the arm curl, arm press, knee flexion, and knee extension. Each exercise lasted for 3 seconds. The concentric movement was performed against a resistance of 80% of the subject's 1-RM strength, and the eccentric movement was against 120% of 1 RM. Both exercise programs resulted in significant gains in strength in all subjects, but neither training procedure produced gains that were significantly different from the other. Interestingly, the subjects felt that the eccentric training movements were easier to perform than the concentric movements.

Jones and Rutherford[41] included a group of subjects who trained by eccentric and isometric procedures as well. In each case subjects trained knee extensor muscles three times per week for 12 weeks. The isometric group held a contraction of 80% of maximum for 4 seconds, the concentric group trained at an intensity of 6 RM, and the eccentric subjects employed a resistance of 145% of the concentric strength. A large and significant increase in isometric force occurred, and these gains were significantly greater than found for both concentric and eccentric training. Even though there was no significant difference between concentric and eccentric training regimens, both programs resulted in significant increases in strength, approximately 15% for the concentric training and 11% for eccentric.

The perception that eccentric exercise is easier to perform would seem to lead subjects to greater compliance and acceptability of such training. However, present equipment and common training habits do not permit isolation of eccentric contractions. Moreover, since a muscle can resist greater force in an eccentric contraction than in a concentric contraction, considerably greater tension is required in the eccentric movement in order to promote strength gains. Thus, in a regular isotonic exercise encompassing both concentric and eccentric contractions, the eccentric phase contributes relatively little to strength development, since the amount of force is undoubtedly well below the training stimulus during that phase of the exercise.

ISOKINETIC EXERCISE

The newest form of exercise used for training is isokinetic exercise. It is often referred to as "accommodating resistance exercise," because, as explained earlier, it has the unique feature of adjusting to the ability of the muscles throughout the range of motion, so that weak spots are eliminated and the muscles remain under constant tension throughout the movement. Actually, few activities produce and maintain isokinetic tension, the arm strokes in swimming and oar strokes in rowing being the major exceptions. Properly designed equipment offers exercise at any one of a range of fixed speeds; the subject determines the resistance by the applied force. Thus, it is possible to exercise maximally throughout a full range of motion using any one of several speeds. In isokinetic exercise, increased force does not produce increased acceleration but simply increased resistance.

One of the earlier studies[42] compared isokinetic training with isotonic and isometric training over an 8-week period. The isokinetic group increased in total muscular ability by 35%, the isotonic group increased 28%, and the isometric group increased approximately 9%. Employing quadriceps and hamstring muscle exercises on 12 male and 48 female subjects, Moffroid and associates[43] studied groups that exercised isometrically, isotonically, and isokinetically for a 4-week period. Significant increases in isometric strength occurred for all groups, with one exception: when the isotonic group was tested at 90 degrees rather than 45 degrees, no significant improvement was noted. None of the groups improved significantly in the quadriceps muscles when tested for isokinetic work, but all were significantly better when the hamstring muscles were tested.

Lesmes and colleagues[44] trained male subjects isokinetically on knee extensors and flexors four times per week for 7 weeks, at maximal intensity and at a constant velocity of 180 degrees/sec. One leg was trained at 6-second work bouts and the other leg at 30-second work bouts, the ratio of work to rest providing a method of keeping workloads equal. Isokinetic testing was accomplished at various intervals between 60 and 300 degrees/sec. Increased peak torque occurred at both 6 and 30 seconds at all intensities except those between approximately 180 and 300 degrees/sec. It apparently makes some difference to train isokinetically, but it depends upon the velocity at which one trains and the speed at which testing occurs.[45] In general, training at slow speed (60 degrees/sec) does not cause significant peak torque increases, and training at fast speed (240 degrees/sec) does not enhance peak torque at slow speeds. This is another example of the specificity of strength training.

Thus, isokinetic exercises are effective in increasing muscular strength but probably not more so than isotonic training. The ability of isokinetic movements to create maximum tension throughout the range of motion is clearly desirable, but methods of measuring strength may not illustrate this advantage. Perhaps future studies using more refined methods to measure gains in strength may show increased gains in strength with isokinetic training compared with isotonic and isometric training. However, the specificity of training and the bias inherent in that situation make it difficult to compare results.

HYPERTROPHY OF SKELETAL MUSCLE

Based on the evidence presented so far, heavy resistance exercise unquestionably results in increases in muscular strength for men. While some of the experimentation has included women, the extent of strength development and muscle hypertrophy for women has not been studied as extensively. One of the most striking occurrences for men engaged in weight training over an extended period of time is the obvious evidence of hypertrophy, as shown by changes in muscle size accompanying increases in strength. The extent of these changes depends on a number of factors surrounding the strengthening regimen. However, for men, high blood levels of androgens account for the increased muscle size.

One of the reasons for the reluctance of women to engage in serious weight training in the past has been a fear that they would develop the same hypertrophy that men do and would look "masculine." Wilmore[12] examined the strength and body composition of 47 women and 26 men before and after a 10-week intensive weight-training program. Men were found to be stronger than women in most measures of strength, but women were stronger in leg strength per unit of lean body weight. Both groups made similar relative gains in strength, but the degree of muscular hypertrophy for women was considerably less than that noted for men.

However, when hypertrophy is assessed in a more direct manner, such as by computed axial tomography (CAT) scan rather than by a more indirect procedure of determining lean body mass, sex differences in muscle hypertrophy apparently disappear or become minimal.[46] Male and female subjects participated in a 16-week training program in which significant strength increases in elbow flexion, elbow extension, knee flexion, and knee extension occurred. Percentage changes in strength were not significantly different between males and females, nor was any significant sex difference found in relative increases in upper arm circumfer-

ence and muscle cross-sectional area. However, male subjects had higher absolute values in strength and hypertrophy than did females. No significant differences occurred in thigh muscle size. Thus, even though men have larger muscles than women, and women normally have low blood concentrations of testosterone, which might be expected to limit the development of muscle size, percentage changes in muscle hypertrophy resulting from heavy-resistance training are similar in men and women. It is also true that anabolic steroid administration during training will promote muscle hypertrophy in women. However, the adverse metabolic effects of anabolic steroid use outweigh their potential desirability for enhancing muscle size.

One of the major issues examined over the years has been to clarify the nature of hypertrophy itself. It is clear that size increases with strength development, and examining the structural changes that take place within the muscle has been of interest to exercise physiologists and biologists. The term "hypertrophy" denotes an increase in the size or bulk of the muscle fibers, rather than an increase in the number of muscle fibers (called hyperplasia). The question of whether the latter actually occurs as a result of systematic weight training has been the subject of a number of investigations. Early studies concentrated on laboratory animals as subjects. Goldspink[47] trained mice by means of an exercise requiring the pulling of a weight to retrieve food. He reported a 30% increase in cross-sectional area of the average fiber. He also reported a threefold or fourfold increase in the number of myofibrils per fiber. In working with guinea pigs, Helander[48] found an increase of some 15% in actomyosin as a result of training. The studies suggest that both hypertrophy and hyperplasia take place.

One of the earliest studies to report the formation of new muscle fibers (hyperplasia) was published by van Linge,[49] who surgically implanted the plantaris muscle of female rats into the calcaneus. He cut the nerve of the other plantar flexors so that the plantaris muscle would provide plantar flexion. The formation of new muscle fibers was observed at the end of a prolonged heavy training period. Several studies have performed muscle tenotomy (severing the muscle tendon at its insertion) to observe the effect of training on the muscle that must take over the function of the cut muscle. A very rapid hypertrophy takes place after this procedure, and fiber splitting and branching have been reported, as well as increases in strength and fiber diameter.

If a muscle is examined repeatedly for several months after removal of its synergists, hyperplasia is noted.[50] Gonyea[51] subjected 20 cats to a conditioning program involving lifting of weights with the right forelimb against increasing resistance to receive a food reward. The program lasted for 34 weeks, and the flexor carpi radialis muscle was examined to determine any increase in fiber number as a result of low-resistance and high-resistance training. The control group experienced no difference in the number of fibers in either the left or right limb, and no difference in the number of fibers was found in those that lifted a "light-resistance" weight. There was a significant increase in fiber number (20.5%) for those lifting the heavy load. This was attributed to muscle fiber splitting.

Male albino rats were trained by Ho and co-workers[52] in a progressive training program against high resistance for 8 weeks. The number of fibers per unit of cross-sectional area increased significantly in the weight-lifting animals. The authors suggested that the fiber splitting appeared to be due to some sort of "pinching off" of a small segment from the parent fiber or to an invagination of the sarcolemma deep into the muscle fiber in a plane parallel to the sarcomeres.

Under certain conditions, fiber splitting seems to occur, but hypertrophy still remains the major mechanism for the size increase that results from intense weight training. In addition to the structural changes evident from hypertrophy and hyperplasia, a number of enzymatic changes

occur in skeletal muscle. Many of these enzymatic changes are important for the attainment of muscle endurance, and many occur during weight training. The biochemical changes that take place for the weight-lifting individual are those that are involved primarily in anaerobic metabolism.

AGING AND STRENGTH DEVELOPMENT

It is agreed that aging results in a decrease in muscular strength. The greatest decline, however, usually does not take place until after the age of 50. On the other hand, strength increases markedly during the adolescent years and reaches its highest value in the early 20s.[53] Klein and colleagues[54] compared physically active subjects of ages 25 and 66 and found the maximal voluntary isometric contraction to be 31% greater in the young subjects. Similar results are found with isokinetic torque. A study of young and old tennis players[55] found that at all speeds, ranging from 30 to 240 degrees/sec, the young subjects generated significantly more torque than the older subjects. When compared with inactive subjects, those who were active were significantly stronger, and men were stronger than women at all speeds. When the data were presented as a percentage of maximum rather than as absolute values, women exhibited a larger relative decline in torque at high speeds than men. It should also be noted that when isokinetic torque is adjusted for fat-free muscle mass or muscle mass itself, age-related differences between men and women are no longer significant.[56]

Strength increases for older men as a result of resistance training have been clearly identified within 12 weeks.[57–59] The same holds true for older women. Charette and co-workers[60] trained women aged 64 to 86 years on lower extremity exercises for 12 weeks, exercising three times a week, performing three sets of each exercise at 6-RM intensity. All seven of the exercises resulted in significantly greater increases in strength than control subjects who did not train. The average gain was 11.5%. When combined aerobic and anaerobic training was examined over 50 weeks, Cress and associates[61] found that the exercise subjects, aged 72 years, responded to regular exercise training of the leg muscles some 12% more than nontraining control subjects. It is significant to note that the control subjects curtailed their normal independent activities by some 34% over the winter months, ostensibly because of a fear of falling in inclement weather.

Further examination of the relative distribution and size of fiber types of muscles that have undergone such training reveals important clues regarding muscle hypertrophy. If one considers that human muscle is composed of a combination of essentially two types of fibers, it helps to understand the response to a functional overload. One type responds rapidly to stimulation, and one responds more slowly. The fast type are called fast-twitch fibers (FT) and fatigue fairly quickly. On the other hand, the slow-twitch fibers (ST) are better adapted to endurance activities, and thus fatigue less quickly. Age-related changes in men reveal the atrophy of FT fibers,[53] but during strength training the relative area of the FT fibers has been shown to increase significantly.[57] The same phenomenon occurs with women. Charette's 12-week training program[60] caused a 20.1% increase in FT fiber area, and Cress's 50-week program[61] revealed an increase of 46%. No evidence indicates any change in the percentage of the fiber types as a result of training, so the conclusion can be reached that not only can elderly women safely engage in a resistance training program, but they can expect changes to occur as a result of muscle hypertrophy.

SUMMARY

The unmistakable conclusion to be drawn is that training for strength is a goal that can be pursued by both men and women. An op-timal regimen of exercises seems to be six to nine repetitions maximum undertaken for three sets at least three times a week. Most individuals will be working with a system that is at the very least an isotonic one. However, because some of the equipment currently available is specifically designed to maximize the tension throughout the full range of motion, many people now use what are called variable-resistance machines (for example, Universal, Keiser, Nautilus). It seems reasonably clear that both isotonic and isokinetic exercises can be used successfully for developing muscle strength. Less effective are isometric exercises and eccentric contractions. Gains are greater for untrained than for trained individuals. Most athletes, male or female, find increases in strength to come more slowly near the peak of training.

Many of the changes associated with muscle hypertrophy are cellular and thus are not associated with noticeable enlargement. With training, men develop greater muscle hypertrophy than women, because they have much higher levels of androgenic hormones, but women can become very strong through weight training and still not develop markedly enlarged muscles. The average woman should find a number of advantages in being physically strong as she carries out normal activities and engages in other fitness exercise. This may have special significance with increasing age.

The principles outlined, not the type of equipment available, should form the basis for exercise selection. Selecting appropriate exercises and establishing an acceptable routine are more important to strength development than the use of certain commercial fitness machines. Training with free weights can accomplish the same gains in strength as training with machines. However, free weights are more likely to cause injury, since the weights are unsupported and require somewhat greater skill to use. The individual should choose the appropriate exercises and engage in a systematic and progressive program. Early gains are due to an increase in motor coordination. Those gains that occur after several months of training are due to greater muscle strength. Expecting great gains in strength after a few weeks of training is unrealistic, since the acquisition of strength is a slow and progressive process. Such unrealistic expectations about improvement are a common cause of attrition among novices. Qualified instruction may be beneficial to many seeking gains in muscular strength.

REFERENCES

1. Ralston HJ, Pollissar MJ, Inman, VT, et al: Dynamic features of human isolated voluntary muscle in isometric and free contractions. J Appl Physiol 1:526, 1949.
2. DeLorme TL, and Watkins AL: Technics of progressive resistance exercise. Arch Phys Med 29:263, 1948.
3. Houtz SJ, Parrish AM, and Hellebrandt FA: The influence of heavy resistance exercise on strength. Physiother Rev 26:299, 1946.
4. Berger RA: Optimum repetitions for the development of strength. Res Q 33:334, 1962.
5. Berger RA: Effect of varied weight training programs on strength. Res Q 33:168, 1962.
6. Berger RA: Comparative effects of three weight training programs. Res Q 34:396, 1963.
7. Berger RA, and Hardage B: Effect of maximum loads for each of ten repetitions on strength improvement. Res Q 38:715, 1967.
8. Anderson T, and Kearney JT: Effects of three resistance training programs on muscular strength and absolute and relative endurance. Res Q Exerc Sport 53:1, 1982.
9. Staron RS, et al: Muscle hypertrophy and fast fiber type conversions in heavy resistance-trained women. Eur J Appl Physiol 60:71, 1990.
10. Graves JE, et al: Effect of reduced training frequency on muscular strength. Int J Sports Med 9:316, 1988.
11. Montoye HJ, and Lamphiear DE: Grip and arm strength in males and females. Res Q 48:109, 1977.
12. Wilmore JH: Alterations in strength, body composition and anthropometric measurements consequent to a 10-week weight training program. Med Sci Sports 6:133, 1974.
13. Heyward V, and McCreary L: Analysis of the static strength and relative endurance of women athletes. Res Q 48:703, 1977.
14. Clarke DH: Sex differences in strength and fatigability. Res Q Exerc Sport 57:144, 1986.
15. Morrow JR, and Hosler WW: Strength comparisons in untrained men and women athletes, age 10 to 69. Med Sci Sports 13:194, 1981.
16. Yates JW, et al: Static lifting strength and maximal isometric voluntary contractions of back, arm and shoulder muscles. Ergonomics 23:37, 1980.
17. Hettinger TL, and Muller EA: Muskelleistung und muskeltrainung. Arbeitsphysiol 15:111, 1953.
18. Muller EA: Physiology of muscle training. Rev Can Biol 21:303, 1962.
19. Muller EA, and Rohmert W: Die geschwindigkeit der muskelkraft zunahme bei isometrischen trainung. Int Z Angew Physiol 19:403, 1963.
20. Josenhans WKT: An evaluation of some methods of improving muscle strength. Rev Can Biol 21:315, 1962.
21. Rose DL, Radzyminski SF, and Beatty RR: Effect of brief maximal exercise on the strength of the quadriceps femoris. Arch Phys Med Rehabil 38:157, 1957.
22. Morehouse CA: Development and maintenance of isometric strength of subjects with diverse initial strengths. Res Q 38:449, 1967.
23. Rarick GL, and Larsen GL: Observations on frequency and intensity of isometric muscular effort in developing static muscular strength in post-pubescent males. Res Q 29:333, 1958.
24. Cotten D: Relationship of the duration of sustained voluntary isometric contraction to changes in endurance and strength. Res Q 38:366, 1967.
25. Meyers CR: Effects of two isometric routines on strength, size, and endurance in exercised and nonexercised arms. Res Q 38:430, 1967.
26. Kitai TA, and Sale DG: Specificity of joint angle in isometric training. Eur J Appl Physiol 58:744, 1989.
27. Thepaut-Mathieu C, Van Hoecke J, and Maton B: Myoelectrical and mechanical changes linked to length specificity during isometric training. J Appl Physiol 64:1500, 1988.
28. Hansen JW: The training effect of repeated isometric muscle contractions. Int Z Angew Physiol 18:474, 1961.
29. Hansen JW: The effect of sustained isometric muscle contraction on various muscle functions. Int Z Angew Physiol 19:430, 1963.
30. Jackson A, et al: Strength development: Using functional isometrics in an isotonic strength training program. Res Q Exerc Sport 56:234, 1985.
31. Rasch PJ, and Morehouse LE: Effect of static and dynamic exercises on muscular strength and hypertrophy. J Appl Physiol 11:29, 1957.
32. Berger RA: Comparison of static and dynamic strength increases. Res Q 33:329, 1962.

33. Berger RA: Comparison between static training and various dynamic training programs. Res Q 34:131, 1963.
34. Coleman AE: Effect of unilateral isometric and isotonic contractions on the strength of the contralateral limb. Res Q 40:490, 1969.
35. Salter N: The effect on muscle strength of maximum isometric and isotonic contractions at different repetition rates. J Physiol 130:109, 1955.
36. Chui EF: Effects of isometric and dynamic weight-training exercises upon strength and speed of movement. Res Q 35:246, 1964.
37. Lawrence MS, Meyer HR, and Matthews NL: Comparative increase in muscle strength in the quadriceps femoris by isometric and isotonic exercise and effects on the contralateral muscle. J Am Phys Ther Assoc 42:15, 1962.
38. Bonde Petersen F: Muscle training by static, concentric and eccentric contractions. Acta Physiol Scand 48:406, 1960.
39. Singh M, and Karpovich PV: Effect of eccentric training of agonists on antagonistic muscles. J Appl Physiol 23:742, 1967.
40. Johnson BL, et al: A comparison of concentric and eccentric muscle training. Med Sci Sports 8:35, 1976.
41. Jones DA, and Rutherford OM: Human muscle strength training: The effects of three different regimes and the nature of the resultant changes. J Physiol 391:1, 1987.
42. Thistle HG, et al: Isokinetic contraction: A new concept of resistive exercise. Arch Phys Med Rehabil 48:279, 1966.
43. Moffroid M, et al: A study of isokinetic exercise. Phys Ther 49:735, 1969.
44. Lesmes GR, et al: Muscle strength and power changes during maximal isokinetic training. Med Sci Sports 10:266, 1978.
45. Ewing JL, et al: Effects of velocity of isokinetic training on strength, power, and quadriceps muscle fibre characteristics. Eur J Appl Physiol 61:159, 1990.
46. Cureton KJ, et al: Muscle hypertrophy in men and women. Med Sci Sports Exerc 20:338, 1988.
47. Goldspink G: The combined effects of exercise and reduced food intake on skeletal muscle fibers. J Cell Comp Physiol 63:209, 1964.
48. Helander EAS: Influence of exercise and restricted activity on the protein composition of skeletal muscle. Biochem J 78:478, 1961.
49. van Linge B: The response of muscle to strenuous exercise. J Bone Joint Surg 44-B:711, 1962.
50. Reitsma W: Some structural changes in skeletal muscles of the rat after intensive training. Acta Morphol Neerl Scand 7:229, 1970.
51. Gonyea WJ: Role of exercise in inducing increases in skeletal muscle fiber number. J Appl Physiol 48:421, 1980.
52. Ho KW, et al: Skeletal muscle fiber splitting with weight-lifting exercise in rats. Am J Anat 157:433, 1980.
53. Larsson L, and Karlsson J: Isometric and dynamic endurance as a function of age and skeletal muscle characteristics. Acta Physiol Scand 104:129, 1978.
54. Klein C, et al: Fatigue and recovery contractile properties of young and elderly men. Eur J Appl Physiol 57:684, 1988.
55. Laforest S, et al: Effects of age and regular exercise on muscle strength and endurance. Eur J Appl Physiol 60:104, 1990.
56. Frontera WR, et al: A cross-sectional study of muscle strength and mass in 45- to 78-year-old men and women. J Appl Physiol 71:644, 1991.
57. Aniansson A, and Gustafsson E: Physical training in elderly men with special reference to quadriceps muscle strength and morphology. Clin Physiol 1:87, 1981.
58. Brown AB, McCartney N, and Sale DG: Positive adaptations to weight-lifting in the elderly. J Appl Physiol 69:1725, 1990.
59. Frontera WR, et al: Strength conditioning in older men: Skeletal muscle hypertrophy and improved function. J Appl Physiol 64:1038, 1988.
60. Charette SL, et al: Muscle hypertrophy response to resistance training in older women. J Appl Physiol 70:1912, 1991.
61. Cress ME, et al: Effect of training on VO_{2max}, thigh strength, and muscle morphology in septuagenarian women. Med Sci Sports Exerc 23:752, 1991.

CHAPTER 4

Endurance Training

THOMAS D. FAHEY, Ed.D.

Until recently, systematic studies of female endurance athletes were limited. This is understandable because, before passage of Title IX of the Civil Rights Act in 1972, the number of women competing in endurance sports was small.[1] This legislation mandated equal opportunity for sports participation in the schools.

The American College of Sports Medicine is perhaps the premier organization for the study of sports medicine in the world. In 1971 it published the *Encyclopedia of Sport Sciences and Medicine*.[2] This monumental work consisted of over 1700 pages, but fewer than 10 pages were devoted to women and sports medicine. Until 1958, the longest event in women's track and field in competitions hosted by the Amateur Athletic Union of the United States was 440 yards. In 1965, top female runners were threatened with banishment from international competition if they ran in a race longer than 1.5 miles. In 1984, the first Olympic marathon for women was held in Los Angeles. Now, it is common for women to compete in endurance events such as ultramarathons, triathlons, and long-distance swimming and cycling.

FACTORS THAT DETERMINE SUCCESS IN ENDURANCE EVENTS

Important factors in endurance performance include maximal oxygen consumption ($\dot{V}O_2$max), mitochondrial density, performance efficiency, and body composition.[3] Sex differences exist in endurance performance. However, the relative changes that occur with training and the basic underlying mechanisms that determine performance are the same in men and women.

Maximal Oxygen Consumption

Maximal oxygen consumption ($\dot{V}O_2max$) is considered to be the best measure of cardiovascular capacity. Many sports medicine experts think of it as the single most important measure of physical fitness. It is defined as the point at which O_2 consumption fails to rise despite an increased exercise intensity or power output. The greater ability of trained people to sustain a high exercise intensity is largely due to a greater $\dot{V}O_2max$.

$\dot{V}O_2max$ is equal to the product of maximum cardiac output and maximum arteriovenous oxygen difference (Eq. 5–1):

$$\dot{V}O_2max = \dot{Q}max\ (a - v)O_2max$$

where $\dot{V}O_2max$ is the maximal rate of O_2 consumption (in $L \cdot min^{-1}$), $\dot{Q}max$ is the maximum cardiac output ($L \cdot min^{-1}$), and $(a - v)O_2max$ is the maximum arterial-venous O_2 difference ($mL\ O_2 \cdot 100\ mL^{-1}$). Thus, $\dot{V}O_2max$ is a function of the maximum rate of oxygen transport and oxygen utilization.

During the transition from rest to maximal exercise, there is a linear increase in $(a - v)O_2$. Arterial oxygen partial pressure (PaO_2) is well maintained in most athletes during exercise. The increase is due to the decrease in venous oxygen partial pressure (PvO_2). There is only a limited capacity to increase oxygen extraction through endurance training. The venous blood draining the active muscles of both trained and untrained people during maximal exercise contains relatively little oxygen.

To be successful in competition, athletes in sports that require endurance must have a large cardiac output capacity. Maximum cardiac output is the product of maximum heart rate (HR) and maximum stroke volume (SV) (Eq. 5–2):

$$\dot{Q}max = (HRmax)(SVmax)$$

Maximum heart rate is largely determined by heredity and age. It is not appreciably affected by training. Because HRmax and $(a - v)O_2max$ are stable, changes in $\dot{V}O_2max$ with training are mostly due to changes in stroke volume.

Stroke volume is affected by hemodynamic and myocardial factors. It is closely linked to venous return of blood to the heart. The ability of the heart to contract with increased force as its chambers are stretched (a phenomenon known as preload) is described by the Frank-Starling principle.[4] Many factors affect preload. These include total blood volume, body position, intrathoracic pressure, atrial contribution to ventricular filling, pumping action of skeletal muscle, venous tone, and intrapericardial pressure.[4] These hemodynamic factors can have acute and chronic effects on stroke volume, oxygen transport capacity, and perception of fatigue. An example is during endurance exercise where there is a decrease in blood volume due to dehydration or a decrease in venous tone. There is a compensatory increase in heart rate and an increase in perceived exertion. Increased blood volume resulting from endurance training also causes an increase in stroke volume.

Stroke volume is also affected by myocardial contractility. The contractile force of the myocardium changes in response to circulating catecholamines, the force-frequency relationship of the muscle, sympathetic nerve impulses, intrinsic depression, loss of myocardium, pharmacologic depressants, and inotropic agents. Positive inotropic agents include digitalis, and negative inotropic agents include hypoxemia, hypercapnia, and acidosis.[4] Endurance training increases myocardial contractility by increasing Ca^{++}-myosin ATPase activity.[5,6] The combination of increased preload and contractility is responsible for the increase in stroke volume that occurs with endurance training. Both of these factors are limited by ventricular volume, which is affected by genetic and environmental factors during growth and development. It can be changed to some extent through endurance training.[7,8]

The relative importance of genetics and environment for success in endurance exercise is not known. Roost[9] examined cardiac dimensions in trained and untrained school children. All of the trained children were classified as talented, with potential for eventual success in endurance events. He could find no children with congenitally enlarged hearts. Thus, considering left ventricular diameter and wall size, the importance of genetic predisposition for success may have been overstated.

The oxygen consumption capacity of a muscle varies according to fiber type.[10] The ability of the mitochondria to extract oxygen from blood is approximately three to five times greater in slow-twitch red than in fast-twitch white fibers. Training can double the mitochondrial mass.[11] It is possible for elite endurance athletes to have 10 times the muscle oxygen-extracting capacity in their trained muscles as sedentary people. Several studies have demonstrated a high correlation ($r \approx 0.80$) between $\dot{V}_{O_2}max$ and leg muscle mitochondrial activity.[12,13] Cardiac output and muscle mitochondrial capacities are important determinants of the upper limits of $\dot{V}_{O_2}max$.

There is a strong genetic component for $\dot{V}_{O_2}max$.[14-17] The well-known exercise physiologist Per-Olaf Åstrand has stated that to become an Olympic-level endurance athlete requires choosing one's parents carefully! Genetic studies typically show less variance in $\dot{V}_{O_2}max$ and muscle fiber type between monozygous twins than between dizygous twins. However, these studies also show that training is critical for success, but the ability to improve performance in response to an endurance training program depends on genetic factors.

Intense endurance training results in a maximum increase in $\dot{V}_{O_2}max$ of approximately 20%.[18-21] However, greater increases are possible if the initial physical fitness of the subject is low.[22,23] Only certain types of exercise promote the cardiac alterations necessary for increased $\dot{V}_{O_2}max$. Maximal stroke volume can be increased in response to a volume overload induced by participation in sports such as running, cycling, and swimming. In pressure-overload sports such as weight lifting, however, left ventric-

ular wall thickness increases, with no increase in left ventricular volume.[24,25] Changes in $\dot{V}_{O_2}max$ and in endurance capacity are not the same. Endurance performance can be improved by much more than 20%. This is possible by improving mitochondrial density, speed, running economy, and body composition.

Factors Limiting $\dot{V}_{O_2}max$

The limiting factor of $\dot{V}_{O_2}max$ has been a source of debate for many years. Proposed limiting factors include cardiac output, pulmonary ventilation, lung diffusion, and oxygen utilization.

A basic experimental design for determining if oxygen supply or utilization is the limiting factor involves artificially increasing the supply of oxygen to the working muscle. If maximal oxygen consumption does not change, it implies that the ability of the tissues to utilize oxygen is the limiting factor. On the other hand, if $\dot{V}_{O_2}max$ increases with an artificial increase in O_2 to the muscles, cardiac output probably is the limiting factor. Considerable evidence suggests that cardiac output is the limiting factor for maximal aerobic capacity. $\dot{V}_{O_2}max$ is increased if the rate of oxygen supply to the muscle is increased through induced erythrocythemia (blood doping) or breathing 100% oxygen during exercise.[26-28]

Another technique for investigating this question is to vary the amount of active tissue requiring increased oxygen during exercise.[29-31] Adding active arm work during maximal treadmill exercise does not increase $\dot{V}_{O_2}max$. This type of exercise increases the amount of tissue that requires oxygen. Several studies have found that $\dot{V}_{O_2}peak$ in isolated quadriceps muscle was much higher than when the muscle was exercised as part of a whole body maximum effort.[29-31]

Many exercisers use expressions such as "I was winded" or "my wind gave out on me." There is little evidence that pulmonary function limits aerobic capacity at sea level in healthy people. The lungs have a very large reserve that enables them to meet most of the body's requirements for gas exchange and acid-base balance during heavy exercise. Considerable direct and indirect evidence exists for this:

- The alveolar and capillary surface areas of the system are approximately 140 and 125 m^2, respectively. The alveolar-capillary diffusion distance is no more than a few microns thick. Thus, the lung has an extremely large diffusion capacity.
- Low pulmonary resistance to blood flow allows pulmonary blood volume to increase during heavy exercise by three times the value at rest.
- During exercise, the ventilation-perfusion ratio increases four to five times above rest.
- The sigmoid shape of the oxyhemoglobin dissociation curve allows the maintenance of resting values of hemoglobin oxygen saturation even when Pa_{O_2} drops slightly.
- Pa_{O_2} changes very little during heavy exercise. A constant Pa_{O_2} suggests that the lungs do not limit $\dot{V}_{O_2}$max, because Pa_{O_2} is an important indicator of lung function.[3,32]

Dempsy and Fregosi[32] presented evidence that the lungs may be limiting in some elite male endurance athletes. No such evidence has been presented for elite female athletes. In their subjects, Pa_{O_2} dropped as low as 65 mm Hg. There was a significant widening in the difference between alveolar oxygen partial pressure (PA_{O_2}) and Pa_{O_2}. They hypothesized that there was a diffusion limitation as well as increased airway impedance at high levels of ventilation in these athletes.

Others have argued that oxygen supply does not limit either $\dot{V}_{O_2}$max or endurance.[33-36] Rather, the limiting factors are biochemical. Suggested limiting factors include decreases in the rate and force of myofibrillar cross-bridge cycle activity. Contributing factors may be failure of calcium transport mechanisms or decreased myofibrillar ATPase activity.

The critical mitochondrial P_{O_2} is thought to be 1 mm Hg.[37] Indirect estimates of mitochondrial P_{O_2} during maximal exercise suggest that it is above the critical level.[33-35]

$\dot{V}_{O_2}$max as Predictor of Endurance Performance

If $\dot{V}_{O_2}$max were the only predictor of endurance performance, then endurance contests could be decided in the laboratory. Research scientists could administer treadmill tests. The person with the highest $\dot{V}_{O_2}$max would be the winner. This might be easier and more precise than conducting athletic contests on the track, road, or swimming pool. However, $\dot{V}_{O_2}$max is only one factor that determines success in endurance events.

In a heterogeneous sample, women with a high $\dot{V}_{O_2}$max tend to run faster in the marathon.[38] This relationship does not exist when the sample is homogeneous (i.e., the runners are of the same ability level).[39] For example, Grete Waitz and Derek Clayton had $\dot{V}_{O_2}$max values of 73 and 69 mL·kg^{-1}·min^{-1}, respectively. These values were measured shortly after they set world records for the women's and men's marathons. Yet, Clayton's time was over 15 minutes faster than Waitz's. Other factors important for success include speed, the ability to continue exercising at a high percentage of $\dot{V}_{O_2}$max, lactic acid clearance capacity, maximal muscle blood flow, and performance economy.

A high $\dot{V}_{O_2}$max is a prerequisite to performing at elite levels in endurance events. The minimum values for elite female endurance athletes are approximately 65 mL·kg^{-1}·min^{-1} for runners and cross-country skiers. Appropriate values for swimmers are 55 to 60 mL·kg^{-1}. Cyclists require approximately 60 mL·kg^{-1}. The evidence for a minimum aerobic capacity requirement is circumstantial:

- All elite endurance athletes have high aerobic capacities. Even though $\dot{V}_{O_2}$max is a poor predictor of performance among athletes at the same level of competition, the variance in maximal aerobic power between them is small.

- Oxygen consumption increases as a function of velocity in all endurance events. Although athletes vary somewhat in their efficiencies, the variance between them is small.

Even though a high $\dot{V}O_2$max is important for achieving superior levels of endurance, it is not the only requirement for success.

Noakes[36] has questioned the validity of $\dot{V}O_2$max as a predictor of endurance performance. His reservations are based on these observations:

- Much of the evidence of an oxygen limitation during exercise is circumstantial. Noakes analyzed the data of the classic studies that established $\dot{V}O_2$max as a laboratory benchmark for cardiovascular performance.[40-42] He found that most subjects did not show that $\dot{V}O_2$ leveled off with increasing intensity of exercise at maximum.
- Studies have used transfusion or O_2 breathing in an attempt to show that O_2 transport is limiting. None of these studies have demonstrated that their subjects reached a plateau in $\dot{V}O_2$ during normal exercise. There was no evidence of an O_2 transport limitation before the experimental intervention.
- In blood doping studies, there is a dissociation between changes in $\dot{V}O_2$max and performance. Performance changes last only a few days, while changes in $\dot{V}O_2$max last longer.
- Exercise at extreme altitudes is not limited by high blood lactate levels or by indications of central limitations in cardiac or respiratory function.
- Exhaustion during maximal exercise occurs at a lower oxygen consumption during cycling than during running in the same subjects.
- Blood lactate levels at exhaustion during progressive treadmill exercise testing are lowest in elite athletes.

- Changes in running performance with training occur without equivalent changes in $\dot{V}O_2$max.

Noakes's data suggest that a good predictor of endurance performance is peak treadmill velocity. He hypothesized that maximum speed may be related to the muscles' capacity for high cross-bridge cycling and respiratory adaptations. Respiratory adaptations may make it possible to prevent the onset of exercise-induced dyspnea.

Mitochondrial Density

Mitochondrial density is a better predictor of endurance capacity than $\dot{V}O_2$max. Endurance is the ability to sustain a particular submaximal level of physical effort. Davies and co-workers[43] showed that cytochrome oxidase activity (which is directly dependent upon mitochondrial mass) had a correlation coefficient of 0.92 with running endurance but only 0.70 with $\dot{V}O_2$max. With training, $\dot{V}O_2$max increases by less than 20% in most people, but the ability to sustain a given submaximal exercise intensity may increase by much more. Endurance performance by athletes in sports such as cycling, running, swimming, and cross-country skiing requires intense effort and maintenance of that intensity for a long time. Increased mitochondrial density may be the key factor in endurance. It may allow some athletes to run, cycle, or swim at high velocities for longer than others, even though their maximal oxygen uptakes are similar to those of slower athletes.

Endurance training results in an increased mitochondrial density in both fast-twitch and slow-twitch muscle fibers.[44] This probably plays a major role in improving endurance. There are several possible mechanisms. Increased mitochondrial mass may increase fat utilization during exercise and thus spare muscle glycogen. It also may improve muscle lactic acid clearance capacity, allowing exercise at a higher intensity.[44,45]

A fundamental purpose of energy metabolism during exercise is to generate ATP to meet the demands of the exercise intensity. A deficit in ATP causes the athlete to fatigue quickly. The rate of ATP formation is critical. Fat provides the most energy per gram. Carbohydrate is the most important fuel for high-intensity endurance exercise, however, because it provides the most ATP per liter of oxygen. Thus, carbohydrate provides ATP more quickly than does fat.[46]

At least two problems are associated with the use of carbohydrates during endurance exercise:

- The supply of carbohydrates is limited.
- The rapid use of carbohydrates during high-intensity exercise results in a rate of lactic acid production greater than its rate of clearance. Accumulation of lactic acid may interfere with muscle contraction and energy metabolism.[47,48]

Increasing muscle mitochondrial mass may help the body to cope with both of these problems.

The glycogen content of muscle is important in endurance capacity. When glycogen is depleted, fatigue results. During sustained exercise, muscle glycogen is the muscle's principal source of carbohydrate.[45] In addition, the rate of glycogen utilization increases as a function of exercise intensity. It is very important, then, for the athlete to conserve glycogen to maintain the intensity of exercise at the desired level. Endurance training, which results in an increased mitochondrial mass, increases the capacity of the muscle to oxidize fat.[49] This slows the rate of glycolysis and the catabolism of glucose and glycogen. Thus, glycogen is spared and fatigue delayed.

The increased mitochondrial mass accompanying training may also increase the muscle's ability to remove lactate through oxidation. For more than 50 years, lactic acid has been thought of by many as a metabolic pariah. However, research using radioactive tracer methodology has demonstrated that lactate is an important substrate during exercise:[45,50]

- During sustained exercise, lactate production and removal occur simultaneously within active muscle.
- Most lactic acid produced during exercise is oxidized.
- During endurance exercise, the turnover and oxidation rates of lactate exceed those of glucose.
- Lactate production during both rest and exercise is not necessarily associated with muscle anaerobiosis.
- Training mainly affects the rate of lactate removal rather than its production.

The effects of the increased mitochondrial mass with training are complex but elegant. Glycogen is the critical fuel for endurance exercise. However, its use increases the risk of its own depletion and lactic acid accumulation due to an excess of lactic acid production over clearance. The increased mitochondrial mass that results from training prevents lactic acid accumulation. It does this by providing the muscles with an increased capacity for lactic acid oxidation. It also prevents glycogen depletion by allowing an increased use of fats as fuel.

Nevertheless, training is probably not as important as genetics for obtaining a high mitochondrial mass in the muscles required for endurance exercise.[50] Studies of successful male endurance athletes have shown that they often have a high percentage of slow-twitch muscle fibers. A high mitochondrial density is a characteristic of these fibers. Tesch and Karlsson[51] suggest, however, that the greater percentage of slow-twitch fibers in the active muscles of endurance athletes may be an adaptive response. As discussed, $\dot{V}O_2max$ and mitochondrial density are highly related. Athletes whose muscles have a high mitochondrial mass also have high $\dot{V}O_2max$ values.

Performance Efficiency

Although exercise intensity is the most important determinant of metabolic rate, individual differences in performance efficiency can be responsible for the difference between winning and losing. When power output can be measured accurately, efficiency can be calculated with the following equation (Eq. 5–3):[52]

ulating ventilation, changing body composition, improving training status, and improving running style.[55]

Other than metabolic considerations,

$$\text{Efficiency} = \frac{\text{Change in power output}}{\text{Change in caloric equivalent of } O_2 \text{ consumption (100)}}$$

Efficiency is decreased by energy lost as heat, by wasted movement, and by mechanical factors such as wind resistance, friction, and drag. The efficiency of walking and cycle ergometry is slightly less than 30%.[52,53] It is probable that the efficiency of running, cycling, swimming, and cross-country skiing at competitive exercise intensities is less than that.

High-intensity exercise is not performed at a steady rate. $\dot{V}O_2$ does not account for all of the ATP supplied during exercise; a portion is supplied through anaerobic glycolysis. Consequently, efficiency cannot be accurately calculated even when power output can be measured.

The relative change in efficiency can be estimated by measuring changes in oxygen consumption under different conditions. $\dot{V}O_2$ measurements can measure the effects of wind resistance, mechanical aids (e.g., toe clips in cycling and wax in cross-country skiing), and technique. A fundamental problem is determining how much of the efficiency is due to mechanical factors (i.e., technique and equipment) and how much to physiologic factors (i.e., mitochondrial density). For example, if one runner seems more efficient than another, it is difficult to identify whether the greater efficiency is due to a more efficient running style or to a superior lactic acid clearance capacity.

In women, running economy (the oxygen cost of running at a specific speed) has not been shown to be a good predictor of performance.[54] However, when the subject population is homogeneous, running economy aids in the prediction of running performance.[55,56] At present, the effect of running economy on performance is not well understood. The most promising methods for improving running economy may be manip-

technique is probably the most important factor affecting performance efficiency. In swimming, athletes should develop good hydrodynamics, using strokes that employ efficient propulsive force and minimize drag. This may contribute almost as much to success as improving the physiologic aspects of endurance. Likewise, the frequent use of "skating" in cross-country skiing has revolutionized the sport. Efficient runners are thought to have a lower vertical component in their technique. Efficient cyclists pedal smoothly at high revolutions per minute without engaging muscle groups that do not contribute to pedaling speed.[57,58] Wind resistance is also a factor in running and cycling. It is reduced by wearing clothing that enhances aerodynamics.

Body Composition

The importance of body composition for endurance varies with the sport. In distance running, gravity places a greater load on the athlete than in swimming or cycling. Runners are usually leaner than other endurance athletes, and there is less variance in body fat among elite performers.[59–62] Typical fat percentages for female endurance athletes are shown in Table 4–1. Although the data are limited, all categories of female endurance athletes are leaner than sedentary women of the same age. Swimmers have more body fat than runners, cyclists, and cross-country skiers. In long-distance swimmers, a slightly higher fat percentage decreases drag in the water and provides insulation against the cold.

Tanaka and Matsuura[60] reported that anthropometric factors accounted for 20% to 40% of the variance in male distance runners. This is comparable to the importance

Table 4–1. BODY COMPOSITION OF ELITE
FEMALE ENDURANCE ATHLETES

Sport	Percent Fat
Distance running[65]	15.2
Distance running[62]	16.9
Distance running[38]	15.3
Distance running[54]	15.4
Cross-country skiing[66]	21.8
Cross-country skiing[67]	16.1
Cycling[20]	15.4
Swimming[68]	18.1
Swimming[69]	17.8
Swimming[70]	13.7
Swimming[71]	15.6
Swimming[59]	16.6
Swimming[72]	21.7

of maximal oxygen consumption. However, remember that correlation coefficients describe relationships. They do not mean that one factor causes another. These investigators did not study female athletes. Most studies have found that female distance runners average 16% fat. Levels as low as 6% have been reported. Christensen and Ruhling[38] have found that female marathon runners continue to become leaner the longer they participate in the sport. Novice marathon runners were found to have 18% fat, experienced marathoners had 16.3%, and elite marathoners had 15.3%. The average body fat percentage of a young adult woman in the United States is 25%.

In running, cycling, and cross-country skiing, excess fat increases the energy cost of exercise. The ideal lower limit of body fat is not known. There is a 40% to 60% difference between men and women in $\dot{V}_{O_2}$max expressed in liters per minute, but these sex differences are reduced to less than 10% when $\dot{V}_{O_2}$max is expressed per kilogram lean body mass.[63] Although it appears that low levels of body fat are desirable for peak endurance performance in women, world distance running records have been set by women with greater than 15% fat. Extremely low levels of body fat in female endurance athletes may affect other aspects of physiology. Related are the training and dietary habits necessary to achieve low body fat. Ef-

fects may include endocrine and reproductive function and bone metabolism. These problems are discussed elsewhere in this volume.

It is possible that the higher percentage of body fat found in female swimmers compared with that of other endurance athletes may be an advantage. When swimming at comparable velocities, women demonstrate a lower body drag than men, probably due to more subcutaneous fat. This makes women more efficient at the sport. The ideal fat percentage of the female swimmer is also affected by fitness and stroke mechanics, however. Rennie and co-workers[64] have hypothesized that women could swim faster than men if they could develop comparable physical capacities. The difference between the sexes in the world record in the 1500-meter run is 10%, but there is only a 6% difference between them in the 400-meter swim. The lower drag among women swimmers may account for the reduced sex difference. Top women swimmers today are swimming faster than did 1972 Olympic champion Mark Spitz.

SEX DIFFERENCES IN ENDURANCE PERFORMANCE

Women's performance times are 6% to 15% slower than men's in most endurance sports[73,74] (Table 4–2). However, there is considerable variance in performance in specific events. As mentioned, in the 400-meter swim, the difference between the men's and women's world record is slightly more than 6%. The difference in the 80-km run is almost 44%. Men rode longer distances in the 1988 Olympic cycling road race competition (82 km for women and 196.8 km for men). Yet the average velocity of the winning man was only 5% faster than that of the winning woman. There are slightly larger differences between the sexes in upper-body endurance events, such as canoeing.[75] Men have relatively more muscle in the upper body, which allows them to generate more power.

Table 4–2. COMPARISON BETWEEN MALE AND FEMALE GOLD MEDAL ENDURANCE PERFORMANCE TIMES IN THE 1992 OLYMPICS

Event	Performance Time	
	Male	Female
Track		
800-m run	1:43.66	1:55.54
1500-m run	3:40.12	3:55.30
10,000-m run	27:46.70	31:06.02
Marathon	2:13.23	2:32.41
Swimming		
200-m freestyle	1:46.70	1:57.90
400-m freestyle	3:45.00	4:07.18
200-m butterfly stroke	1:56.26	2:08.67
200-m breaststroke	2:10.16	2:26.65
200-m backstroke	1:58.47	2:07.06

Some events, such as the 80-km run, are not contested very often by women. This makes it difficult to determine true sex differences from performance comparisons. Sex differences in the physiologic responses to exercise are often unclear from the literature, since many studies have compared physically fit male subjects with sedentary female subjects.

Organ size and body mass are probably the most important factors determining the sex differences in endurance performance. Greater size provides a greater power-output capacity. Men have more muscle mass, both in relative and absolute terms, while women have more fat. Greater lean body mass is an asset, while more fat weight is a hindrance. Although muscle fiber composition is similar between the sexes, both fast-twitch and slow-twitch muscle fibers are usually larger in men.[76]

Sex differences in endurance performance increase as sport levels decrease.[75] Thus, there are fewer sex differences between male and female elite athletes than between those of lesser standing. Strength and power differences are major reasons for sexual dimorphism in performance. Males and females make the same relative gains in strength when they are subjected to the same training stimuli.[79,80] At elite levels, the training programs of men and women may be closer to each other in intensity than those of lower-level athletes. With years of training, men and women get closer to their absolute potential. As they approach absolute potential, it becomes possible to make realistic comparisons of true sex differences.

Absolute maximal oxygen consumption $(L \cdot min^{-1})$ is typically more than 40% greater in men than in women. This difference is reduced to approximately 20% when $\dot{V}O_2max$ is expressed per kilogram body weight.[77] It decreases further to less than 10% when expressed per kilogram of lean body weight. Although excess fat is a handicap to women endurance athletes, it does not appear to account for all sex differences in performance. Cureton and Sparling[78] added extra weight to men in an attempt experimentally to equalize fat masses. They were able to completely abolish the differences between men and women in relative $\dot{V}O_2max$, but the following sex differences remained: 30% in distance run in 12 minutes, 31% in maximum treadmill run time, and 20% in running efficiency after the experimental intervention. They estimated that fat percentage accounts for 74% of the sex differences in running performance. The higher $\dot{V}O_2max$ of men $(mL \cdot kg \ LBM^{-1})$ accounted for 20%.

The average man has a larger heart size and heart volume than the average woman (in both absolute and relative terms). This results in a greater stroke volume during maximal exercise and contributes to the sex differences in $\dot{V}O_2max$. Even though women have a higher relative heart rate during exercise, it is not enough to compensate for their lower stroke volume. The resultant smaller cardiac output of women contributes to their lower aerobic capacity. The amount and concentration of hemoglobin also are higher in men, giving male blood greater oxygen-carrying capacity. Women average about 13.7 g $Hb \cdot 100 \ mL^{-1}$, whereas men average 15.8 g $Hb \cdot 100 \ mL^{-1}$. The difference is attributed to the stimulating effect of .

androgens on hemoglobin production and to the effects of menstrual blood loss and differences in dietary intake[3] (see Chapter 6).

There are few sex differences among the factors that account for individual differences in endurance performance. In comparatively trained men and women, the energy cost of running is similar.[8] Bosco and colleagues[82] have shown that the energy cost of running is related to the percentage of fast-twitch fibers. They have hypothesized that many women runners have a higher proportion of slow-twitch fibers than most men. Women thus may have a predisposition for a higher running economy during submaximal exercise.[83] As discussed, other investigators have found no difference between men and women in the distribution of muscle fiber types.

There are differences in running economy in different subject populations. This may partially explain some of the variability in running performance not explained by $\dot{V}O_2$max. Most studies show no sex differences in the percentage of $\dot{V}O_2$max sustained during exercise.[84,85] Although there is some disagreement among researchers, there do not seem to be any appreciable sex differences in performance efficiency in running or cycling.[86]

To date, there are no definitive studies on sex differences in lactate production and clearance rates. No large sex differences in temperature regulation capacity have been found when researchers have made a serious attempt to use subjects of equal fitness. Finally, there are no sex differences in the ability to improve $\dot{V}O_2$max through training or in the ability to improve endurance performance through interval and continuous exercise programs.[87]

Ullyot[88] hypothesized that the higher body fat of women could be an advantage during marathon and ultramarathon endurance events, because they may have a greater capacity for fat metabolism. Ullyot observed that, unlike male runners, many women runners do not "hit the wall" during the marathon. "Hitting the wall" is sudden, extreme fatigue that occurs late in the race and is probably related to glycogen depletion.

Costill and co-workers[89] did not support this hypothesis. They used equally trained male and female subjects who ran for 1 hour on a treadmill and found that the capacity to use fat as fuel during exercise was similar in men and women. Muscle succinate dehydrogenase and carnitine palmitoyl transferase activities were higher in the men, suggesting that the muscle mitochondrial density in the male subjects may have been greater.

TRAINING FOR ENDURANCE

Training is an adaptive process. Unfortunately, athletes often forget this simple fact. They attempt overzealous training programs with no real thought as to how their bodies will respond to them. Consequently, they often become overtrained. They fail to improve at a desirable rate, or they become injured.

Selye[90] formulated a theory of stress adaptation, which has implications for conditioning endurance athletes. Selye called his theory the general adaptation syndrome (GAS). He described three processes involved in the response to a stressor: (1) alarm reaction, (2) resistance development, and (3) exhaustion.

In the alarm reaction, the body mobilizes its resources. During exercise, cardiac output increases, blood is directed to active muscle, and metabolic rate increases. Body balance is upset.

The resistance development stage can also be called the adaptive stage. It occurs when fitness is increased. It is the goal and purpose of the endurance training program. The athlete must exercise at a threshold intensity to get an adaptive response. This threshold is individual and is much higher in elite athletes than in sedentary people.

When a stress cannot be tolerated, the athlete enters the stage of exhaustion. This stress can be either acute or chronic. Symptoms of acute exhaustion include fractures, sprains, and strains. Chronic exhaustion is characterized by stress fractures, staleness, and emotional stress. The basic purpose of the training program is to train hard enough to get an adaptive response and improve fitness, but not so hard as to become injured.

The body adapts specifically to the stress of exercise.[91] Athletes should develop the type of fitness required in their sport; runners should run and weight lifters should lift weights. The training program should also reflect the various components of the activity. For example, if a runner or cyclist must go up hills in competition, then she should include hill-running or hill-cycling in her program.

The varying force requirements encountered during exercise are met by recruiting the number of motor units needed to perform the task. Because a motor unit is trained in proportion to its recruitment,[92] it is critical that the motor units that will be used in competition be trained regularly. Therefore, a runner who hopes to run repeated 6-minute miles in competition must include a portion of her training at race pace or faster. This will condition the motor units that will be recruited during the race. The frequency of different types of training depends upon the relative importance of their target motor units. So, while repeated short sprints may be the central component for a 100-meter runner, they would be much less valuable for a distance runner.

Components of Overload

The amount of overload (training stimulus) in the training program can be varied by manipulating intensity, volume, duration, and rest. Intensity is the speed at which the activity is carried out. Volume is the number of repetitions. Duration is the distance of each repetition. Rest is the amount of time between repetitions; each factor is affected by the others. For example, if the intensity (speed) is increased, volume and duration

will probably have to be decreased and rest, increased. The application of each factor depends on variables such as experience, time of year, health, goals, and environment.

Intensity is perhaps the most critical of the basic overload factors. As discussed, the optimum intensity during endurance exercise is tied to carbohydrate metabolism. If the intensity is too high, lactic acid production exceeds clearance capacity. The athlete fatigues very quickly, and recovery is more difficult. In addition, valuable glycogen stores are rapidly depleted. However, if the pace is too slow, then the athlete does not perform up to potential. She will probably lose the race or will not reach the desired level of physical conditioning.

There have been many attempts by researchers to identify physiologic markers of the ideal exercise intensity. Markers include blood lactate, heart rate, ventilation, perceived exertion, and percentage of maximum effort. Esoteric physiologic measures such as lactate inflection point have not been very useful. Good measures of training load are exercise heart rate, percentages of race pace, and perceived exertion. Exercise heart rate helps select a pace that is proportional to oxygen consumption. Training at different speeds helps to train more motor units, since different motor units are recruited when running fast or slow. Perceived exertion helps the athlete to adjust the training program. She can better respond to injury, illness, glycogen depletion, overtraining, and environmental stress. The most effective programs are those that work the athlete through a range of distances and intensities according to the requirements of the sport.

The program should consist of over-distance training and interval training. The purpose of over-distance training (long, slow distance) is to increase or maintain $\dot{V}O_2$max. It also increases tissue respiratory capacity by increasing muscle mitochondrial density. As discussed, mitochondrial density is better correlated with endurance capacity than is $\dot{V}O_2$max. It is probably the major beneficiary of over-distance conditioning. Because of the principle of specificity, however, a segment of this distance training should be conducted close to race pace.

Interval training involves periods of intense exercise interspersed with rest (see Chapter 1). The nature of the interval training program varies with the distance of competition. Athletes who run shorter races will run shorter, faster distances in training than those who run longer, slower races. Interval training increases $\dot{V}o_2$max. It does this by increasing maximal cardiac output and speed. Interval training also teaches pace, builds speed, and improves lactate removal. It also increases mitochondrial density but is less effective than over-distance training.

Principles of Training

Nine principles of endurance training are listed in Table 4–3. They are explicit instructions for applying the general adaptation syndrome to the training of endurance athletes and will result in improved performance with a minimum risk of injury.

The first principle is to train all year round. Athletes lose much fitness through deconditioning. They are much more susceptible to injury if they try to get in shape rapidly during the competitive season. The next principle is related to the first: Get in shape gradually. The athlete should give her body time to adapt to the stress of exercise. Overzealous training leads to injury and overtraining.

Table 4–3. PRINCIPLES OF ENDURANCE TRAINING

- Train all year round.
- Get in shape gradually.
- Listen to your body.
- Begin with over-distance training before progressing to interval training.
- Cycle your training: Incorporate load, peak, and recovery cycles.
- Do not overtrain; rest the day before competition.
- Train systematically.
- Train the mind.
- Put sport in its proper perspective.

"Listen to your body," the third principle, is familiar to anyone who has ever read a book or article on exercise. While the expression is a bit weathered, it is true nevertheless. The athlete should not adhere to her planned program too dogmatically. Sometimes her body needs rest more than exercise. Most studies show that the absolute intensity is perhaps the most important factor in improving fitness. An overtrained athlete is typically not recovered enough to train at the optimal intensity. A few days' rest sometimes will allow her to recover enough to train more intensely. On the other hand, she should still try to follow a structured program.

Endurance athletes should train first for distance and only later for speed. Soft tissues need time to adjust to the rigors of training. Ligaments and tendons adjust very slowly to the stresses of exercise.[93] The athlete must prepare her body for heavy training, or injury may result.

The fifth training principle suggests that athletes should cycle the volume and intensity of their workouts. The practice of alternating between hard and easy training days is an application of cycle training (also called periodization of training).[3] Cycle training allows the body to recover more fully and to train hard when hard training is required.

Athletes should incorporate base and peak cycles (workouts) into the competitive strategy. These cycles are groups of workouts practiced to improve fitness gradually (base) or to increase sharpness for competition (peak). Base or load cycles are characterized by high volume with varying intensity. Peak cycles employ low volume and high-intensity workouts with plenty of rest. Peak cycles are designed to produce maximum performance. The base or load cycle is the foundation for peak performance. However, peak fitness can be maintained for only a short time, and every peak is gained at the price of deconditioning. Both cycles are thus important. The successes of the peaks make the hard work of the base period worthwhile.

A difficult training principle to adhere to is the sixth, "do not overtrain." It contradicts the work ethic that is ingrained in so many athletes. The athlete should think of conditioning for endurance events as a multiyear process. Adaptations to training take place very gradually. Excessive training tends to lead to overtraining and overuse injuries rather than to accelerated development of fitness. Similarly, athletes should avoid excessive competition because numerous studies have shown that considerable muscle damage occurs during long-distance races.[74] Competing too frequently results in an inability to recover, which decreases the overall level of conditioning.

The seventh training principle tells the athlete to train systematically. The athlete should plan an approximate workout schedule for the coming year (or even the next 4 years), month, and week. Of course, she should not be so rigid that she cannot change the program owing to unforeseen circumstances. She should train in a manner that will produce a consistent increase in fitness. Coaching, training partners, and a training diary will help her workouts become more systematic. Coaching helps the athlete meet her competitive goals. A good coach, who is knowledgeable and experienced, can keep her from repeating common training mistakes made by others. The coach will also help motivate the athlete. Training partners are important for motivation and competition. The training diary will help the athlete to formulate her goals and to identify effective training techniques.

Training the mind is as important as training the body. Successful athletes believe in themselves and their potential; they have goals and know how to achieve them. In endurance training in particular, the athlete must be patient and be content with continuous small improvements over many years.

Finally, sports should be put in their proper perspective. Too often, athletes think of themselves solely as runners, cyclists, or swimmers rather than as human beings who participate in those activities. Although sports are important, the athlete must also have time for her family and other aspects of life that are important to her.

SUMMARY

The determining factors of endurance performance include maximal oxygen consumption, mitochondrial density, performance efficiency, and body composition. Maximal oxygen consumption is the body's maximum ability to transport and use oxygen and is largely determined by the cardiac output capacity. It is improved by about 20% through training. A high initial value is important for success in endurance events. Mitochondrial density is highly related to endurance capacity. It provides a high oxidative capacity and the ability to use fats as fuel during exercise. Efficiency is determined by physiologic factors such as mitochondrial density. Mechanical factors, such as technique and wind resistance, are also important. The importance of body composition for endurance varies with the sport. In sports such as running, cycling, and cross-country skiing, additional fat increases the energy cost of exercise. The ideal lower limit of body fat is not known. In long-distance swimmers, a slightly higher fat percentage decreases drag in the water and provides insulation against the cold.

Sex differences exist in endurance performance. The relative changes that occur with training and the basic underlying mechanisms that determine performance are the same in men and women. Women trail men by 6% to 15% in most endurance sports, but there is considerable variance in performance in specific events. It is difficult to summarize and quantify physiologic sex differences reported in the literature; physically fit male subjects were often compared with sedentary female subjects.

Training is an adaptive process. Athletes should not become involved in overzealous training programs that often lead to injury. Because the body adapts specifically to the stress of exercise, the training program should reflect the various components of the activity. Training overload can be varied by manipulating intensity, volume, duration, and rest. Intensity is most important for achieving high levels of performance. Good measures of intensity are exercise heart rate, percentages of race pace, and perceived exertion. Endurance athletes should use a combination of interval and over-distance training techniques.

REFERENCES

1. Brooks GA (ed): Perspectives on the Academic Discipline of Physical Education. Human Kinetics, Champaign IL, 1981.
2. American College of Sports Medicine: Encyclopedia of Sport Sciences and Medicine. Macmillan, New York, 1971.
3. Brooks GA, and Fahey TD: Exercise Physiology: Human Bioenergetics and Its Applications. Macmillan, New York, 1984.
4. Braunwald E, Ross J, and Sonnenblick EH: Mechanisms of the normal and failing heart. N Engl J Med 277:794, 1967.
5. Bhan A, and Scheuer J: Effects of physical training on cardiac myosin ATPase activity. J Physiol 228:1178, 1975.
6. Scheuer J, and Tipton CM: Cardiovascular adaptations to physical training. Ann Rev Physiol 39:221, 1977.
7. Stromme SB, and Ingjer F: The effect of regular physical training on the cardiovascular system. Scand J Soc Med 29(Suppl):37, 1982.
8. Zeldis SM, Morganroth J, and Rubler S: Cardiac hypertrophy in response to dynamic conditioning in female athletes. J Appl Physiol 44:849, 1978.
9. Roost R: The athlete's heart: What we did learn from Henschen, what Henschen could have learned from us! J Sports Med Phys Fit 30:339, 1990.
10. Tesch PA: Short- and long-term histochemical and biochemical adaptations in muscle. In Komi PV (ed): Strength and Power in Sport. Blackwell Scientific Publications, London, 1992, p 239.
11. Gohil K, Jones DA, Corbucci, GG, et al: Mitochondrial substrate oxidation, muscle composition, and plasma metabolite levels in marathon runners. In Knuttgen HG, Vogel GA, and Poortsman J (eds): Biochemistry of Exercise. Human Kinetics, Champaign, Il, 1982, p 286.
12. Booth FW, and Narahara KA: Vastus lateralis

13. cytochrome oxidase activity and its relationship to maximal oxygen consumption in man. Pflugers Arch 349:319, 1974.
13. Ivy JL, Costill DL, and Maxwell BD: Skeletal muscle determinants of maximal aerobic power in man. Eur J Appl Physiol 44:1, 1980.
14. Klissouras V, Pirnay F, and Petit J-M: Adaptations to maximal effort: Genetics and age. J Appl Physiol 35:288, 1973.
15. Bouchard C, and Lortie G: Heredity and endurance performance. Sports Med 1:38, 1984.
16. Komi PV, and Karlsson J: Physical performance, skeletal muscle enzyme activities, and fiber types in monozygous and dizygous twins of both sexes. Acta Physiol Scand 462(Suppl):462, 1979.
17. Bouchard C: Discussion: Heredity, fitness, and health. In Bouchard C, Shephard RJ, Stephens T, et al (eds): Exercise, Fitness, and Health. Human Kinetics, Champaign, IL, 1990, p 147.
18. Blumenthal JA, Emery CF, Madden DJ, et al: Cardiovascular and behavioral effects of aerobic exercise training in healthy older men and women. J Gerontol 44:M147, 1989.
19. Kearney JJ, Stull GA, Ewing JL, et al: Cardiorespiratory responses of sedentary college women as a function of training intensity. J Appl Physiol 41:822, 1976.
20. Burk EJ: Physiological effects of similar training programs in males and females. Res Q 48:510, 1977.
21. Hanson JS, and Nedde WH: Long-term physical training effect in sedentary females. J Appl Physiol 37:112, 1974.
22. Hickson RC, Bromze HA, and Holloszy JO: Linear increase in aerobic power induced by strenuous exercise. J Appl Physiol 42:372, 1977.
23. Lewis S, Haskell WL, Wood PD, et al: Effects of physical activity on weight reduction in obese middle-aged women. Am J Clin Nutr 29:151, 1976.
24. Schaible TF, and Scheuer J: Response of the heart to exercise training. In Zak R (ed): Growth of the Heart in Health and Disease. Raven Press, New York, 1984, p 381.
25. Longhurst JC, Kelly AR, Gonyea WJ, et al: Echocardiographic left ventricular mass in distance runners and weight lifters. J Appl Physiol 48:154, 1980.
26. Ekblom B, Goldbarg AN, and Gullbring B: Response to exercise after blood loss and reinfusion. J Appl Physiol 33:175, 1972.
27. Gledhill N: Blood doping and related issues: A brief review. Med Sci Sports 14:183, 1982.
28. Fagraeus L: Cardiorespiratory and metabolic functions during exercise in the hyperbaric environment. Acta Physiol Scand 92(Suppl 414):1, 1974.

29. Wagner PD: Central and peripheral aspects of oxygen transport and adaptations with exercise. Sports Med 11:133, 1991.
30. Andersen P, and Saltin B: Maximal perfusion of skeletal muscle in man. J Physiol 366:233, 1985.
31. Rowell LB, Saltin B, Kiens B, and Christensen NJ: Is peak quadriceps blood flow in humans even higher during exercise with hypoxemia? Am J Physiol 251:H1038, 1986.
32. Dempsy JA, and Fregosi RF: Adaptability of the pulmonary system to changing metabolic requirements. Am J Cardiol 55:59D, 1985.
33. Connett RJ, and Honig CR: Regulation of $\dot{V}_{O_2}$ in red muscle: Do current biochemical hypotheses fit in vivo data? Am J Physiol 256:R898, 1989.
34. Gayeski TEJ, Connett RJ, and Honig CR: Minimum intracellular PO_2 for maximum cytochrome turnover in red muscle in situ. Adv Exper Med Biol 200:487, 1987.
35. Stainsby WN, Brechue WF, O'Drobinak DM, and Barclay JK: Oxidation/reduction state of cytochrome oxidase during repetitive contractions. J Appl Physiol 67:2158, 1989.
36. Noakes TD: Implications of exercise testing for prediction of athletic performance: A contemporary perspective. Med Sci Sports Exerc 20:319, 1988.
37. Jones DP, Kennedy FG, and Yee Aw T: Intracellular O_2 gradients. In Sutton J (ed): Hypoxia: The Tolerable Limits. Benchmark Press, Indianapolis, 1988, p 59.
38. Christensen CL, and Ruhling RO: Physical characteristics of novice and experienced women marathon runners. Br J Sports Med 17:166, 1983.
39. Costill DL, and Winrow E: Maximal oxygen intake among marathon runners. Arch Phys Med Rehab 51:317, 1970.
40. Hill AV, and Lupton H: Muscular exercise, lactic acid, and the supply and utilization of oxygen. Q J Med 16:135, 1923.
41. Wyndham CH, Strydom NB, Maritz JS, et al: Maximal oxygen intake and maximum heart rate during strenuous work. J Appl Physiol 14:927, 1959.
42. Åstrand PO: Experimental Studies of Physical Work Capacity in Relation to Sex and Age. Munksgaard, Copenhagen, 1952.
43. Davies KJS, Maguire JJ, Brooks GA, et al: Muscle mitochondria, muscle, and whole-animal respiration to endurance training. Arch Biochem Biophys 209:538, 1981.
44. Holloszy JO: Adaptation of skeletal muscle to endurance exercise. Med Sci Sports 7:155, 1975.
45. Donovan CM, and Brooks GA: Training affects lactate clearance, not lactate production. Am J Physiol 244:E83, 1983.
46. Hill TL: Free Energy Transductions in Biology. Academic Press, New York, 1977.
47. Gollnick PD, Bayly WM, and Hodgson DR: Exercise intensity, training, diet, and lactate concentration in muscle and blood. Med Sci Sports Exerc 18:334, 1986.
48. Brooks GA: The lactate shuttle during exercise and recovery. Med Sci Sports Exerc 18:360, 1986.
49. Gollnick PD, and Saltin B: Hypothesis: Significance of skeletal muscle oxidative enzyme enhancement with endurance training. Clin Physiol 2:1, 1983.
50. Saltin B, Henriksson J, Hygaard E, et al: Fiber types and metabolic potentials of skeletal muscles in sedentary man and endurance runners. NY Acad Sci 301:3, 1977.
51. Tesch PA, and Karlsson J: Muscle fiber types and size in trained and untrained muscles of elite athletes. J Appl Physiol 59:1716, 1985.
52. Gaesser GA, and Brooks GA: Muscular efficiency during steady-rate exercise: Effects of speed and work rate. J Appl Physiol 38:1132, 1975.
53. Donovan CM, and Brooks GA: Muscular efficiency during steady-rate exercise: II. Effects of walking speed on work rate. J Appl Physiol 43:431, 1977.
54. Fay L, Londeree BR, Lafontaine TP, and Volek MR: Physiological parameters related to distance running performance in female athletes. Med Sci Sports Exerc 21:319, 1989.
55. Baily SP, and Pate RR: Feasibility of improving running economy. Sports Med 12:228, 1991.
56. Morgan D, Baldini F, Martin P, and Kohrt W: Ten km performance and predicted velocity at $\dot{V}_{O_2}$max among well trained runners. Med Sci Sport Exerc 21:78, 1989.
57. Margaria R, Cerretelli P, and Aghems P: Energy cost of running. J Appl Physiol 18:367, 1963.
58. Faria IE: Applied physiology of cycling. Sports Med 1:187, 1984.
59. Malina RM, Muellere WH, Bouchard C, et al: Fatness and fat patterning among athletes at the Montreal Olympic Games: 1976. Med Sci Sports Exerc 14:445, 1982.
60. Tanaka K, and Matsuura Y: A multivariate analysis of the role of certain anthropometric and physiological attributes in distance running. Ann Hum Biol 9:473, 1982.
61. Fleck SJ: Body composition of elite American athletes. Am J Sports Med 11:398, 1983.
62. Wilmore JH, and Brown CH: Physiological profiles of women distance runners. Med Sci Sports 6:178, 1974.
63. Sady SP, and Freedson PS: Body composition and structural comparisons of female and male athletes. Clin Sports Med 3:755, 1984.

64. Rennie DW, Pendergast DR, and diPrampero PE: Energetics of swimming in man. In Clarys JP, and Lewillie L (eds): Swimming II. University Park Press, Baltimore, 1975, p 97.

65. Wilmore JH, and Behnke AR: An anthropometric estimation of body density and lean body weight in young women. Am J Clin Nutr 23:7, 1970.

66. Rusko H, Hara M, and Karvinen E: Aerobic performance in athletes. Eur J Appl Physiol 38:151, 1978.

67. Sinning WE, Cunningham LN, Racaniello AP, et al: Body composition and somatotype of male and female Nordic skiers. Res Q 48:741, 1977.

68. Tittle K, and Wutscherk H: Sportanthropometrie. Johann Ambrosius Barth, Leipzig, 1964, p 1.

69. Farmosi I: Az úszónök testalkatának és teljesítményének összefüggése. In Lásló N (ed): A Sport és Testnevelés Időszerű Kérdései—23. Sport, Budapest, 1980, p 77.

70. Dessein M: Studie van enkele zwemtechnisch gebonden componenten en in het bijzonder van somatische karakteristieken. Licentiaat. Katholieke Universitait te Leuven, Leuven, 1981, p 66.

71. Meleski BW, Shoup RF, and Malina RM: Size, physique and body composition of competitive female swimmers 11 through 20 years of age. Hum Biol 54:609, 1982.

72. Vallières F, Tremblay A, and St-Jean L: Study of the energy balance and the nutritional status of highly trained female swimmers. Nutr Res 9:699, 1989.

73. International Olympic Committee: Games of the XXIIIrd Olympiad Los Angeles 1984 Commemorative Book. International Sport Publications, Salt Lake City, 1984.

74. Noakes T: Lore of Running. Oxford University Press, Capetown, 1985.

75. Drabik J: Sexual dimorphism and sports results. J Sports Med Phys Fit 28:287, 1988.

76. Wells CL, and Plowman SA: Sex differences in athletic performance: Biological and behavioral. Phys Sports Med 11:52, 1983.

77. Sparling PB: A meta-analysis of studies comparing maximal oxygen uptake in men and women. Res Q 51:542, 1980.

78. Cureton KJ, and Sparling PB: Distance running performance and metabolic responses to running in men and women with excess weight experimentally equated. Med Sci Sports Exerc 12:288, 1980.

79. Cureton KJ, Collins MA, Hill DW, and McElhannon FM: Muscle hypertrophy in men and women. Med Sci Sports Exerc 20:338, 1988.

80. Holloway JB, and Baechle TR: Strength training for female athletes. Sports Med 9:216, 1990.

81. Brunc V, and Heller J: Energy cost of running in similarly trained men and women. Eur J Appl Physiol 59:178, 1989.

82. Bosco C, Montanari G, Ribacchi P, et al: Relationship between the efficiency of muscular work during jumping and the energetics of running. Eur J Appl Physiol 56:138, 1987.

83. Bosco C, Komi PV, and Sinkkonen K: Mechanical power, net efficiency, and muscle structure in male and female middle distance runners. Scand J Sports Sci 2:47, 1980.

84. Davies CTM, and Thompson MW: Aerobic performance of female marathon and male ultra-marathon athletes. Eur J Appl Physiol 41:233, 1979.

85. Conley DL, Krahenbuhl GS, Burkett LN, et al: Physiological correlates of female road racing performance. Res Q 52:544, 1981.

86. Pate RR, and Kriska A: Physiological basis of the sex difference in cardiorespiratory endurance. Sports Med 1:87, 1984.

87. Eddy DO, Sparks KL, and Adelizi DA: The effects of continuous and interval training in women and men. Eur J Appl Physiol 37:83, 1977.

88. Ullyot J: Women's secret weapon. In Van Aaken E: Van Aaken Method. World Publications, Mountain View, CA, 1976.

89. Costill DL, Fink WJ, Getchell LH, et al: Lipid metabolism in skeletal muscle of endurance-trained males and females. J Appl Physiol 47:787, 1979.

90. Selye H: The Stress of Life. McGraw-Hill, New York, 1976.

91. Henry FM: The evolution of the memory drum theory of neuromotor reaction. In Brooks GA (ed): Perspectives on the Academic Discipline of Physical Education. Human Kinetics, Champaign, IL, 1981.

92. Edgerton VR: Mammalian muscle fiber types and their adaptability. Am Zool 18:113, 1976.

93. Zernicke RF, and Loitz BJ: Exercise-related adaptations in connective tissue. In Komi PV (ed): Strength and Power in Sport. Blackwell Scientific Publications, London, 1992, p 77.

CHAPTER 5

Bone Concerns

EVERETT L. SMITH, Ph.D., and CATHERINE GILLIGAN, B.A.

INCIDENCE AND COST OF
OSTEOPOROSIS

EFFECTS OF CALCIUM INTAKE

MECHANISM OF EXERCISE
BENEFITS

EFFECTS OF INACTIVITY

EFFECTS OF EXERCISE

ATHLETIC AMENORRHEA AND
BONE

PROBLEMS IN STUDYING EXERCISE
EFFECTS

The skeleton is a dynamic tissue, constantly responding to conditions relative to its two major functions: providing structural support and acting as a mineral reservoir. Two interacting homeostatic mechanisms control plasma calcium and skeletal mineral: hormones and mechanical stress. The structural support function of the skeleton permits movement and protects vital organs. As a reservoir, the skeleton responds to changes in hormone levels and helps to maintain blood calcium at about 9.8 mg/dL (Table 5-1).[1] Because of the skeleton's dual role, structural integrity is jeopardized when the demands on the reservoir to maintain serum homeostasis are too high. When dietary calcium is inadequate, calcium is mobilized from the bone to maintain serum calcium. If the dietary inadequacy is chronic, calcium will be pulled continually from the bone reservoir, resulting in a negative calcium balance and a net loss of calcium and phosphorus. Mechanical strain through weight bearing and muscle contraction play a significant role in maintaining skeletal structural integrity, as bone mineral content (BMC) changes in response to the mechanical stressors applied. Under balanced conditions, the hormonal and mechanical homeostatic mechanisms maintain both skeletal integrity and serum calcium. With aging, however, multiple factors decline (involving diet, hormonal levels, and mechanical strain), precipitating bone involution that results in bone more susceptible to fracture and osteoporosis.

Hormones and mechanical strain interact in maintaining body and skeletal functions. If stress to specific skeletal segments or to the skeleton as a whole is significantly reduced, bone mass declines. In severe disuse, such as in bed rest or spinal cord injury, the mobilization of calcium from bone increases serum levels, decreases parathyroid levels and 1,25-$(OH)_2$ vitamin D, and thus decreases calcium absorption in the intestinal tract and increases calcium elimination from

Table 5–1. SERUM CALCIUM HOMEOSTASIS

Condition	Hormonal Response	Metabolic Adaptation to Condition
Low serum calcium	Increased PTH	Increased fractional calcium absorption Decreased renal excretion of calcium Increased active form of vitamin D Increased bone resorption
High serum calcium	Decreased PTH Increased calcitonin	Decreased fractional calcium absorption Increased renal excretion of calcium Decreased active form of vitamin D Decreased bone resorption
Decreased gonadal function	Decreased gonadal hormones	Decreased fractional calcium absorption Increased sensitivity of bone to PTH

PTH = parathyroid.
Source: Adapted from Smith and Raab,[1] with permission.

the kidneys. Generally, the decline in activity with age and the resultant bone and biochemical changes are subtle. Over a long term, however, inactivity can significantly reduce bone mass and threaten the integrity of skeletal structure.

INCIDENCE AND COST OF OSTEOPOROSIS

Osteoporosis is a major public health problem, affecting more than 20 million people in the United States. Osteoporosis causes 1.3 million fractures at a cost of 3.8 billion dollars each year.[2] A major cause of osteoporosis is age-related bone loss. Peak bone mass is reached at about age 35 in both men and women. After age 35, women lose up to 1% per year, and they may lose as much as 4% to 6% per year during the first 4 to 5 years after menopause (Fig. 5–1). Men maintain bone mass until about age 50, after which they lose approximately 0.4% to 0.5% per year. Both peak bone mass and rate of loss are involved in the likelihood of developing osteoporosis. In cortical bone, loss occurs primarily on the endosteal surface,

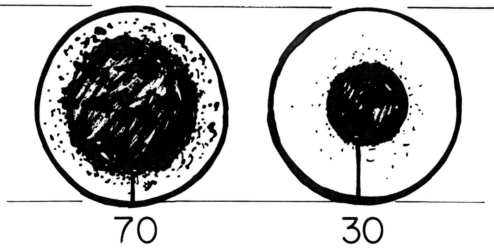

Figure 5–1. Cross-sections of long bones of women aged 30 and 70 years. Note the enlarged medullary cavity and increased porosity of the cortical bone at age 70.

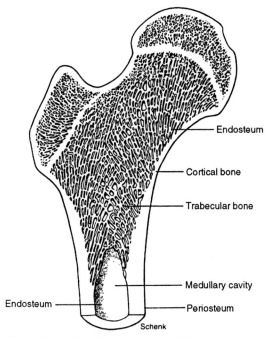

Figure 5-2. A longitudinal section of the proximal end of a femur, showing the trabecular structure within the bone that provides maximum strength in the direction of greatest applied pressure. The periosteum is a highly vascular layer covering the surface of the bone; the endosteum lines all interbone surfaces. (Adapted from Van De Graff, KM: Human Anatomy, ed 2. Dubuque IA, William C. Brown Publishers, 1988, p 158.)

with some loss on the periosteal surface (Fig. 5-2). In trabecular bone, the trabeculae are thinned and may be entirely resorbed (see Fig. 11-2). In the spine, horizontal support trabeculae are lost preferentially, which reduces bone strength more than indicated by the density alone (Fig. 5-3). In conjunction with this decreased bone mass, the internal structure of bone also changes. Osteons are decreased in size and increased in number. Micropetrosis increases with lacunae filled by calcium depositions. These qualitative bone changes, in addition to the decreased BMC, contribute to a greater fracture potential.

Although bone mass plays a significant role in determining bone strength, it is not the sole determinant. The geometric structure of the tissue, determined by habitual stresses, collagen orientation, ligaments, and muscle tone, is also important.

EFFECTS OF CALCIUM INTAKE

Both cross-sectional and longitudinal studies of the effect of calcium intake on bone density or bone loss have produced mixed results. In a cross-sectional study, Matkovic and colleagues[3] compared bone mass and fracture incidence in two Yugoslavian populations, one with high (947 mg/d) and one with low (424 mg/d) calcium intake based on dietary histories. The two groups were otherwise similar in heredity and environment. The high-calcium group had a significantly greater skeletal mass at maturity and a lower fracture incidence in old age. The loss of bone mass with age was similar in the two groups; therefore, the greater incidence of fractures in the low-calcium group was attributed to lower peak bone mass. Other cross-sectional studies have reported slight or nonsignificant correlations of habitual calcium intake with bone mass or fracture incidence.[4,5]

Studies of the effects of calcium supplementation on bone loss have not consistently demonstrated a positive effect. In 3- and 4-year studies, we found that calcium supplementation reduced cortical bone loss in the arm (radius, ulna, and humerus) of elderly and middle-aged postmenopausal women, but did not affect bone loss in premenopausal women.[6,7] Horsman and colleagues[8] also reported that calcium supplementation reduced bone loss over 2 to 3 years at cortical forearm sites. In a 2-year study, Prince and associates[9] found that calcium supplementation combined with exercise decreased forearm bone loss significantly compared to exercise alone. Other 2-year studies, however, failed to detect a significant difference in radius bone loss between calcium-supplemented and control groups.[10–12] Riis[13] reported that calcium supplementation reduced cortical bone loss in the proximal forearm but did not retard trabecular bone loss in the distal radius or spine in women who were recently postmenopausal. Similarly, Ettinger and coworkers[14] found no effect of calcium supplementation for 1 year on spine bone loss in early postmenopausal women.

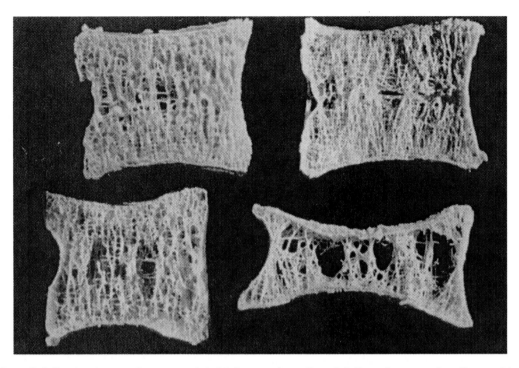

Figure 5–3. Varying degrees of osteoporosis in lumbar vertebrae. *Upper left:* Normal structure in a 63-year-old man. *Lower left:* The longitudinal trabeculae are narrowed and some broken ones are seen in the center of this vertebra, showing mild osteoporosis in a 65-year-old woman; the horizontal trabeculae are conspicuously reduced. *Upper right:* Pronounced osteoporosis in a 70-year-old woman. There is clear-cut breaking off of numerous longitudinal trabeculae on the right and the left. *Lower right:* High-grade osteoporosis in a 71-year-old woman. The vertebral body has almost completely collapsed; there are several gaps in the trabecular structure, and the restraining bone is transformed, with formation of new longitudinal trajectories. (From Remagen, W: Osteoporosis. Sandoz Ltd., Basle, Switzerland, 1989, Fig. 31, with permission.)

Recent studies have investigated the effects of calcium supplementation on bone loss in premenopausal and early and late postmenopausal women. Premenopausal women who increased their dietary calcium by an average of 610 mg/d (n = 20) did not change significantly in spine bone mineral density (BMD), while control subjects decreased significantly (n = 17). Calcium subjects thus had significantly greater spine BMD after 30 and 36 months than did control subjects.[15] Dawson-Hughes and colleagues[16] studied 301 women with self-selected diets low in calcium (<650 mg/d), who were divided into placebo, calcium citrate malate (CCM) supplement, and calcium carbonate (CC) supplement groups and followed for 2 years. In early postmenopausal women (≤5 years since menopause), the groups did not differ in BMD loss in the spine, femur, or ra-

dius. In late postmenopausal women (>5 years since menopause), however, the CCM group did not change significantly at any site measured; those taking CC declined significantly in spine BMD; and the placebo group declined significantly in spine and femur BMD. Radius BMD declined significantly less in the CCM than in the placebo group. When subgroups of the late postmenopausal groups were formed on the basis of calcium intake (<400 mg or 400 to 650 mg), differences in change between groups were apparent only for the lower-calcium subgroup. After 2 years, CCM had significantly reduced loss in spine, femur, and radius BMD compared to the placebo group, and CC had significantly reduced loss in radius BMD compared to the placebo group. Elders and associates[17] found that calcium supplementation retarded spine bone loss in early postmenopausal women during the first year, but not the second year, of their trial. Finally, a team led by Nelson[18] randomly assigned postmenopausal women (mean age 60, mean years since menopause 11) to a high-calcium (831 mg) or placebo (41 mg calcium) drink over a 1-year period. Half of the subjects in each group participated in a 1-year walking program. Calcium supplementation significantly reduced loss in femur BMD but did not affect loss in the spine, radius, or total body calcium.

Some of the differences among calcium intervention studies may be due to the wide variety of forms and doses of calcium used, along with differences in study length, subject selection criteria, menopausal age, self-selected dietary intake, sites measured, and sample sizes. It is reasonable to hypothesize that calcium supplementation affects mainly cortical bone in the early postmenopause[19] but may affect other sites in premenopausal and late postmenopausal women. Calcium supplementation may be most beneficial for women with a self-selected diet low in calcium and can be expected to avert only that portion of bone loss due to inadequate calcium intake.[20]

MECHANISM OF EXERCISE BENEFITS

While evidence is accumulating that physical activity increases bone mass, research on the mechanisms by which bone is affected by mechanical stress is still in its early stages.

In 1892, Wolff[21] hypothesized that increased weight bearing compresses and bends the long bones, increases mineral content, and consequently strengthens bones, making them less liable to fracture under similar loads. Weight bearing (gravity) and muscle contraction are the two major mechanical forces applied to bone. Both hypodynamic and hyperdynamic states affect bone balance. Bone mass increases with greater weight-bearing activity or muscle contraction or both and decreases with immobilization or weightless-

ness. The degree of bone hypertrophy or atrophy is proportional to the difference in magnitude and frequency of the mechanical stimulus from normal. The habitual stimulus to weight-bearing segments (legs and spine) is much greater than that to the non–weight-bearing areas (ribs, arms, and skull). For example, the impact of the heel during walking (1.2 to 1.5 times body weight) is much greater than the stress applied by muscle contractions in the arm during activities of daily living. Therefore, the calcaneus is normally under greater stress than the radius, so when both bones are free of stress (as in the case of the astronauts in space), more bone is lost from the calcaneus than from the radius.[22,23]

Numerous models of the mechanism by which bone responds to mechanical forces have been proposed. Bassett[24] indicated that bone functions as a piezoelectric crystal, generating an electric charge in proportion to the forces applied to the bone. Carter[25] hypothesized that mechanical forces produce microfractures, which stimulate osteoclastic remodeling coupled with osteoblastic activity. A recent study, however, did not detect evidence of microfracture in rats subjected to 20,000 loading cycles per day for 5 or 6 days.[26] Other ways in which exercise may stimulate osteoclastic and osteoblastic activity include increased hydrostatic pressure and streaming potentials.

Whereas dynamic loading produces hypertrophy, static loading of bone produces little or no hypertrophy.[27] For a bone to hypertrophy, dynamic stimuli must exceed a threshold magnitude and frequency. Lanyon[28] demonstrated that both the rate and magnitude of strain influenced bone remodeling. He monitored BMC in the radii of sheep under artificial stimulation. No change occurred with a strain magnitude less than that of the animal's normal walking load. With higher strain magnitude and normal strain rates, periosteal bone deposition increased slightly on both convex and concave surfaces. When both magnitude and rate were higher than in normal walking, periosteal bone increased substantially. Other studies have applied more precisely quantified stress to bone. Rubin and Lanyon[29] applied controlled mechanical loads, using a pneumatically operated device, to rooster ulnae isolated from muscular stress. Bone mass decreased if no load was applied, remained fairly constant at 4 cycles per day of normal (2000 microstrain) magnitude, and hypertrophied at a normal magnitude loading for 36 cycles per day (each cycle about 2 seconds). The hypertrophy from 3600 cycles per day and 36 cycles per day did not differ. In a similar study, the number of loading cycles was held constant, and the magnitude of the strain varied.[30] Bone change was directly proportional to the strain. Bone atrophied at strains below 1000 microstrain, and cross-sectional area increased with strains over 1000 microstrain. It appears that the magnitude of the strain is more important than the frequency of application.

Recent studies have investigated the biochemical and histologic sequelae of bone loading. The mechanism by which strain produces an osteogenic cellular response has not been delineated. Histomorphometric data show increased osteoclastic function with disuse and increased osteoblastic function with increased activity. Neither mature osteoclasts nor osteoblasts, however, seem to respond directly to changes in skeletal strain. Osteocytes (that number up to 20,000 per cubic millimeter), however, may respond to changes in skeletal strain by the production of chemical transmitters acting on bone precursor cells. Using an in vitro core biopsy model in the presence of [3H]uridine, El Haj and colleagues[31] observed an increase in radioactive osteocyte RNA compared to nonloaded specimens. Pead and Lanyon[32] reported that within 5 days after a single period of skeletal loading, quiescent surface-lining cells were transformed into active, bone-forming osteoblasts.

Cellular activity at the femur midshaft increased significantly in sows training on a motor-driven treadmill for 20 weeks.[33] Trained sows had a 27% greater active peri-

osteal surface than did untrained sows. Mineral apposition rate was also higher, at both the periosteal (76%) and intracortical osteonal (23%) levels. Similarly, evidence of altered cellular activity was found in trained adult rats.[34] Bone density and trabecular number, thickness, and density were significantly higher in trained animals than in controls after 18 and 26 weeks of exercise. The mineral apposition rate and bone formation rate were significantly higher in trained animals, while the percentage of eroded and labeled perimeter tended to be lower in the trained animals. This study supports the concept of Frost[35] that increased activity stimulates modeling and depresses remodeling.

Bone requires a specific magnitude and rate of stimulus in order to hypertrophy. Within a normal range of stimulus specific to the individual's activities and genotype, bone neither atrophies nor hypertrophies. Beyond or below this range, bone will change, as shown in Figure 5–4. Increased hypertrophy with increased stress will occur only to a point, however. Severe, repetitive loading may result in fatigue damage such as that seen in the metatarsals, calcaneus, tibia, and femur of some soldiers and distance runners. Fatigue damage may also occur in untrained persons who increase their activity levels more rapidly than the bone can adapt. At the other end of the spectrum, bone atrophies with lessened mechanical stress due to bed rest and weightlessness.

EFFECTS OF INACTIVITY

Donaldson and associates[36] observed three men for 30 to 36 weeks of bed rest, and Hulley and colleagues[37] observed five men for 24 to 30 weeks of bed rest. Calcium balance was negative throughout bed rest, with 0.5% to 0.7% of total body calcium lost per month. In the weight-bearing calcaneus, bone loss was magnified; 25% to 45% was lost after 36 weeks. After remobilization, calcium balance became positive within a month, and BMC was regained at a rate sim-

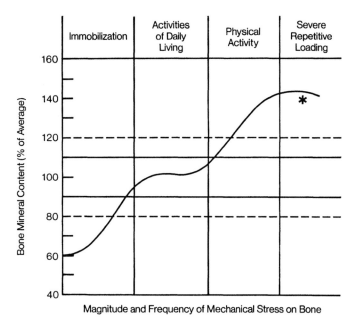

Magnitude and Frequency of Mechanical Stress on Bone

*Point at which the magnitude and duration of the load approach the elastic limits of the bone and osteoclast activity is greater than osteoblast.

Figure 5–4. Effect of mechanical loading on bone mineral content. (Adapted from Carter.[25])

ilar to the rate of loss, reaching baseline levels in about 36 weeks. Krolner and Toft[38] observed a 0.9% per week loss from the lumbar spine in individuals at bed rest for an average of 27 days because of a disk protrusion. LeBlanc and co-workers[39] recently reported the effects of 17 weeks of bed rest and 6 months of recovery at various skeletal sites. During bed rest, subjects lost significantly in BMD at the calcaneus (10%), femur trochanter (5%), lumbar spine (4%), femur neck (4%), tibia (2%), and total body (1.4%). The lumbar spine, femur trochanter, and tibia BMD tended to increase during the recovery period, but only calcaneus BMD increased significantly. The distal and proximal radius and ulna BMD did not decrease significantly during bed rest or increase significantly during recovery. Regional analysis of total body scans showed significant decreases in lumbar spine, total spine, pelvis, trunk, and legs during bed rest, with a significant increase in head BMD during bed rest. Pelvis and trunk BMD increased significantly in the recovery period. In the average woman, the usual decline in activity is more gradual and

less severe than that of a patient at bed rest, but extended over 10 to 20 years, the resultant bone loss can be a major contributor to the development of osteoporosis.

Human studies of immobilization are rare, but a number of animal studies have been performed. Kazarian and Von Gierke[40] immobilized 16 rhesus monkeys in full body casts for 60 days. Bone from the immobilized animals had fewer and thinner trabeculae, smaller trabecular plates, reduced trabecular surfaces, and reduced cortical thickness compared with bones of control animals. Remodeling occurred in the trabeculae of the femoral neck, which "corresponded in position and curvature to the lines of maximum compressive stress," so that only those trabeculae necessary for structural integrity were retained. The compressive strength of the immobilized bones was two to three times less than that in control animals. Cortical bone at the sites of muscle and tendon attachments also was significantly weaker than in control animals.

Young[41] and Niklowitz[42] and their co-workers investigated changes in the tibias of monkeys during 7 months of immobilization and up to 40 months of recovery and remobilization. Remodeling was obvious within 1 month of immobilization. After 10 weeks, they observed endosteal resorption, subperiosteal loss, striations in the cortex (indicative of resorptive cavities), surface erosion in the juxta-articular areas (patella and femoral condyles), and thin, irregular external lamellar bone. During 6 months of immobilization, BMC decreased 23% to 31% and bending stiffness, 36% to 40%. Normal bending properties of the bone were restored within 8½ months of recovery and remobilization, but BMC did not return to normal even after 15 months. New primary haversian systems were generated during that time, and by 40 months the cortex contained many secondary and tertiary osteons and approached normal BMC.

EFFECTS OF EXERCISE

Numerous studies indicate that bone density is responsive to mechanical loading. The effect appears to be primarily local and proportional to the level of strain placed on the bone. The most convincing evidence that bone hypertrophy is localized appears in studies of both young and old tennis players, whose dominant humerus was up to 35% higher in BMD than was the nondominant arm.[43-45] In studies of athletes, the amount of hypertrophy was related to the loading applied by the sports activity. For example, weightlifters had higher bone density in the spine and femur than aerobic athletes,[46-49] whereas swimmers did not have significantly higher spine density than did sedentary subjects.[48-50] In one study, male swimmers had significantly higher vertebral BMD than sedentary subjects, but no difference could be detected between swimming and sedentary women.[51]

Intervention studies have confirmed the beneficial effect of exercise at various skeletal sites, including the spine, radius, calcaneus, and tibia. Femur BMD, however, was not significantly affected by exercise in any of the studies in which it was measured. Aerobic weight-bearing activities increased spine bone density in middle-aged postmenopausal women[18,52] and women with osteoporosis.[53] In two of these studies,[52,53] the total BMD of L2 to L4 was increased significantly compared to controls, while in the third study,[18] trabecular (L1 to L3) but not total BMD was affected. Physical activity programs incorporating arm exercises increased BMD or decreased bone loss in the radius and ulna.[6,54-56] In our study[56] of middle-aged women, the response to exercise appeared to be independent of menopausal status. A few studies that used primarily aerobic weight-bearing training reported no effects on radius[9,57,58] or spine[59] bone density.

The bone hypertrophy observed in weightlifters, along with animal studies showing a linear relationship between strain and bone hypertrophy, have led to several studies utilizing resistance training to promote BMD. In studies comparing general aerobic training with and without additional resistance training, groups performing the strength training tended nonsignificantly to increase more in calcium bone index (bone mass of the central third of the skeleton adjusted for body size) and radius BMD than those in aerobic training alone.[54,60] Resistance training alone, however, has not consistently altered BMD. In studies of premenopausal and early postmenopausal women, exercise subjects increased in vertebral BMD relative to controls.[61,62] Calcaneus, femur, and distal forearm BMD, however, were not significantly affected in these studies. Postmenopausal women receiving estrogen replacement therapy (ERT) and assigned to a resistance-training group increased significantly in spine, total body, and radius BMD; only in the radius, however, did the change differ significantly from that in the women receiving ERT alone.[63] In contrast to these positive findings, premenopausal women in a resistance-training program lost significantly more vertebral BMD than did controls.[64] Postmenopausal women who performed back extensions with light weights for 2 years did not differ significantly in vertebral BMD change from controls.[65]

ATHLETIC AMENORRHEA AND BONE

Whereas exercise is associated with an increase in bone density, *excessive* exercise leading to amenorrhea is associated with a *decrease* in bone density. Investigators have found that unlike hyperprolactinemic, anorexic, and premature menopausal women, amenorrheic athletes do not have significantly lower cortical (radius) BMD,[66-74] but they are significantly lower than eumenorrheic athletes in vertebral BMD[67-69,73,75] and vertebral trabecular density.[72,75-79] Menstrual history is an important determinant of vertebral density even among currently eumenorrheic athletes.[68,77] Athletes with menstrual disorders also appear more prone to injury and stress fractures.[68,80-82]

A few longitudinal studies have demonstrated that subjects with menstrual disturbances lose more vertebral bone. Prior and colleagues[83] studied 66 women without overt menstrual irregularities, who varied widely in their exercise patterns. They found that ovulatory disturbances accounted for 24% of the variance in vertebral bone loss: spinal bone density tended to increase in women with normal cycles but decreased significantly in women with two or more short luteal phases and in those with anovulatory cycles. Cann and associates[84] reported that loss of vertebral bone with amenorrhea was biphasic. In one year, women who had been amenorrheic 3 years or less lost 4.2% in vertebral trabecular mineral content, while those who had been amenorrheic for longer periods did not change significantly.

In most of these studies of bone density, the athletes were runners or involved in other aerobic sports that did not particularly stress the back musculature. On the other hand, Snyder and co-workers[74] reported that oarswomen, regardless of menstrual status, did not differ significantly in vertebral BMC from sedentary eumenor-

rheic controls; in fact, oarswomen tended to be higher in vertebral BMC. Regular, oligomenorrheic and amenorrheic oarswomen did not differ significantly. This may have been the result of small sample sizes, however, since a nonsignificant trend toward lower density in groups with menstrual disturbances was apparent. The authors speculated that the increased muscular work of the back involved in rowing and weightlifting exerted a protective effect on vertebral bone. Wolman and colleagues,[85] however, did not confirm this protective effect on vertebral trabecular bone density. A two-way analysis of variance incorporating menstrual status and sports activity showed a significant (negative) factor for amenorrhea and a significant (positive) factor for rowers but no significant interactive effect.

The apparent immunity of the radius and susceptibility of the spine to menstrual disorders indicates that there may be a differential responsiveness of cortical and trabecular bone. A recent study included additional sites of varying trabecular composition.[68] Ninety-seven athletes were graded for menstrual history, and BMD was measured at the spine (L1 to L4), femur neck and shaft, radius (10% and 20% distal), tibia, and fibula. Spine and femur shaft BMD were higher in subjects who had always been regular than in subjects with some history of menstrual irregularity. Currently amenorrheic subjects with a history of oligomenorrhea or amenorrhea were significantly lower in vertebral BMD than subjects with other patterns of irregularity. No differences were detected at other sites. The authors concluded that deficits in bone density from previous menstrual irregularity appeared to be confined to the vertebrae. Weight was significantly correlated with BMD at all sites, and the association became stronger as the severity of menstrual disorder increased.

An important question is whether bone deficits due to amenorrhea can be corrected or averted. Seven subjects who regained menses following a reduction in training increased significantly (6.3%) in vertebral BMD, while matched eumenorrheic subjects did not change significantly over 1 year.[86] Bone density increased more slowly the following year, and then plateaued. After 4 years of normal menses, vertebral density remained well below normal. Further evidence of the persistence of vertebral loss was provided by a study of 208 runners. Subjects with past or current untreated amenorrhea had significantly lower spinal density than subjects who had always been regular. Women with current or past oligomenorrhea but no amenorrhea, and women with treated (by estrogen or oral contraceptives) amenorrhea for less than 3 years were similar in bone density to the always-regular subjects.

PROBLEMS IN STUDYING EXERCISE EFFECTS

In animal studies, exercise and mechanical loading have consistently benefitted bone density. Although the mechanisms have not been fully elucidated, loading produces increased cellular activity and bone formation rates. In humans, athletes had greater bone density than sedentary subjects, but few cross-sectional studies of non-athletes have been able to detect a difference in bone density between moderately active and sedentary subjects. It could be that many moderately active subjects do not exceed the threshold for stimulating bone hypertrophy. Intervention studies generally, but not always, increased bone density or reduced bone loss. A confusing aspect of bone research is the failure of intervention with weight training to increase bone mass in some studies. Some of the negative results in human studies can be attributed to measurement sites not stressed by the exercise, exercise programs of insufficient intensity, or lack of adequate control groups. One general difference between human and animal studies is human diversity in genetics, lifestyles, and implementation of the exercise program (intensity, attendance, etc.). Another problem in interpreting exercise intervention studies is the wide range of training programs used. At this time, we are still at-

tempting to delineate the exercise programs most effective in stimulating bone hypertrophy.

SUMMARY

Bone is a dynamic tissue performing two functions: providing structural support and acting as a mineral reservoir. Two homeostatic mechanisms act on bone at the same time: hormones and mechanical stress.

Researchers have evaluated the relationship of weight-bearing and non–weight-bearing forces on bone to bone mass and bone strength. Bone adjusts locally to support the structural demands of weight-bearing and muscular activity. Inactivity results in bone involution, whereas increased activity induces bone hypertrophy. Subjects at bed rest or in weightless conditions lose bone rapidly. Conversely, athletes have greater bone mass than their sedentary counterparts. Exercise intervention slows or reverses bone loss in middle-aged and elderly women. Bone response is specific to the area stressed, as seen in the selective hypertrophy of the dominant arm in tennis players. Very intense levels of exercise coupled with amenorrhea may reduce skeletal mass, especially in the spine.

More research is needed to understand the precise mechanisms by which exercise affects bone, and the optimum type and intensity of physical activity for preventing osteoporosis.

REFERENCES

1. Smith EL, and Raab DM: Osteoporosis and exercise. In Åstrand PO, and Grimby G (eds): Proceedings, Second Acta Medica Scandinavica International Symposium: Physical Activity in Health and Disease. Almqvist and Wiksell Trycheri, Uppsala, Sweden, 1986, p 149.
2. National Institutes of Health: Consensus Development Conference on Osteoporosis. Vol 5, No 3. US Government Printing Office, pub no 421-132:46, Washington, DC, 1984.
3. Matkovic V, Kostial K, Simonovic I, et al: Bone status and fracture rates in two regions of Yugoslavia. Am J Clin Nutr 32:540, 1979.

4. Freudenheim JL, Johnson NE, and Smith EL: Relationships between usual nutrient intake and bone-mineral content of women 35–65 years of age: Longitudinal and cross-sectional analysis. Am J Clin Nutr 44:863, 1986.

5. Mazess RB, and Barden HS: Bone density in premenopausal women: Effects of age, dietary intake, physical activity, smoking, and birth-control pills. Am J Clin Nutr 53:132, 1991.

6. Smith EL, Reddan W, and Smith PE: Physical activity and calcium modalities for bone mineral increase in aged women. Med Sci Sports Exerc 13:60, 1981.

7. Smith EL, Gilligan C, Smith PE, et al: Calcium supplementation and bone loss in middle-aged women. Am J Clin Nutr 50:833, 1989.

8. Horsman A, Gallagher JC, Simpson M, et al: Prospective trial of oestrogen and calcium in postmenopausal women. Br Med J 2:789, 1977.

9. Prince RL, Smith M, Dick IM, et al: Prevention of postmenopausal osteoporosis: A comparative study of exercise, calcium supplementation, and hormone-replacement therapy. N Engl J Med 325:1189, 1991.

10. Recker RR, Saville PD, and Heaney RP: Effects of estrogen and calcium carbonate on bone loss in postmenopausal women. Ann Intern Med 87:649, 1976.

11. Recker RR, and Heaney RP: The effect of milk supplements on calcium metabolism, bone metabolism and calcium balance. Am J Clin Nutr 41:254, 1985.

12. Polley KJ, Nordin BEC, Baghurst PA, et al: Effect of calcium supplementation on forearm bone mineral content in postmenopausal women: A prospective, sequential controlled trial. J Nutr 117:1929, 1987.

13. Riis B, Thomasen K, and Christiansen C: Does calcium supplementation prevent postmenopausal bone loss? A double-blind, controlled clinical study. N Engl J Med 316:173, 1987.

14. Ettinger B, Genant HK, and Cann CE: Postmenopausal bone loss is prevented by treatment with low-dosage estrogen with calcium. Ann Intern Med 106:40, 1987.

15. Baran D, Sorensen A, Grimes J, et al: Dietary modification with dairy products for preventing vertebral bone loss in premenopausal women: A three-year prospective study. J Clin Endocrinol Metab 70:264, 1989.

16. Dawson-Hughes B, Dallal GE, Krall EA, et al: A controlled trial of the effect of calcium supplementation on bone density in postmenopausal women. N Engl J Med 3223:878, 1990.

17. Elders PJM, Netelenbos JC, Lips P, et al: Calcium supplementation reduces perimenopausal bone loss. J Bone Min Res 4(Suppl):1128, 1989 (abstr).

18. Nelson ME, Fisher EC, Dilmanian FA, et al: A 1-y walking program and increased dietary calcium in postmenopausal women: Effects on bone. Am J Clin Nutr 53:1304, 1991.

19. Dawson-Hughes B: Calcium supplementation and bone loss: A review of controlled clinical trials. Am J Clin Nutr 54:274S, 1991.

20. Heaney RP: Effect of calcium on skeletal development, bone loss, and risk of fractures. Am J Med 91:23S, 1991.

21. Wolff J: Das Gesetz der Transformation Knochen. A. Hirschwald, Berlin, 1892.

22. Vogel JM, and Whittle MW: Bone mineral changes: The second manned skylab mission. Aviat Space Environ Med 47:396, 1976.

23. Smith MC, Rambaut PC, Vogel JM, et al: Bone mineral measurement-experiment M078. In Johnston RS, and Dietlein LF (eds): Biomedical Results from Skylab. National Aeronautics and Space Administration, Washington, DC, 1977, p 183.

24. Bassett CA: Biophysical principles affecting bone structure. In Bourne GH (ed): The Biochemistry and Physiology of Bone, ed 2. Vol III. Academic Press, New York, 1971, p 1.

25. Carter DR: Mechanical loading histories and cortical bone remodeling. Calcif Tissue Int 36S:19, 1984.

26. Forwood MR, and Parker AW: Repetitive loading, in vivo, of the tibiae and femora of rats: Effects of repeated bouts of treadmill-running. Bone Min 13:35, 1991.

27. Lanyon LE, and Rubin CT: Static vs. dynamic loads as a stimulus for bone remodeling. J Biomech 15:767, 1984.

28. Lanyon LE: Bone remodeling, mechanical stress and osteoporosis. In DeLuca HF, Frost HM, Jee WSS, et al (eds): Osteoporosis: Recent Advances in Pathogenesis and Treatment. University Park Press, Baltimore, 1981, p 129.

29. Rubin CT, and Lanyon LE: Regulation of bone formation by applied dynamic loads. J Bone Joint Surg 66a:397, 1984.

30. Rubin, CT and Lanyon, LE: Regulation of bone mass by mechanical strain magnitude, Calcif Tissue Int 37:411, 1985.

31. El Haj AJ, Minter SL, Rawlinson SCF, et al: Cellular responses to mechanical loading in vitro. J Bone Min Res 5:923, 1990.

32. Pead MJ and Lanyon LE: Indomethacin modulation of load-related stimulation of new bone formation in vivo. Calcif Tissue Int 45:44, 1989.

33. Raab DM, Crenshaw TD, Kimmel DB, et al: A histomorphometric study of cortical bone activity during increased weight-bearing exercise. J Bone Min Res 6:741, 1991.

34. Jee WSS and Li XJ: Adaptation of cancellous bone to overloading in the adult rat: A single

photon absorptiometry and histomorphometry study. Anat Rec 227:418, 1990.

35. Frost, HM: A new direction for osteoporosis research: A review and proposal. Bone 12:429, 1991.

36. Donaldson CL, Hulley SB, Vogel JM, et al: Effect of prolonged bed rest on bone mineral. Metabolism 19:1071, 1970.

37. Hulley SB, Vogel JM, and Donaldson CL: Effect of supplemental calcium and phosphorus on bone mineral changes in bed rest. J Clin Invest 50:2506, 1971.

38. Krolner B, and Toft B: Vertebral bone loss: An unheeded side effect of therapeutic bed rest. Clin Sci 64:537, 1983.

39. LeBlanc AD, Schneider VS, Evans HFJ, et al: Bone mineral loss and recovery after 17 weeks of bed rest. J Bone Min Res 8:843, 1990.

40. Kazarian LE, and Von Gierke HE: Bone loss as a result of immobilization and chelation: Preliminary results in macaca mulatta. Clin Orthop 65:57, 1969.

41. Young DR, Niklowitz WJ, and Steele CR: Tibial changes in experimental disuse osteoporosis in the monkey. Calcif Tissue Int 35:304, 1983.

42. Niklowitz WJ, Bunch TE, and Young DR: The effects of immobilization on cortical bone in monkeys (m nemestrina). Physiologist 26(Suppl):S115, 1983.

43. Huddleston AL, Rockwell D, Kulund DN, et al: Bone mass in lifetime tennis athletes. JAMA 44:1107, 1980.

44. Jones HH, Priest JS, Hayes WC, et al: Humeral hypertrophy in response to exercise. J Bone Joint Surg 59A:204, 1977.

45. Montoye HJ, Smith EL, Fardon DF, et al: Bone mineral in senior tennis players. Scandinavian Journal of Sports Science 2:26, 1980.

46. Block J, Genant HK, Black D, et al: Greater vertebral bone mineral in exercising young men. Western J Med 145:39, 1986.

47. Davee AM, Rosen CJ, and Adler RA: Exercise patterns and trabecular bone density in college women. J Bone Min Res 5:245, 1990.

48. Heinrich CH, Going SB, Pamenter RW, et al: Bone mineral content of cyclically menstruating female resistance and endurance trained athletes. Med Sci Sports Exerc 22:558, 1990.

49. Nilsson BE, and Westlin NE: Bone density in athletes. Clin Orthop Rel Res 77:179, 1971.

50. Jacobson PC, Beaver W, Grubb SA, et al: Bone density in women: College athletes and older athletic women. J Orthop Res 2:328, 1984.

51. Orwoll ES, Ferrant J, and Owatt SK: The relationship of swimming exercise to bone mass in men and women. Arch Intern Med 149:2197, 1989.

52. Dalsky GP, Stocke KS, Ehsani AA, et al: Weight-bearing exercise training and lumbar bone mineral content in postmenopausal women. Ann Intern Med 108:824, 1988.

53. Krolner B, Toft B, Nielson SP, et al: Physical exercise as prophylaxis against involutional vertebral bone loss: A controlled trial. Clin Sci 64:541, 1983.

54. Rikli RE, and McManis BG: Effects of exercise on bone mineral content in postmenopausal women. Res Q Exerc Sport 61:243, 1990.

55. Simkin A, Ayalon J, and Leichter I: Increased trabecular bone density due to bone-loading exercises in postmenopausal osteoporotic women. Calcif Tissue Int 40:59, 1986.

56. Smith EL, Smith PE, Ensign CJ, et al: Bone involution decrease in exercising middle-aged women. Calcif Tissue Int 36:S129, 1984.

57. Aloia JF, Cohn SH, Ostuni JA, et al: Prevention of involutional bone loss by exercise. Ann Intern Med 89:356, 1978.

58. Sandler RB, Cauley JA, Hom DL, et al: The effects of walking on the cross-sectional dimensions of the radius in postmenopausal women. Calcif Tissue Int 41:65, 1987.

59. Cavanaugh DJ, and Cann CE: Brisk walking does not stop bone loss in postmenopausal women. Bone 9:201, 1988.

60. Chow RK, Harrison JE, and Notarius C: Effect of two randomised exercise programmes on bone mass of healthy postmenopausal women. Br Med J 292:607, 1987.

61. Gleeson PB, Protas EJ, LeBlanc AD, et al: Effects of weight lifting on bone mineral density in premenopausal women. J Bone Min Res 5:153, 1990.

62. Pruitt LA, Jackson RD, Bartels RL, et al: Weight-training effects on bone mineral density in early postmenopausal women. J Bone Min Res 7:179, 1992.

63. Notelovitz M, Martin D, Tesar R, et al: Estrogen therapy and variable-resistance weight training increase bone mineral in surgically menopausal women. J Bone Min Res 6:583, 1991.

64. Rockwell JC, Sorenson AM, Baker S, et al: Weight training decreases vertebral bone density in premenopausal women: A prospective study. J Clin Endocrinol Metab 71:988, 1990.

65. Sinaki M, Wahner HW, Offord KP, et al: Efficacy of nonloading exercises in prevention of vertebral bone loss in postmenopausal women: A controlled trial. Clin Proc 64:762, 1989.

66. Cann CE, Martin MC, Genant HK, et al: Decreased spinal mineral content in amenorrheic women. JAMA 251:626, 1984.

67. Drinkwater BL, Nilson K, Chesnut CH, et al:

Bone mineral content of amenorrheic and eu-monorrheic athletes. N Engl J Med 311:277, 1984.

68. Drinkwater BL, Bruemner B, and Chesnut, CH: Menstrual history as a determinant of current bone density in young athletes. JAMA 263:545, 1990.

69. Fisher EC, Nelson ME, Frontera WR, et al: Bone mineral content and levels of gonadotropins and estrogens in amenorrheic running women. J Clin Endocrinol Metab 62:1232, 1986.

70. Jones KP, Ravnikar VA, Tulchinsky D, et al: Comparison of bone density in amenorrheic women due to athletics, weight loss, and premature menopause. Obstet Gynecol 66:5, 1985.

71. Linnell SL, Stagger JM, Blue PW, et al: Bone mineral content and menstrual regularity in female runners. Med Sci Sports Exerc 16:343, 1984.

72. Marcus R, Cann C, Madvig P, et al: Menstrual function and bone mass in elite women distance runners. Ann Intern Med 102:156, 1985.

73. Nelson ME, Fisher EC, Catsos PD, et al: Diet and bone status in amenorrheic runners. Am J Clin Nutr 43:910, 1986.

74. Snyder AC, Wenderoth MP, Johnston CC, et al: Bone mineral content of elite lightweight amenorrheic oarswomen. Hum Biol 58:863, 1986.

75. Cook SD, Harding AF, Thomas KA, et al: Trabecular bone density and menstrual function in women runners. Am J Sports Med 15:503, 1987.

76. Buchanan JR, Myers C, Lloyd T, et al: Determinants of peak trabecular bone density in women: The role of androgens, estrogen and exercise. J Bone Min Res 3:673, 1988.

77. Cann CE, Cavanaugh DJ, Schnurpfiel K, et al: Menstrual history is the primary determinant of trabecular bone density in women. Med Sci Sports Exerc 20:S59, 1988 (abstr).

78. Lloyd T, Buchanan JR, Bitzer S, et al: Interrelationships of diet, athletic activity, menstrual status and bone density in collegiate women. Am J Clin Nutr 46:681, 1987.

79. Louis O, Demeirlier K, Kalender W, et al: Low vertebral bone density values in young non-elite female runners. Int J Sports Med 12:214, 1991.

80. Myburgh KH, Hutchins J, Fataar AB, et al: Low bone density is an etiologic factor for stress fractures in athletes. Ann Intern Med 113:754, 1990.

81. Lloyd T, Triantafyllou J, Baker ER, et al: Women athletes with menstrual irregularity have increased musculoskeletal injuries. Med Sci Sports Exerc 18:374, 1986.

82. Warren MP, Brooks-Gunn J, Hamilton LH, et al: Scoliosis and fractures in young ballet dancers. N Engl J Med 314:1348, 1986.

83. Prior JC, Vigna YM, Schechter MT, et al: Spinal bone loss and ovulatory disturbances. N Engl J Med 323:1221, 1990.

84. Cann CE, Martin MC, and Jaffe RB: Duration of amenorrhea affects rate of bone loss in women runners: Implications for therapy. Med Sci Sports Exerc 17:214, 1985 (abstr).

85. Wolman RL, Clark P, McNally E, et al: Menstrual state and exercise as determinants of spinal trabecular bone density in female athletes. Br Med J 301:516, 1990.

86. Drinkwater BL, Nilson K, Ott S, et al: Bone mineral density after resumption of menses in amenorrheic athletes. JAMA 256:380, 1986.

CHAPTER **6**

Nutrition for Sports

GABE MIRKIN, M.D.

With the exception of iron and calcium, nutrient requirements for female athletes are the same as those for their male counterparts. Women suffer far more frequently than men from deficiencies of iron and calcium. Ten percent of healthy, white, middle-class female adolescents are iron deficient, while 5% have iron-deficiency anemia.[1] Athletes are at greater risk than nonathletes for developing iron deficiency,[2] which, even in the absence of anemia, can limit athletic endurance.

Hypoestrogenic female athletes are at increased risk of developing osteoporotic bone fractures.[3] In addition to hormone replacement, the prevention and treatment of this condition should include ingestion of adequate amounts of calcium.

A proper diet can help female athletes to maximize performance. However, many athletes have nutritional misconceptions that hinder performance rather than help it. For example, many athletes incorrectly believe that a high-protein diet improves performance and increases muscle size and strength, that vitamin requirements are significantly greater for athletes, that fluid requirements during exercise should be dictated by thirst, and that salt tablets should be taken in hot weather.[4,5] All of these myths will be refuted in this chapter.

In 1967, the women's world record for the marathon was 3:15:22, set by Maureen Wilton of Toronto, Canada. By 1985, the world record was lowered to 2:21:06 by Ingrid Kristiansen of Norway. The fantastic improvement in world records in all sporting events is due primarily to superior training methods, but it is also due to improved knowledge about nutrition. In the late 1960s, it was common for athletes to eat high-protein diets, to reduce their intake of food on the days before competition, to ingest no food or liquids during competition, and to eat only a limited amount of food after competition. Today knowledgeable athletes follow none of these old regimens.[6]

This chapter reviews some of the basic physiologic principles that serve as the foundation for advising athletes how to use nutrition to improve sports performance.

NUTRIENTS

Humans require approximately 46 nutrients to be healthy. An *essential nutrient* is one that cannot be produced by the body in adequate amounts and, therefore, must be supplied by the diet (Table 6-1). Lack of an essential nutrient can impair performance, but taking large amounts of any specific nutrient has not been shown to improve performance.

Athletes can improve their performances

Table 6-1. ESSENTIAL NUTRIENTS

Water
Linoleic acid
8 or 9 amino acids
13 vitamins
Approximately 21 minerals
Glucose (for energy)

in competition by following sound scientific nutritional practices. A brief discussion of basic principles of nutrition will precede the sections on the application of such principles to athletic competition.

Carbohydrates

Carbohydrates are composed of sugars. They can be monosaccharides, such as glucose and fructose in fruit; disaccharides, such as lactose in milk or sucrose in candy; and polysaccharides, such as starch in a potato or fiber in celery.

Before carbohydrates can be absorbed, they must first be hydrolyzed into one or more of the following four sugars: glucose, fructose, galactose, and mannose. Of these sugars, only glucose circulates beyond the portal system. The other three are converted to glucose by hepatocytes before they can re-enter the circulation (Fig. 6-1).

Circulating glucose can be used by all cells as a source of energy. Glucose that is not used immediately can be stored as glycogen only in the liver and muscles. When these tissues are saturated with glycogen, excess glucose is then converted to fat. Liver glycogen can yield glucose to the circulation, where it subsequently can be used by other tissues. On the other hand, the glucose from muscle glycogen can be utilized only by that particular muscle.

Proteins

Fifteen percent of ingested protein is hydrolyzed to amino acids and polypeptides in the stomach, while the remaining protein undergoes hydrolysis in the small intestine. These metabolites are actively transported

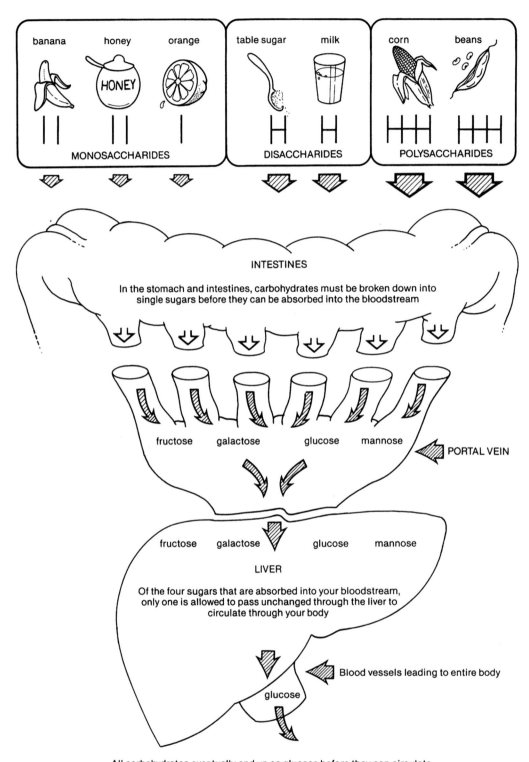

Figure 6–1. Sugar circulation. All carbohydrates are sugars bound together. They can be single sugars, as in fruit and honey; two sugars bound together, as in milk and table sugar; and hundreds and thousands of sugars bound together, as in corn and beans.

into intestinal epithelial cells. Once there, most of the polypeptides are hydrolyzed to form amino acids, which are then absorbed into the general circulation.

The main functions of proteins are to form structural components, enzymes, hormones, neurotransmitters, antibodies, transport molecules, and clotting factors. Protein also can be a source of energy. As much as 10% of energy during exercise can come from protein, with more than half coming from one amino acid, leucine. Since leucine represents only a small fraction of the amino acids in ingested protein, the leucine that is used for energy must come from a source other than ingested protein. It also does not come from muscle sources of leucine. Most of the leucine that is used for energy is formed de novo. The nitrogen for the newly formed leucine comes from other branched-chain amino acids (isoleucine and valine), and most of the carbon comes from glucose and other amino acids.

Before amino acids can be used for energy, deamination or transamination must occur to remove the nitrogen. Athletic training can double the levels of important transaminases, such as SCOT and SGPT, and this increases significantly the body's ability to utilize leucine and other amino acids for energy.

Fats

More than 95% of the fat in foods is in the form of triglycerides. Fat is separated from other foodstuffs in the stomach, but it is not degraded until it is emulsified (dispersed in water) by bile salts in the small intestine. The fat globules are then hydrolyzed by pan-

creatic lipase into monoglycerides, free fatty acids, and glycerol (Table 6–2), which enter the epithelial cells lining the intestines. Once there, the monoglycerides are hydrolyzed to form glycerol and fatty acids. Then, triglycerides are formed again, are combined with cholesterol and phospholipids, and are covered with a lipoprotein coating to form chylomicron particles, which pass through the lymphatic system into the general circulation. Short-chain fatty acids can be absorbed directly into the circulation. Excess fat is stored primarily in fat cells and muscles.

ENERGY STORAGE

Only fats and carbohydrates are stored for future use as an energy source. The human body cannot store extra protein. Fat stores energy in the most economic way, as it provides 14 times as much energy per given weight as stored liver glycogen, which must be stored with other liver tissue. One pound of stored fat will yield 3500 kcal, whereas 1 lb of liver contains only enough glycogen to yield 250 kcal. This great disparity in energy storage is explained by the fact that fat occupies 85% of the space in fat cells, while liver glycogen is diluted by other cellular elements and occupies less than 15% of the space in liver cells.

The body of the average athlete contains only enough stored fat to support exercise for 119 hours, enough stored muscle glycogen for 1½ hours, and enough stored liver glycogen for 6 minutes. Table 6–3 shows how limited the stores of carbohydrates are and how extensive the fat stores are.

Table 6–2. GLYCEROL AND FATTY ACIDS

C–C–C–C · · · C–C–COOH | C–C–C–C · · · C–C–COOH ---------→ | C–C–C–C · · · C–C–COOH TRIGLYCERIDE ----------------------→	C–OH | C–OH | C–OH GLYCEROL	 + +	C–C–C · · · C–C–COOH C–C–C · · · C–C–COOH C–C–C · · · C–C–COOH FATTY ACIDS	

Table 6-3. MAXIMAL BODY STORAGE
CAPACITY FOR CARBOHYDRATES AND
FATS[7]

Storage Site	Weight of Tissue (g)	Available Energy (kcal)
Muscle glycogen	125–300	500–1200
Liver glycogen	50–100	200–400
Body fat	6000–15,000	50,000–140,000

Comparing Women and Men

At the same level of fitness, the average woman has 7% to 10% more body fat than the average man. For example, top female marathon runners have 12% to 20% body fat, compared with 5% to 10% for their male counterparts.

Muscles use primarily fats and carbohydrates as their energy sources. At rest, muscles use mostly fats for energy. During exercise, muscles use more carbohydrates, with a higher percentage of carbohydrates and a lower percentage of fat being used as the intensity of the exercise is increased. In spite of their increased percentage of body fat, women use the same percentage of fat as men through all intensities of exercise. For example, at race pace for the marathon, top male and female runners have been shown to derive the same 50% of their energy from fat,[8] and top female athletes have not demonstrated greater endurance than male athletes.

In running events from 100 to 1500 meters, world records for women are 7% to 10% slower than those for men.[9,10] In running events from 1500 meters to the marathon, world records for women are 13% to 15% slower than those for men.[11] The extra fat that most women carry slows them down during running. However, having extra fat is an advantage during swimming. Penny Dean of California set the world's record for men and women for a single crossing of the English Channel in 7 hours and 40 minutes (in 1978), and Cynthia Nichols of Canada set the record for a double crossing at 19 hours and 12 minutes (in 1977). Their extra fat may well be the reason for their great endurance

swimming performances. It is likely that the insulating properties of fat, rather than the glycogen-sparing effect, gave them an advantage. Loss of body heat is a major problem in distance swimming. Furthermore, having extra fat raises a swimmer higher out of the water and reduces drag (see Chapter 4).

ENDURANCE

Endurance is the ability to continue exercising muscles for an extended period of time. To continue exercising, muscles require energy, the major sources of which are triglycerides and glycogen in muscles and triglycerides and glucose in blood.

The main advantage of fats is that the body can store vast amounts. The main advantage of carbohydrates is that they can be utilized under anaerobic conditions. Fat metabolism always requires oxygen. As exercise intensity increases, the percentage of energy derived from muscle glycogen also increases. Much of the exercise during most competition events is done at maximum or near-maximum intensity. The limiting factor for exercising at an intensity greater than 70% of $\dot{V}O_2$max is the amount of glycogen that muscles can store.[12]

"Hitting the Wall": Depletion of Muscle Glycogen

Muscle endurance depends on the adequacy of muscle glycogen stores. Depletion of muscle glycogen causes pain and fatigue and causes an athlete to lose much of her strength and to have difficulty coordinating muscle movements. Athletes refer to this as *hitting the wall*, a common occurrence in marathon runners after they have raced more than 18 miles. The more glycogen that can be stored in a muscle, the longer it can be exercised. Recent research has called into question this explanation. Since bicycle racers run out of their muscle glycogen after 2 hours of racing and do not "hit the wall," another explanation would be more feasible.

The most likely cause is that hard running damages the fibrous connective tissue in muscles, while the smooth rotary motion of pedalling does not.

"Bonking": Depletion of Liver Glycogen

Brain endurance depends on circulating glucose. More than 98% of the energy for the brain is derived from blood glucose, which depends on hepatic glycogen stores for maintenance. When the blood concentration of glucose falls to low levels, the athlete may feel very tired and can suffer from a syncopal episode or seizures or both. Athletes refer to this as "bonking." Bicyclists who do not eat during endurance races may experience this after 4 or more hours of cycling.

INCREASING ENDURANCE

An athlete can improve endurance by using training methods and dietary manipulations that increase muscle glycogen storage and decrease muscle glycogen utilization by increasing fat utilization.[13]

Training to Increase Endurance

To improve the ability of muscles to store increased amounts of glycogen[13] and utilize increased amounts of fat (and less glycogen),[14] athletes use a training technique called *depletion*. They exercise until muscle glycogen has been nearly depleted (Table 6–4). This causes muscle cells to increase production of glycogen synthetase, which increases glycogen synthesis and, in turn, glycogen storage.[15]

Table 6–4. AVERAGE TIMES FOR MUSCLE GLYCOGEN DEPLETION IN ELITE ATHLETES

Marathon runner	1½–2½ h
Bicycle racer	4–6 h
Cross-country skier	10–12 h

After the athlete eats, her muscles fill with glycogen, and this reduces production of glycogen synthetase. Therefore, the effects of depletion training are short-lived, and depletion training should be repeated at frequent intervals. However, athletes usually do not perform depletion training more frequently than once a week, because depletion of muscle glycogen leads to increased utilization of muscle protein for energy. This damages the muscle, delays recovery, and limits the amount of intense training the athlete can accomplish.

Many recreational athletes do not appreciate the importance of depletion training and enter marathons before they have put this training technique to adequate use. As a result, they have inadequate muscle glycogen stores to enable them to run the necessary distance.

UTILIZING FAT INSTEAD OF GLYCOGEN

In addition to depletion training, other techniques that have been promoted to decrease glycogen utilization by muscles during exercise include eating a high-fat diet for several days prior to competition, taking nutritional supplements, and taking sympathomimetic agents.

At least one study showed that eating a high-fat diet for several days prior to competition will increase muscle utilization of fat. However, endurance was not improved by this technique.[16,17] It is not unusual for blood glucose concentrations to fall as low as 30 mg/dL during vigorous exercise. Eating a high-fat diet does not reduce muscle glycogen utilization or prevent the development of hypoglycemia (with or without symptoms) during exercise.[17]

There is no evidence that taking large amounts of any vitamin, mineral, protein, or carbohydrate will cause muscles to increase their utilization of fat.[18]

Claims have been made that carnitine supplements enhance endurance. Carnitine is a protein that transports fat into mitochondria, where fat is catabolized for energy. However, there is no evidence that any supplement will increase mitochondrial fat content enough to increase fat utilization. Myocytes and hepatocytes synthesize large amounts of carnitine from lysine and methionine, and human myocytes contain enough carnitine to support fat metabolism even under extreme exercise conditions.[19] The fact that most athletes include meat, fish, or chicken—rich sources of carnitine—in their diets provides another reason why athletes do not need carnitine supplements.

Caffeine raises blood triglyceride levels by increasing catecholamine production and sensitivity. Catecholamines increase triglyceride utilization by promoting free fatty acid release from adipocytes and uptake by myocytes. Taking caffeine prior to workouts has been shown to increase endurance in training sessions by increasing muscle utilization of fat,[20] but it has not been shown to increase endurance in competition. A possible explanation for this difference in responses is that caffeine may be effective in prolonging endurance only when endogenous catecholamine levels are low. In a laboratory setting, athletes may be relaxed and have low circulating levels of catecholamines. Raising catecholamines in this situation may enhance performance. However, prior to competition most athletes have very high levels of catecholamines. Raising their levels further may not help them and, indeed, may harm them. Large amounts of catecholamines can cause tremors and irritability.

Seven days of supplementation of a high-carbohydrate diet with dihydroxyacetone and pyruvate has been shown in one study to increase endurance.[21] Further studies are needed before this practice can be accepted as an effective means of increasing endurance.

DIET AND ENDURANCE

Female athletes should follow the same nutritional principles as men, since their bodies process foods in the same ways. An athlete can increase her endurance by eating the right meals 3 days before, the night before, or several hours before competition.

Food Intake during the Week before Competition

In 1939, Scandinavian researchers showed that eating a high-carbohydrate diet for several days before a competitive event increases muscle glycogen stores and endurance, while a low-carbohydrate diet decreases muscle glycogen stores and endurance.[22] In the mid-1960s, other investigators proposed a method of "carbohydrate loading" that was practiced by many endurance athletes throughout the world.[23,24]

1 Seven days prior to competition, the athlete performs a long depletion workout.
2 For the next 3 days, she keeps the glycogen content of her exercised muscles low by eating a low-carbohydrate diet.
3 For the next 3 days, she eats her regular diet plus extra carbohydrate-rich foods.

Athletes should not ingest extra carbohydrate for more than 3 consecutive days. In that time, muscles and liver will be at their maximum capacity for storing glycogen, so no additional glycogen can be stored. In addition, carbohydrate packing should not be used in events lasting less than 60 minutes, because it will not be helpful and may even be harmful.[25] The muscles of trained athletes are not depleted of glycogen in so short a time. Carbohydrate packing may *reduce* performance in events requiring great speed over short distances, since each gram of glycogen is stored with almost three additional grams of water, making the muscles much heavier than usual.

Few top athletes practice this 7-day regimen today because it can hinder performance. During the depletion phase, the athlete cannot train properly and usually is irritable and unable to perform mental tasks effectively. During the high-carbohydrate phase, the ingestion of vast amounts of carbohydrates has been reported to cause chest pain,[26] myoglobinuria, and nephritis.[27] However, these side effects are rare. Marked overeating raises blood lipid levels, and this can lead to occlusion of the coronary arteries in exercisers who already have significant arteriosclerosis. Furthermore, this regimen has not been shown to be more effective than simply reducing the workload and ingesting some extra carbohydrates.[28]

As a result of all of these concerns, most top athletes in endurance sports avoid the low-carbohydrate phase and modify the high-carbohydrate phase. The runner can maximize muscle glycogen by a combination of reducing her workload and eating a regular diet that contains at least 55% of its calories from carbohydrates.[29] The 7-day carbohydrate-packing regimen thus is changed to eating a high-carbohydrate diet and stopping intense exercise 4 days prior to competition.

Eating the Night before Competition

On the night before a competitive event, many athletes eat a high-carbohydrate meal. The primary purpose of this meal is to increase muscle glycogen stores (Table 6–5). The pregame meal cannot serve this function, since it takes at least 10 hours to replenish muscle glycogen stores.[30]

It is controversial whether muscle glycogen storage is promoted more by ingestion of starch or monosaccharides and disaccharides. One recent study showed that a high-monosaccharide and high-disaccharide diet caused more muscle glycogen to be stored than did a high-starch diet.[31] Based on these findings, ingestion of simple sugars on the

Table 6–5. PRIMARY FUNCTION OF MEALS BEFORE AN AFTERNOON COMPETITION

Supper (the day before): To increase muscle glycogen stores
Breakfast: To increase hepatic glycogen stores

evening prior to competition does not seem to hinder performance and may actually help it. However, more research is needed to resolve this question.

Eating the Meal before Competition

The major function of the precompetition meal is to maximize hepatic glycogen (see Table 6–5). Serum glucose is sufficient to support brain function for only 3 minutes. To prevent hypoglycemia, hepatocytes must release glucose constantly. However, there is enough glycogen in hepatocytes to last only 12 hours when the athlete is at rest.[32] Obviously, during exercise, liver glycogen is depleted much faster than that.

Timing of Meal

To maximize hepatic glycogen stores, the precompetition meal should be ingested 5 or fewer hours before competition. If the meal is eaten more than 5 hours before competition, the hepatocytes will be depleted of a considerable amount of stored glycogen and will have less than maximal glycogen stores when the athlete starts competition. Several previous studies showed that eating sugared food just before competition increased an athlete's chances of developing postprandial hyperinsulinemia, which can cause hypoglycemia.[33] However, the vast majority of recent reports conclude that pre-event glucose consumption can cause reduced blood glucose levels during exercise, but it has no effect on endurance.[34,35] The brains of well-conditioned athletes can continue to function at lower blood sugar levels than those of unfit individuals.

At rest, blood glucose levels as low as 25 mg/dL usually cause a deterioration in brain function and loss of consciousness. However, physically fit individuals can usually tolerate such levels during exercise without developing any symptoms at all,[36] even though they are using up their muscle glycogen stores at an accelerated rate[37] and will feel fatigue sooner than usual.[38]

Composition of Meal

Precompetition meals should be high in carbohydrates. It does not make any difference whether the meal is also high in fat. A combination of a high-carbohydrate meal 4 hours before exercise and around 50 g of carbohydrate 5 minutes before exercise can increase glycogen stores and maximize endurance.[39] The athlete can eat any foods she likes, as long as she suffers no discomfort and has an empty stomach by the time she starts to exercise (Table 6-6).

Theoretically, fat and protein are poor choices for the precompetition meal. Fat delays stomach emptying, and the urea and ketones released by the catabolism of protein can promote diuresis. However, no controlled studies have demonstrated adverse effects from fat or protein in precompetition meals, and many athletes can tolerate high-fat and high-protein precompetition meals without having their performances hindered.

Eating Before Exercising

Provided that the exercise is not too intense and the amount of food eaten is not too great, most exercisers will not suffer from abdominal pain or discomfort when they eat

Table 6-6. EXAMPLES OF PRECOMPETITION MEALS THAT PASS RAPIDLY FROM THE STOMACH

Breakfast # 1

Breakfast cereal with milk
A few small pieces of fruit
Toast with butter
1 cup of coffee
1 glass of milk
No more than ½ glass of orange juice

Breakfast # 2

Pancakes
A small pat of jelly
Breakfast cereal
Milk or coffee
Glass of water
½ glass of fruit juice or a small piece of fruit

just prior to exercising. It is speculated that, when pain does occur, it is due to stomach muscle spasms, which result from ischemia caused by the shunting of blood from the stomach muscles to the exercising muscles.[40] During exercise, gastric motility increases,[41-43] and splanchnic blood flow decreases.[44]

A drug company has advertised that taking fructose before exercise, compared to glucose, results in a much lower rate of muscle glycogen depletion, because fructose does not cause a rapid rise in either blood sugar or insulin.[45] However, there is no evidence that eating fructose prior to exercising offers any advantage over eating nothing at all, and there is evidence that eating fructose is less advantageous than eating nothing at all. It is true that fructose ingestion may cause a *lower* rise than glucose in blood glucose and insulin levels,[46,47] but eating fructose does cause an increase in circulating glucose and insulin levels, whereas eating nothing does not. Fructose ingestion also causes a greater rate of muscle glycogen utilization, compared with eating nothing.[48,49] The fact that fructose costs 15 times as much as glucose offers an added disadvantage.

Eating During Competition

It is not necessary for most conditioned athletes to eat during events that last less than 2 hours. However, athletes can benefit from eating during events lasting longer than that. The ability of exercising muscles to utilize ingested carbohydrates in place of muscle glycogen is dependent on conditioning. The higher the level of fitness, the better able the athlete is to utilize ingested carbohydrates during exercise.[50]

In contrast to ingestion of food before exercising, ingestion of food *during* exercise does not cause significant pancreatic output of insulin. At rest, eating causes hyperglycemia, which promotes insulin release. However, during exercise, muscles remove glucose so rapidly from the circulation that blood levels of glucose rarely rise high enough to induce significant insulin release from the pancreas.[51] Insulin-induced hypoglycemia caused by eating during intense exercise does not occur.[52]

Almost any food can be used for energy. When taken during exercise, glucose has not been shown to be more effective than table food in prolonging endurance. Studies comparing glucose with fructose offer conflicting results. One study showed that neither glucose nor fructose is better than placebo in reducing muscle glycogen utilization.[43] Another study showed that fructose has a greater muscle-glycogen–sparing effect,[53] while a third study showed that glucose has a greater glycogen-sparing effect.[54]

Any maneuver that causes muscles to increase the rate at which they utilize fat for energy theoretically should help to conserve muscle glycogen and prolong endurance. A high-fat diet has been shown to increase endurance in rats,[55] but neither a fatty meal nor glycerol has been shown to prolong endurance in humans.[56,57]

Ten years ago, maltodextrin glucose polymer solutions, Exceed (Ross Laboratories, Columbus, Ohio) and MAX (Coca-Cola), appeared to enhance endurance in events lasting longer than 2 hours.[58] The polymers in these drinks are composed of five glucose molecules and seemed to supply calories at a low osmotic pressure, thereby not delaying absorption and resultant glucose utilization. However, recent data show that they are not superior to free glucose for maintaining hydration and blood glucose levels, and they have not been shown to increase endurance.[59]

DRINKING BEFORE COMPETITION

The maximal amount of fluid that can be absorbed during exercise is 600 to 800 mL/h. No matter how much fluid an athlete ingests during competition, she will not be able to absorb enough to keep up with her losses. She can increase hydration during the week prior to competition by doubling her daily intake of fluid for 1 week. An increase from 1 L to 2 L can increase blood volume by 10%.[60] The extra fluid is not lost completely as urine.

She can also increase her intake of fluids during exercise by distending her stomach with a large amount of fluid just before she competes. If she drinks 600 mL of water just before competition, almost 400 mL will pass into the intestines in 20 minutes.[61] Then she should try to ingest 3 oz (about 90 mL) of water every 10 minutes.

DRINKING DURING COMPETITION

Although most fit athletes do not gain any advantage from eating during competition in events lasting less than 2 hours, they can always benefit from keeping themselves adequately hydrated. Competitive runners and swimmers can lose approximately 1½ L of fluid during an intense 1-hour workout. Although athletes exercising in warm, humid environments can see their sweat and appreciate their obvious fluid loss, those exercising in water sports may not be able to perceive that this loss has occurred.

Dehydration and "Heat Cramps"

As the athlete becomes progressively more dehydrated, her blood volume decreases. There may not be an adequate volume of circulating blood to carry heat from exercising muscles to the skin, where the heat can be dissipated, and, at the same time, to carry oxygen to heavily exercising muscles. Reduced cutaneous blood flow will raise body temperature, and this will impair performance. The decreased blood volume can also limit the amount of blood that flows to the most heavily exercising muscles. The resultant hypoxia can cause sustained painful muscle contractions, known as heat cramps.[62]

Women May Need Less Fluid than Men

Earlier studies showed that men have better tolerance than women for exercising in the heat. However, these studies did not compare men and women exercising at comparable percentages of their $\dot{V}O_2$max. More recent studies have shown that women are able to tolerate exercise in the heat as well as men, provided that they both have the same $\dot{V}O_2$max.[63]

During exercise, women perspire less than men of the same fitness level,[63] but there is no evidence that women tolerate exercise in the heat better than men. Therefore, female athletes should take the same precautions as men to ensure that they are adequately hydrated during hot-weather exercise.

When to Drink

The athlete should drink before she feels thirsty. By the time that she perceives thirst, she already will have lost 1 to 2 L of fluid and will not be able to replace that deficit while she exercises. During intense exercise, it is impossible to absorb fluids as fast as they are lost. The maximum rate of gastric emptying is about 800 mL/h. It is common for competing athletes to perspire as much as 2000 mL/h.

Thirst is a late sign of dehydration during exercise because osmoreceptors in the brain will not signal a thirst sensation until the blood sodium concentration rises considerably. The primary mode of fluid loss during exercise is sweating. Sweat contains some sodium, although it is hypotonic in comparison to blood. As sodium is secreted into sweat, the serum sodium level rises more slowly than if water alone were lost. As a result, significant amounts of fluid are lost before hypernatremia develops enough to cause thirst. Therefore, on a warm day, the athlete should drink a cup of cool water just before she starts to exercise and every 15 minutes during exercise.

What to Drink

Adequate hydration will usually prevent heat cramps and hyperthermia. Water is the preferred drink to be taken during exercise lasting less than 1 hour. Extra calories[64] and minerals[65] are usually not needed. With adequate dietary intake, the athlete will store enough hepatic and muscle glycogen to last 1 hour.[64,65] Athletes who exercise longer than that need energy sources and minerals also. The rules for energy-containing fluids have changed dramatically in the last few years. In 1968, studies showed that 2.5% was the highest concentration of sugar that could be contained in an exercise drink and still be absorbed.[66,67] This posed a problem because drinks taste best when they contain a 7% to 10% concentration of sugar. Soft drinks and fruit juices contain 7% to 10% sugar. Soon after these studies, many exercise drinks containing 2.5% sugar appeared on the market. They did not taste good because the concentration of sugar was too low, so some of the manufacturers added saccharin to sweeten the taste.

Twenty years later, new studies refuted the 1968 report. The 1968 data were collected on resting subjects. Exercise increases gastric emptying for both solid meals and liquids.[68] When the same studies were repeated using people who were exercising, 7% to 10% sugared drinks were absorbed rapidly. Based on the most recent evidence, special exercise drinks are not necessary, although many athletes prefer them. All 10% drinks are equally effective in supplying energy. A basic 10% sugared drink may be prepared by dissolving 8 tablespoons of sugar in 1 L of water. Each tablespoon of sugar contains 12 g of sucrose.

Drinks with low levels of minerals are absorbed slightly more quickly than pure water, but the difference is not significant. Mineral loss through sweat occurs so slowly that conditioned athletes rarely develop hyponatremia, hypokalemia, or hypocalcemia during exercise.[65] In fact, the opposite is more likely to occur. Serum sodium and potassium levels rise during exercise and do not fall unless the exercise is intense and prolonged. Increased serum sodium levels are due to the loss of sweat, which is hypotonic in relation to blood. Increased serum potassium levels are due to release of potassium from myocytes, preventing overheating of muscles during exercise. Blood calcium levels usually are not altered during exercise. Magnesium levels in blood decrease slightly during exercise, but this is due primarily to cellular uptake of magnesium and not to a significant loss of magnesium from the body.[69,70]

Cold or Warm?

In the 1960s, studies showed that cold drinks (4°C) are absorbed faster and are less likely to cause abdominal cramps than warm ones.[67] The theory was that cold water causes the stomach to contract and push fluids rapidly into the intestines. However, more recent studies show that temperature does not make much difference.[71,72] Furthermore, carbonated drinks are absorbed as rapidly as noncarbonated ones.[73]

EATING AND DRINKING AFTER COMPETITION

Much of postcompetition tiredness is due to depletion of muscle glycogen stores and dehydration. Recovery from vigorous exercise depends on muscle glycogen replenishment and rehydration.[74] It makes no difference whether such replacement is accomplished by eating simple sugars or complex carbohydrates.[75,76] Fructose offers no advantage over other carbohydrates, as glucose causes more rapid muscle glycogen restoration than fructose does.[77] Carbohydrate intake in athletes averages around 250 g/d. This is far too little to afford maximal glycogen replacement. It takes at least 600 g/d of carbohydrate for maximum compensation. Therefore, it is important for athletes to eat carbohydrate-rich meals *after* competition.[78]

Table 6–7. IMMEDIATE POSTCOMPETITION MEAL TO PREPARE FOR ANOTHER COMPETITION WITHIN A FEW HOURS*

Food	Carbohydrate
1 orange	10 g
1 slice of bread	13 g
2 chocolate chip cookies	12 g
1 banana	30 g
1 12-ounce soft drink	35 g
No fluid restriction	

*A 50-kg woman needs 75 to 100 g of CHO.

In events such as gymnastics, track and field, wrestling, and swimming, athletes may be scheduled to compete in several events on the same day. It is very important for them to drink and eat immediately after they finish each event. Even if they rehydrate completely (as evidenced by a return to normal weight), it will still take 4 to 5 hours for the water to redistribute among the body fluid compartments.[79] Delaying carbohydrate ingestion ½ hour markedly delays muscle glycogen replenishment.[80] The recommended amount of carbohydrate ingestion for immediate maximal rate of replenishment is 1.5 g/kg of body weight[81] (Table 6–7). Doubling that amount does not increase glycogen replenishment further.

PROTEIN REQUIREMENTS

When adjusted for weight, protein requirements are the same for men and women. The protein requirement of 0.8 g/kg body weight per day is based on body mass. It is increased significantly by reduced caloric intake, but had previously been felt to be increased only slightly during exercise.[82–84] However, several recent studies using leucine turnover measurements seem to show an increase of up to 20% in protein turnover during aerobic exercise.[85,86] The case for increased protein needs during exercise is supported further by other studies showing increased excretion of 3-methyl histidine,[87] increased urea nitrogen losses,[87] and depression of protein synthesis.[88]

Further research is necessary before protein can be considered a significant source of energy during exercise.[89] Studies show an increased utilization of only the branched-chain amino acids, leucine, isoleucine, and valine. This does not make a strong case for increased protein utilization during exercise. The branched-chain amino acids are degraded by active skeletal muscles to release nitrogen, which is combined with pyruvate in muscles to form alanine. The liver removes nitrogen from alanine to form glucose, as a source of energy. However, turnover rates for amino acids that are not branched chain, such as lysine, are unaffected by exercise,[90] nitrogen losses are not consistently elevated during and after exercise,[90] and no loss of muscle mass can be detected during exercise.[90]

Taking extra protein does not increase protein turnover rates in exercisers,[91] but when combined with a heavy resistance program, it was shown to increase protein retention slightly.[92] In that study, an extra 2 g of protein supplements per kilogram per day was added to the subjects' usual intake of 1.3 g. The vast majority of the extra protein was oxidized for energy, with only a small amount retained in lean tissue.

The sole stimulus to make a muscle stronger is to exercise that muscle against resistance. This stimulus is so strong that muscles can be enlarged and strengthened by proper resistance training, even if a subject is fasting or losing weight and if all of her other muscles are becoming smaller.[93]

It does not take much *extra* protein to supply amino acids for enlarging muscles. An athlete with an excellent strength-training program may gain 1 lb of muscle in a week. Since muscle is 72% water, 1 lb of muscle contains only about 100 g of protein. However, the loss of efficiency in high-quality protein utilization is around 30% and in poorer-quality protein, around 60%. Therefore, to build 100 g of extra protein, the athlete must consume 130 g of high-quality protein (1.3 × 100) or 160 g of lower-quality protein in a week. This is accomplished by eating the equivalent of only 2 cups of corn and beans per day.

Since the body cannot store extra protein, the excess is catabolized into ammonia and organic acids, much of which is excreted in the urine. These compounds act as diuretics and, during exercise in hot weather, can cause dehydration and increase the risk of heat stroke.[94] Ingesting excessive amounts of protein can also increase calcium requirements by increasing urinary loss.[95] While this is probably of little significance to most women, it may accelerate bone loss in hypoestrogenic female athletes. Taking more than 4 g of extra protein per kilogram per day can also cause loss of appetite and diarrhea.

VITAMINS

Sixty million Americans, or 37% of the adult population, take vitamin supplements.[96] More women (42%) than men (31%) take vitamins, presumably because they are more health conscious than men. Three out of four Americans think that taking extra vitamins will give them more energy.[97] One out of five believes that lack of vitamins causes arthritis and cancer,[98] and one out of 10 does not know that vitamin requirements can be met without taking supplements.[99] Although 10% may seem like a small part of the population, this figure signifies that 25 million Americans believe that they have to take vitamin supplements to be healthy.

Mechanism of Function

A vitamin is an organic compound that the body requires in small amounts for health. While the exact mechanisms of function for several vitamins are not completely understood, much is known about the function of the B vitamins, which are parts of enzymes. Because the enzymes containing these vitamins are required in only small amounts, they catalyze reactions without being depleted.

The B vitamins enter the cells that are to use them. Such cells produce apoenzymes, which combine with the vitamins to form holoenzymes. Cells produce only limited amounts of apoenzymes, leaving unbound B vitamins in excess. The Recommended Dietary Allowances (RDAs) for B vitamins, determined by the Food and Nutrition Board (FNB) of the National Research Council of the National Academy of Sciences, "are the levels of intake . . . adequate to meet the known nutritional needs of practically all healthy persons."[100] It also represents the amount of B vitamins that will saturate the apoenzymes of the target cells.[100] Ingesting more vitamins does not increase the rate of reactions, because cellular apoenzymes are the limiting factor.

To help your patients understand why excess dosages of B vitamins are not needed, you can use the following analogy offered by Herbert and Barrett.[101] Consider the human body to be like a traffic intersection. Many cars (chemical reactions) pass through the intersection, but only one police officer (vitamin) is necessary to direct traffic. Bringing in many police officers (excess vitamins) will not cause more cars (chemical reactions) to pass through the intersection.

Vitamin Needs of Female Athletes

The diets of athletes who take in more than 2000 calories per day usually supply vitamins in amounts greater than their RDAs.[102] People who try to control their weight usually restrict their intake of food, and this can lead to an intake of vitamins that is less than the RDA. However, the RDAs are set so far above minimum requirements that dieters rarely develop signs or symptoms of vitamin deficiency, even if they do not meet the RDAs.[103]

Prolonged exercise can increase requirements for thiamine, niacin, riboflavin, and pantothenic acid beyond their RDAs.[104]

These four vitamins catalyze the reactions that convert carbohydrates and protein to energy.[105] For example, heavy exercise can increase riboflavin requirements by as much as 17%,[105] but the total daily needs for riboflavin can be met by drinking three glasses of milk. The total needs for all four "energy" vitamins can be met by eating a varied diet that contains more than 2000 calories per day, because all four of these vitamins are found in meat, fish, chicken, milk, and whole grains.

Although the refining process removes thiamine, niacin, riboflavin, and pantothenic acid from flour, most manufacturers routinely add these vitamins in order to comply with interstate shipping laws. Thus, athletes who eat breads made from refined flour rarely need supplements containing these "energy vitamins."

Vitamin C and Colds

Some athletes take large doses of vitamin C in the hope that it will help to protect them from developing upper respiratory infections. However, virtually all double-blind studies on the subject show that vitamin C does not prevent colds.[106]

Vitamins and Birth Control Pills

Whether women who take oral contraceptives require vitamin supplementation remains controversial.[107-109] A review of the literature shows that, on the average, women who take birth control pills have lower serum levels of riboflavin, pyridoxine, folacin, cyanocobalamin, and ascorbic acid and higher body levels of vitamin K.[109] However, their tissue levels[110] and blood levels[111] are still within the normal range. There is no evidence that such women are more likely to develop clinical symptoms of vitamin deficiency. Since birth control pills increase the need for these vitamins only a small percentage, if at all, it seems unlikely that vitamin requirements change appreciably because of oral contraceptive use.

Vitamins and Premenstrual Syndrome

Strength, speed, endurance, and coordination have not been shown to vary consistently throughout the menstrual cycle. Female athletes report greater perceived exertion premenstrually. Premenstrual syndrome (PMS) is discussed more thoroughly in Chapter 13.

Several investigators have suggested that nutritional factors play a role in PMS and have proposed dietary therapy for this syndrome. Pyridoxine has been touted as a treatment for PMS, because it is claimed to raise serotonin levels in the brain. Pyridoxine is a coenzyme for 5-hydroxy-tryptophan decarboxylase, which catalyzes tryptophan's conversion to serotonin. High levels of serotonin are associated with mood elevation; low levels are associated with depression. There is no evidence, however, that PMS sufferers have low brain levels of serotonin or that giving extra pyridoxine will raise brain levels. Two studies showed that taking pyridoxine improves PMS symptoms,[112,113] while another showed no improvement.[114] Although many women consider pyridoxine, in any dosage, to be harmless, large doses of pyridoxine have been reported to cause neural toxicity.[115,116]

MINERALS

The major minerals are listed in Table 6–8. Iron and calcium are the only supplements that healthy female athletes may need to take. An adequate diet can provide adequate amounts of all minerals, but many diets are deficient in these two.

Iron

Because of the high prevalence of iron deficiency among female athletes and because of its detrimental effect upon performance, I recommend that female athletes who have ferritin levels below 25 take daily supplements containing 30 to 60 mg of elemental iron. All others should avoid all supple-

Table 6–8. Minerals

Major	Trace
Calcium	Fluorine
Phosphorus	Silicon
Chlorine	Vanadium
Potassium	Chromium
Sulfur	Manganese
Sodium	Iron
Magnesium	Cobalt
	Nickel
	Copper
	Zinc
	Selenium
	Molybdenum
	Tin
	Iodine

ments which contain iron. Most healthy people can take iron supplements without developing obvious toxicity.[124] However, a recent study from Finland[124a] showed that high stored iron levels may increase a person's chances of developing a myocardial infarction. It is proposed that free iron catalyzes free radical production which converts LDL cholesterol to oxidized LDL to form arteriosclerotic plaques in arteries. Iron supplements can harm people who have hereditary disorders of iron metabolism, such as hemochromatosis and porphyria.

As many as one out of every four female athletes is iron deficient.[117] Men and non-menstruating women need about 12 mg of iron per day. The average man ingests adequate iron from dietary sources alone. The average woman ingests around 12 mg of iron per day, but menstruating women need 18 mg of iron per day, the extra 6 mg needed to replace the iron that is lost through menstrual bleeding. Birth control pills reduce iron requirements by decreasing menstrual blood loss and increasing iron absorption.[118]

Iron deficiency, even in the absence of anemia, can impair endurance.[119] Approximately 40% of the iron in the body is in the iron reserves, such as the liver, bone marrow, and spleen. The rest is contained in hemoglobin. Iron-deficiency anemia does not occur until almost all of the iron reserves are depleted. Iron deficiency reduces the concentration of α-glycerophosphate oxidase in muscle, and this impairs glycolysis and leads to lactic acid accumulation in muscle and blood.[120] An increase in lactate causes a lowering of pH, and this reduces muscular endurance.[121] People who have iron deficiency, even without anemia, have a reduced rate of lactic acid clearance from the blood, and they tire earlier during exercise. Restoring their iron reserves to normal increases their endurance.[122]

The most accurate test for detecting iron deficiency is a microscopic examination of bone marrow for stained iron. However, obtaining marrow is painful, invasive, and expensive. A simple, noninvasive screening test for iron deficiency is the measurement of serum ferritin. Caution must be used in interpreting the results, since inflammation anywhere in the body can raise ferritin levels. A person who has an inflammatory process may have normal serum ferritin levels despite having iron deficiency. Furthermore, exercise raises serum ferritin levels. Patients who have a microcytic, hypochromic anemia with normal ferritin levels without elevated fetal hemoglobin should have their serum ferritin levels repeated after they stop exercising for a week.[123]

Up to 30% of heme iron, found in meat, fish, and chicken, is absorbed, while less than 10% is absorbed from nonheme iron sources. Acidity enhances iron absorption from nonheme sources but not from heme sources. Thus, eating an orange with spinach enhances iron absorption from the spinach, but taking vitamin C with meat does not increase absorption of iron from meat. On the other hand, alkalinity, fiber, and tannins reduce iron absorption from both heme and nonheme sources. For example, taking antacids, eating fibrous vegetables, or drinking tea or coffee decreases iron absorption from all sources.

Calcium

Estrogen, androgenic hormones, exercise, dietary calcium, etidronate, calcitonin,

and vitamin D all help to prevent osteoporosis. Estrogen appears to be the most important. With adequate calcium intake, estrogen replacement, and exercise, even osteoporotic bones can increase in density.[125] Low bone density of any cause increases a woman's chances of developing stress fractures during exercise.[126]

Exercise can enlarge bones and increase bone density.[127,128] The bones in the racquet-holding arm of a tennis player are larger and denser than those in the other arm. Runners have denser femoral shafts than rowers, dancers, and sedentary controls.[129] However, exercise will not maintain bone density effectively in women who lack estrogen.[130] For example, exercise-associated amenorrhea is associated with decreased bone density,[131] and estrogen replacement helps to maintain bone density in hypoestrogenic women.[132] Birth control pills do not affect bone density in women whose bodies produce estrogen.[133] Women who have higher-than-normal levels of androgens have denser bones.[134]

Nevertheless, adequate calcium intake is essential for maintenance of bone density. Children who do not ingest adequate amounts of calcium during growth have smaller bones with reduced amounts of calcium, and develop osteoporosis at an increased rate as adults.[135,136] Increasing dietary calcium can improve calcium balance in women who lack estrogen.[137] Hypoestrogenic women require 1500 mg of calcium per day to maintain zero calcium balance, whereas euestrogenic women require 1000 mg to do so.[138] However, estrogen is far more effective than dietary calcium in maintaining bone density.[139] Hypoestrogenic, amenorrheic women who do not have a contraindication to estrogen replacement therapy should be treated with estrogen and, if dietary calcium is inadequate, calcium supplements.

The best dietary sources of calcium are dairy products and soft-boned fish, such as canned salmon and sardines (Table 6–9). Dairy products provide 72% of dietary calcium for the average American.[140] Those who

Table 6–9. FOODS THAT CONTAIN
APPROXIMATELY 250 MG CALCIUM

1 glass milk
1 cup yogurt
1¾ cups cottage cheese
1¾ cups ice cream
1½ oz hard cheese
2 oz sardines with bones
4 oz canned salmon with bones

do not meet their calcium requirements
from diet alone should take calcium supplements (Table 6–10), unless they are predisposed to nephrolithiasis.

The Food and Drug Administration has
found significant amounts of lead in some
samples of bone meal and dolomite.[141] Dolomite is most frequently harvested from the
shells of shellfish at the bottom of harbors.
Dolomite taken from polluted harbors can
contain toxic amounts of lead, mercury, arsenic, and other heavy metals. Bone meal
also may contain significant amounts of
toxic metals, since it usually comes from the
bones of older animals.[142] With aging, toxic
metals accumulate in the bones of all animals, including humans. Because dolomite
and bone meal are usually sold as food supplements rather than drugs, manufacturers
are not required by the government to list
the heavy metal content of their products.
Therefore, labels on packages containing
these products do not list their heavy metal
content.

Table 6–10. CALCIUM CONTENT IN 600-
MG SUPPLEMENT

Content of Pill	Mg	% Calcium	Number of Pills Required to Ingest 1 G
Calcium carbonate	240	40	4
Calcium lactate	78	13	12
Calcium gluconate	54	9	18.5
Calcium phosphate (dibasic)	171	28	6

Sodium

Most people do not need to consume extra
sodium when they exercise. The requirement for sodium for people at rest is 0.2 g/d.
With prolonged exercise in very hot
weather, the maximal requirement for sodium is approximately 3 g/d. The average
American diet contains between 6 and 18 g
of sodium chloride per day, of which 40% is
sodium (2.4 to 7.2 g). Manufacturers add sodium chloride to foods as a preservative,
and some people add sodium chloride to
foods to improve the taste. Athletes who try
to limit sodium intake by avoiding salty-tasting foods and by adding no sodium to foods
still take in about 3 g of sodium each day.

Sodium chloride tablets should not be
given routinely to exercising athletes. Besides being unnecessary, they can cause
gastric irritation, nausea, and, in very large
doses, potassium deficiency.

Sodium deficiency can occur in healthy
people because of an inadequate intake of
sodium or excessive use of diuretics. It can
also occur in people with hormonal or renal
defects. Any exerciser who feels tired and
weak or develops painful muscle cramps
should have serum levels of sodium measured. If present, hyponatremia requires a
thorough evaluation to determine the cause
(e.g., diabetes insipidus, diabetes mellitus,
water intoxication, and so on).

Many women who experience premenstrual fluid retention as part of PMS may
benefit from dietary sodium restriction at
the times of symptoms during each cycle.
Despite anecdotal reports of the success of
this regimen, no scientific studies have assessed its effectiveness.

Potassium

Potassium deficiency is an extremely rare
condition in trained athletes. The kidney
and sweat glands are highly efficient in conserving potassium in response to low body
levels. Even with prolonged exercise in very
hot weather, potassium needs can be met by
an intake of only 3 to 4 g/d.[143] However, po-

tassium deficiency can occur as the result of potassium restriction and sodium loading.[144]

The only way that one researcher could create a low-potassium diet for athletes and still provide enough calories for exercise was to feed them candy and little else throughout the day. Even then, the athletes did not develop potassium deficiency.[145] Almost all foods are rich in potassium. Since potassium is found primarily within cells, any food that contains cells also contains potassium.

Hypokalemia always requires a thorough evaluation to determine the cause. Potassium deficiency can be caused by drugs, such as diuretics and corticosteroids, and certain foods, such as licorice. Prolonged diarrhea and vomiting also can cause potassium deficiency (Table 6–11). With diarrhea, potassium is lost in the stool. With vomiting, loss of hydrogen ions causes a metabolic alkalosis, which increases potassium loss in the urine to conserve renal hydrogen ions.

Bulimia can present in athletes as weakness and tiredness with laboratory evidence of potassium deficiency. If blood samples show reduced potassium levels, and 24-hour urine collections contain increased amounts of potassium, suspect vomiting as the cause.

Trace Minerals

Humans require approximately 14 trace minerals in small amounts. There is no evidence that athletes need trace mineral supplements, with the exception of iron, because trace mineral deficiencies are extremely rare in healthy athletes.

Some lay publications for athletes claim incorrectly that trace mineral deficiencies are common causes of fatigue in athletes.

Table 6–11. MECHANISM BY WHICH VOMITING CAUSES HYPOKALEMIA

Loss of hydrogen ions
Raised blood pH
Renal hydrogen retention
Renal potassium loss

They argue that repeated harvesting of crops depletes the soil of essential minerals. When the soil in a certain region is deficient in a mineral, the plants and animals that grow in that region will suffer from a deficiency of that mineral also. That may have been possible in the past, but it is extremely unlikely to occur now. Although it is possible that some soils lack certain minerals, our transportation system is so extensive and efficient that very few Americans eat foods grown only in a single locality. It is impossible for all soils to be deficient in the same single mineral.

Oral contraceptive agents may reduce requirements for copper slightly and raise those for zinc, but there is no evidence that the latter is enough to require supplementation. Women who take birth control pills have higher serum levels of copper and lower levels of zinc than those who do not take such pills.[146,147] Estrogen is thought to raise serum copper levels by increasing serum ceruloplasmin levels.[148] The mechanism by which oral contraceptives lower serum zinc levels is not known.[149]

THE ATHLETE'S DIET

Of course, your patients cannot become great athletes just by altering their diets. They have to choose their parents wisely and train harder than their competitors. From the foregoing discussion, it is obvious that they can get all the nutrients their bodies need from the foods they eat. With the possible exceptions of iron and calcium, a female athlete's requirement for nutrients is the same as it is for male athletes. The only supplements that are required commonly are iron and calcium. Taking large doses of vitamin and mineral supplements can be toxic. Adverse side effects have been reported from large doses of even the relatively harmless water-soluble vitamins, such as niacin, pyridoxine, and folic acid. To help your patients perform sports more effectively, you should recommend that they eat a varied diet that is rich is carbohydrates and that they follow the rules for eating and timing foods and drinks that are outlined in this chapter.

Several lay books claim that a high-fiber, low-fat diet will improve athletic performance. There is no evidence to support this. In fact, one study showed that exercisers who ate a diet that contained 10% fat had the same improvement in $\dot{V}O_2$max as those who obtained 45% of their calories from fat.[150] Nevertheless, you may want to recommend restricting dietary fat, saturated fat, and cholesterol because it may help to reduce a woman's chances of developing coronary artery disease and certain types of cancers in the future.

Taking into account that foods have nutrients in different combinations and that foods in similar groups have similar nutrient content, the Department of Agriculture developed a simple plan for eating a varied diet that will supply all nutrients. The four food groups are

1 Fruits and vegetables
2 Grains and cereals
3 Milk and milk products
4 High-protein foods, which include meat, fish, fowl, and beans

The athlete should make sure that she eats a wide variety of foods from all four groups each day.

SUMMARY

With the exception of iron and calcium, nutrient requirements for female athletes are the same as those for their male counterparts and can be met by consuming foods that contain energy sources that are adequate to maintain exercise. Iron deficiency, even in the absence of anemia, can impair endurance. Amenorrhea can be associated with exercise and can increase calcium requirements.

Endurance can be enhanced by maximizing muscle and liver glycogen stores by reducing the volume of training 4 days before competition, by eating a high-carbohydrate meal on the night before competition, and by eating an easily absorbed meal 5 or fewer hours prior to competition. Maintaining adequate hydration, even before experiencing thirst, will also improve endurance. The rate of recovery following intense exercise can be hastened by eating extra carbohydrates and drinking large amounts of fluids soon after exercising.

Vitamin supplementation is not necessary, since requirements can be met through diet. Healthy athletes do not need to increase their intake of sodium, potassium, or trace minerals because the body can usually compensate for increased loss or decreased intake by increasing retention.

REFERENCES

1. Cook JD, Clement AF, and Smith NJ: Evaluation of the iron status of a population. Blood 48:449, 1976.
2. Smith NJ, Stanitski CL, Dyment PC, et al: Decreased iron stores in high school female runners. Am J Dis Child 139:115, 1985.
3. Lloyd T, Triantaflou SJ, Baker ER, et al: Women athletes with menstrual irregularity have increased musculoskeletal injuries. Med Sci Sports Exerc 18:374, 1986.
4. Wolf EMB, Wirth JC, and Lohman TG: Nutritional practices of coaches in the Big Ten. The Physician and Sportsmedicine 7:113, 1979.
5. Grandjean AC, Hursh LM, Majure WC, et al: Nutrition knowledge and practices of college athletes. Med Sci Sports Exerc 13:82, 1981.
6. Mirkin GB, and Shangold MM: Sports Medicine. JAMA 254:2340, 1985.
7. Davison AJ, Banister E, and Tauton J: Rate limiting processes in energy metabolism. In Taylor AW (ed): Application of Science and Medicine to Sport. Charles A Thomas, Springfield, IL, 1975, p 105.
8. Costill DL, Fink WJ, Getchell LH, et al: Lipid metabolism in skeletal muscle of endurance-trained males and females. J Appl Physiol 47:787, 1971.
9. Dyer KF: Making up the difference: Some explanations for recent improvements in women's athletic performance. Search 16:264, 1985.
10. Dyer KF: The trend of the male-female differential in various speed sports 1936–84. J Biosoc Sci 18:169, 1986.

11. Costill DL: Inside Running: Basics of Sports Physiology. Benchmark Press, Indianapolis, 1986, p 154.

12. Hultman E: Studies on muscle metabolism of glycogen and active phosphate in man with special reference to exercise and diet. Scand J Clin Lab Invest 19:94, 1967.

13. Mirkin GB: Food and nutrition for exercise. In Bove AA, and Lowenthal DT (eds): Exercise Medicine: Physiological Principles and Clinical Applications. Academic Press, New York, 1983.

14. Koivisto V, Hendler R, Nadel E, et al: Influence of physical training on the fuel-hormone response to prolonged low-intensity exercise. Metabolism 31:192, 1982.

15. Karlsson J, Nordesjo LO, and Saltin B: Muscle glycogen utilization during exercise after physical training. Acta Physiol Scand 90:210, 1974.

16. Maughan RJ, Williams C, Campbell DM, et al: Fat and carbohydrate metabolism during low-intensity exercise: Effects of the availability of muscle glycogen. Eur J Physiol 39:7, 1978.

17. Miller JM, Coyle EF, Sherman WM, et al: Effect of glycerol feeding on endurance and metabolism during prolonged exercise in man. Med Sci Sports Exerc 15:237, 1983.

18. Askew EW: Role of fat metabolism in exercise. Clin Sports Med 3:605, 1984.

19. Askew EW, Dohm GL, Weiser PC, et al: Supplemental dietary carnitine and lipid metabolism in exercising rats. Nutr Metab 24:32, 1980.

20. Ivy JL, Costill DL, and Fink WI: Influence of caffeine and carbohydrate feedings on endurance performance. Med Sci Sports Exerc 11:6, 1979.

21. Stanko RT, Robertson RJ, Galbreath RW, et al: Enhanced leg exercise endurance with a high-carbohydrate diet and dihydroxyacetone and pyruvate. J Appl Physiol 69:1651, 1990.

22. Christensen EN, and Hansen O: Hypoglykamie, Arbeitsfahigkeit und Ermudung. Scand Arch Physiol 81:172, 1939.

23. Hultman E: Studies on muscle metabolism of glycogen and active phosphate in man with special reference to exercise and diet. Scand J Clin Lab Invest 19:94, 1967.

24. Åstrand PO: Something old and something new—very new. Nutr Today 3:9, 1968.

25. Lamb DR, Rinehardt KF, Bartels RL, et al: Dietary carbohydrate and intensity of interval swim training. Am J Clin Nutr 52:1058, 1990.

26. Mirkin GB: Carbohydrate loading: A dangerous practice. JAMA 223:1511, 1973.

27. Banks WJ: Myoglobinuria in marathon runners: Possible relationship to carbohydrate and lipid metabolism. Ann NY Acad Sci 301:942, 1977.

28. Sherman WM, Costill DL, Fink WJ, et al: The effect of exercise-diet manipulation on muscle glycogen and its subsequent utilization during performance. Int J Sports Med 2:114, 1981.

29. Costill DL, Sherman M, Fink W, et al: The role of dietary carbohydrates in muscle glycogen resynthesis after strenuous running. Am J Clin Nutr 34:1831, 1981.

30. Piehl K: Time course for refilling of glycogen stores in human muscle fibers following exercise-induced glycogen depletion. Acta Physiol Scand 90:297, 1974.

31. Roberts KM, Noble EG, Hayden DB, et al: The effects of simple and complex carbohydrate diets on skeletal muscle glycogen and lipoprotein lipase of marathon runners. Clin Physiol 5:41, 1985.

32. Hultman E, and Nilson LH: Liver glycogen in man: Effect of different diets on muscular exercise. In Saltin B, and Pernow B (eds): Muscle Metabolism During Exercise. Plenum, New York, 1971, p 143.

33. Costill DL, Coyle E, Dalsky G, et al: Effects of elevated plasma FFA and insulin on muscle glycogen usage during exercise. J Appl Physiol 43:695, 1977.

34. Fielding RA, Costill DL, Fink WJ, et al: Effects of pre-exercise carbohydrate feedings on muscle glycogen use during exercise in well-trained runners. Eur J Appl Physiol 56:225, 1987.

35. Neufer PD, Costill DL, Flynn MG, et al: Improvement in exercise performance: Effects of carbohydrate feedings and diet. J Appl Physiol 62:983, 1987.

36. Felig P, Cherif A, Minagawa A, et al: Hypoglycemia during prolonged exercise in normal men. N Engl J Med 306:895, 1982.

37. Costill DL, Coyle E, Dalsky G, et al: Effects of elevated plasma FFA and insulin on muscle glycogen usage during exercise. J Appl Physiol 43:695, 1977.

38. Karlsson J, and Saltin B: Diet, muscle glycogen and endurance performance. J Appl Physiol 31:203, 1971.

39. Neufer PD, Costill DL, Flynn MG, et al: Improvement in exercise performance: Effects of carbohydrate feedings and diet. J Appl Physiol 62:983, 1987.

40. Fogoros RN: Runners' trots: Gastrointestinal disturbances in runners. JAMA 243:1743, 1980.

41. Nielsen AA: Roentgenological examinations of the motility of the stomach in healthy individuals during rest and motion. Acta Radiol 1:379, 1921.

42. Helebrandt FA, and Tepper RH: Studies on

the influence of exercise on the digestive work of the stomach. Am J Physiol 107:355, 1934.

43. Fordtran JS, and Saltin B: Gastric emptying and intestinal absorption during prolonged severe exercise. J Appl Physiol 23:331, 1967.

44. Clausen JP: Effect of physical training on cardiovascular adjustments to exercise in man. Physiol Rev 57:779, 1977.

45. American Health April, 1985, p 27 (advertisement).

46. Decombaz J, Sartori D, Arnaud MJ, et al: Oxidation and metabolic effects of fructose or glucose ingested before exercise. Int J Sports Med 6:282, 1985.

47. Koivisto VA, Karvonen S-L, and Nikkila EA: Carbohydrate ingestion before exercise: Comparison of glucose, fructose and sweet placebo. J Appl Physiol 51:783, 1981.

48. Hargreaves M, Costill DL, Fink WJ, et al: Effect of pre-exercise carbohydrate feedings on endurance in cyling performance. Med Sci Sports Exerc 19:33, 1987.

49. Bjorkman O, Sanlin K, Hagenfeldt L, et al: Influence of glucose and fructose ingestion on the capacity for long-term exercise in well-trained men. Clin Physiol 4:483, 1984.

50. Krzentowski G, Pirnay F, Luyckx AS, et al: Effect of physical training on utilization of a glucose load given orally during exercise. Am J Physiol 246:E412, 1984.

51. Ivy JL, Costill DL, Fink WJ, et al: Influence of caffeine and carbohydrate feedings on endurance performance. Med Sci Sports Exerc 11:6, 1979.

52. Koivisto VA, Harkonen M, Karonen S-L, et al: Glycogen depletion during prolonged exercise: Influence of glucose, fructose or placebo. J Appl Physiol 58:731, 1985.

53. Levine L, Evans WJ, Cadarette ES, et al: Fructose and glucose ingestion and muscle glycogen use during submaximal exercise. J Appl Physiol 55:1767, 1983.

54. Bjorkman O, Sahlin K, Hagenfeldt L, et al: Influence of glucose and fructose on the capacity for long-term exercise in well-trained men. Clin Physiol 4:483, 1984.

55. Simi B, Sempore B, Mayet MH, and Favier RJ: Additive effects of training and high-fat diet on energy metabolism during exercise. J Appl Physiol 71:197, 1991.

56. Miller JM, Coyle EF, Sherman WM, et al: Effect of glycerol feeding on endurance and metabolism during prolonged exercise in man. Med Sci Sports Exerc 15:237, 1983.

57. Murray R, Eddy DE, Paul GL, et al: Physiological responses to glycerol ingestion during exercise. J Appl Physiol 71:144, 1991.

58. Coyle EF, Hagberg JM, Hurley BF, et al: Carbohydrate feeding during prolonged stren-

uous exercise can delay fatigue. J Appl Physiol 55:230, 1983.

59. Massicotte D, Peronnet F, Brisson G, et al: Oxidation of a glucose polymer during exercise: Comparison with glucose and fructose. J Appl Physiol 66:179, 1989.

60. Kristal-Boneh E, et al: Improved thermoregulation caused by forced water intake in human desert dwellers. Eur J Appl Physiol 57:220, 1988.

61. Rehrer N, et al: Gastric emptying with repeated drinking during running and bicycling. Int J Sports Med 11:238, 1990.

62. Mirkin GB, and Shangold MM: Muscle cramps during exercise. JAMA 253:1634, 1985.

63. Eddy DO, Sparks KL, and Adelizi DA: The effects of continuous and interval training in women and men. Eur J Appl Physiol 37:83, 1977.

64. Hargreaves M, Costill DL, Cogan A, et al: Effects of carbohydrate feeding on muscle glycogen utilization and exercise performance. Med Sci Sports Exerc 16:219, 1984.

65. Costill DL, Cote R, Fink WJ, et al: Muscle water and electrolyte distribution during prolonged exercise. Int J Sports Med 3:130, 1981.

66. Costill DL, and Saltin B: Factors limiting gastric emptying during rest and exercise. J Appl Physiol 37:679, 1974.

67. Fordtran JS, and Saltin B: Gastric emptying and intestinal absorption during prolonged severe exercise. J Appl Physiol 23:331, 1967.

68. Moore JG, Datz FL, and Christian BS: Exercise increases solid meal gastric emptying in men. Dig Dis Sci 35:428, 1990.

69. Wolfswinkel JM, Van Der Walt WH, and Van Der Linde A: Intravascular shift in magnesium during prolonged exercise. South Afr J Sci 79:37, 1983.

70. Refsum HE, Meen HD, and Stromme SB: Whole blood serum and erythrocyte magnesium concentrations after repeated heavy exercise of long duration. Scand J Clin Invest 32:123, 1973.

71. McArthur KE, and Feldman M: Gastric acid secretion, gastric release and gastric emptying in humans as affected by liquid meal temperature. Am J Clin Nutr 49:51, 1989.

72. Maughan RJ, and Lambert CP: Effects of beverage temperature on the appearance of a deuterium tracer in the blood. Med Sci Sports Exerc 23:S84, 1991.

73. Zachwieja JJ, Costill DL, Widrick JJ, et al: The effects of carbonation on the gastric emptying characteristics of water. Med Sci Sports Exerc 23:S84, 1991.

74. Costill DL, Sherman WM, Fink WJ, et al: Role of dietary carbohydrate in muscle glycogen

resynthesis after strenuous running. Am J Clin Nutr 34:1831, 1981.

75. Costill DL, and Miller JM: Nutrition for endurance sport: Carbohydrate and fluid balance. Int J Sports Med 1:2, 1980.

76. Williams C, Patton A, and Brewer J: Influence of diet on recovery from prolonged exercise. Proc Nutr Sec 44:28A, 1985.

77. Conlee RK, Lawler RM, and Ross PE: Effects of glucose or fructose feeding on glycogen repletion in muscle and liver after exercise or fasting. Ann Nutr Metab 31:126, 1987.

78. Costill DL, Sherman WM, Fink WJ, et al: The role of dietary carbohydrate in muscle glycogen resynthesis after strenuous running. Am J Clin Nutr 34:1831, 1982.

79. McCutcheon ML: The athlete's diet: A current view. J Fam Pract 16:529, 1983.

80. Ivy JL, Katz AL, Cutler CL, et al: Muscle glycogen synthesis after exercise: Effect of time of carbohydrate ingestion. J Appl Physiol 64:1480, 1988.

81. Ivy JL, Lee MC, Brozinick JT Jr, and Reed MJ: Muscle glycogen storage after different amounts of carbohydrate ingestion. J Appl Physiol 65:2018, 1988.

82. Consolazio CF, Johnson HL, Nelson RQ, et al: Protein metabolism of intensive physical training in the young adult. Am J Clin Nutr 28:29, 1975.

83. Wilson HEC: The influence of work on muscular metabolism. J Physiol (Lond) 75:67, 1932.

84. FAO/WHO: Energy and protein requirements: A report of a joint ad hoc expert committee, serial number 522. FAO/WHO, Rome, 1973, p 5.

85. Fielding RA, Meredith CN, O'Reilly KP, et al: Enhanced protein breakdown after eccentric exercise in young and older men. J Appl Physiol 71:674, 1991.

86. Henderson SA, Balck AL, and Brooks GA: Leucine turnover and oxidation in trained rats during exercise. Am J Physiol 249:E137, 1985.

87. Dohm GL, Williams RT, Kasperek GJ, Van Rij AM: Increased excretion of urea and NT methylhistidine by rats and humans after a bout of exercise. J Appl Physiol 52:27, 1982.

88. Wolfe RR, Goodenough RD, Wolfe MH, et al: Isotopic analysis of leucine and urea metabolism in exercising humans. J Appl Physiol 52:548, 1982.

89. Layman DK: Energy and protein metabolism during exercise. Cereal Foods World 32:178, 1987.

90. Wolfe RR, Wolfe MH, Nadel ER, and Shaw JHF: Isotopic determination of amino acid-urea interactions in exercise in humans. J Appl Physiol 56:221, 1984.

91. Carraro F, Hartl WH, Stuary CA, et al: Whole body protein synthesis in exercise and recovery in human subjects. Am J Physiol 258:E821, 1990.

92. Fern EB, Bielinski RN, and Schutz Y: Effects of exaggerated amino acid and protein supply in man. Experimentia 47:168, 1991.

93. Goldberg AL, Etlinger JD, Goldspink PF, et al: Mechanism of work-induced hypertrophy of skeletal muscle. Med Sci Sports Exerc 7:185, 1975.

94. Serfass RC: Nutrition for athletes. Contemp Nutr 12:1, 1977.

95. Anand CR, and Linkswiler HM: Effect of protein intake on calcium balance of young men given 500 mg calcium daily. J Nutr 104:695, 1974.

96. The Gallop Study of Vitamin Use in the United States: Survey VI, Vol I. The Gallop Organization, Princeton, NJ, 1981, p 1.

97. US Department of Health, Education and Welfare, Food and Drug Administration, Bureau of Foods: Consumer nutrition knowledge survey: Report II, 1975. US Government Printing Office, Washington, DC, 1976.

98. National Analysts, Inc: A study of health practices and opinions. Contract number FDA 66-193. National Technical Information Service, Springfield, VA, 1972.

99. Herbert V: Nutrition Cultism: Facts and Fictions. George F. Stickly Co, Philadelphia, 1980, p 145.

100. Food and Nutrition Board: Recommended Dietary Allowances, ed 9. National Academy of Sciences, Washington, DC, 1980, p 1.

101. Herbert V, and Barrett S: Vitamins and "Health Foods": The Great American Hustle. George F. Stickly Co, Philadelphia, 1981, p 6.

102. Short SH, and Short WR: Four-year study of university athlete's dietary intake. J Am Diet Assoc 82:632, 1983.

103. Hickson J, Schrader J, and Cunningham L: Female athletes' energy and nutrient intakes. Fed Proc 42:803, 1983.

104. Belko AZ, Obarzanek E, Kalkwarf HJ, et al: Effects of exercise on riboflavin requirements of young women. Am J Clin Nutr 37:509, 1983.

105. Shills ME: Food and nutrition relating to work and environmental stress. In Goodhart RS, and Shills ME (eds): Nutrition in Health and Disease, ed 5. Lea and Febiger, Philadelphia, p 711.

106. Hodges RE: Food fads and megavitamins. In Hodges RE (ed): Nutrition in Medical Practice. WB Saunders, Philadelphia, 1980, p 293.

107. Prasad AS, Lei KY, and Moghissi KS: The effect of oral contraceptives on micronutri-

ents. In Mosley WH (ed): Nutrition and Human Reproduction. Plenum Press, New York, 1978.

108. Smith JL, Goldsmith GA, and Lawrence JD: Effects of oral contraceptive steroids on vitamin and lipid levels in serum. Am J Clin Nutr 28:371, 1975.

109. Webb JL: Nutritional effects of oral contraceptive use. J Reprod Med 25:150, 1980.

110. Shojania M: Oral contraceptives: Effects on folate and vitamin B₂ metabolism. CMA 126:244, 1982.

111. Roe DA, Eogusz S, Sheu J, et al: Factors affecting riboflavin requirements of oral contraceptive users and nonusers. Am J Clin Nutr 35:495, 1982.

112. Day JE: Clinical trials in the premenstrual syndrome. Curr Med Res Opin 6(Suppl 5):40, 1979.

113. Abraham GE, and Hargrove JT: Effect of vitamin B₆ on premenstrual symptomatology in women with premenstrual tension syndrome: A double-blind cross-over study. Infertility 3:155, 1980.

114. Stokes J, and Mendels J: Pyridoxine and premenstrual tension. Lancet 1:1177, 1972.

115. Schaumberg H, et al: Sensory neuropathy from pyridoxine abuse: A new megavitamin syndrome. N Engl J Med 309:445, 1983.

116. Vasile A, Goldberg R, and Kornberg E: Pyridoxine toxicity: Report of a case. J AOA 83:790, 1984.

117. Margen S, and King J: Effect of oral contraceptive agents on the metabolism of some trace minerals. Am J Clin Nutr 28:392, 1975.

118. de Wijn JF, De Jongste JL, Mosterd W, et al: Hemoglobin, packed cell volume, serum iron and iron-binding capacity of selected athletes during training. Nutr Metab 13:129, 1971.

119. Lukkaski HC, Hall CB, and Siders WA: Altered metabolic response of iron-deficient women during graded, maximal exercise. Eur J Appl Physiol 63:140, 1991.

120. Finch CA, Miller LR, Inamdar AR, et al: Iron deficiency in the rat, physiological and biochemical studies on muscle dysfunction. J Clin Invest 58:447, 1976.

121. Finch CA, Gollnick PD, Hlastala MP, et al: Lactic acidosis as a result of iron deficiency. J Clin Invest 64:129, 1979.

122. Nilson K, Schoene RE, Robertson HT, et al: The effects of iron repletion on exercise-induced lactate production in minimally iron-deficient subjects. Med Sci Sports Exerc 13:92, 1981.

123. Pattini A, Schena F, and Guidi GC: Serum ferritin and serum iron changes after cross-country and roller ski endurance races. Eur J Appl Physiol 61:55, 1990.

124. Finch CA, and Monsen ER: Iron nutrition and the fortification of food with iron. JAMA 219:1462, 1972.

124a. Salonen JT, Nyyssonen K, Korpela H, et al: High iron levels are associated with excess risk of myocardial infarction in eastern Finnish men. Circulation 86:803, 1992.

125. Leblanc A, and Schneider V: Can the skeleton recover lost bone? Exp Gerontol 26:189, 1991.

126. Myburgh KH, Hutchins J, Fataar AB, et al: Low bone density is an etiologic factor for stress fractures in athletes. Ann Int Med 113:754, 1990.

127. Aloia JF: Exercise and skeletal health. J Am Geriatr Soc 29:104, 1981.

128. Smith EL, Gilligan C, McAdam M, et al: Determining bone loss by exercise intervention in premenopausal and postmenopausal women. Calcif Tissue Int 44:312, 1989.

129. Wolman RL, Faulman L, Clark P, et al: Different training patterns and bone mineral density of the femoral shaft in elite, female athletes. Ann Rheum Dis 50:487, 1991.

130. Dhuper S, Warren M, Brooks-Gunn J, and Fox R: Effect of hormonal status on bone density in adolescent girls. J Clin Endocrinol Metab 71:1083–1088, 1991.

131. Drinkwater E, Nilson K, Chesnut CH, et al: Bone mineral content of amenorrheic and eumenorrheic athletes. N Engl J Med 311:277, 1984.

132. Shangold MM: Causes, evaluation, and management of athletic oligo/amenorrhea. Med Clin North Am 69:83, 1985.

133. Lloyd T, Buchanan JR, Ursino GR, et al: Long-term oral contraceptive use does not affect trabecular bone density. Am J Obstet Gynecol 160:402, 1989.

134. Dixon JE, Rodin A, Murby B, et al: Bone mass with androgen excess. Clin Endocrinol 30:271, 1989.

135. Matkovic V: Calcium metabolism and calcium requirements during skeletal remodeling and consolidation of bone mass. Am J Clin Nutr 54:245S, 1991.

136. Sentipal JM, Wardlaw GM, Mahan J, and Matkovic V: Influence of calcium intake and growth indexes on vertebral bone mineral density in young females. Am J Clin Nutr 54:425, 1991.

137. Recker RR, Saville PD, and Heaney RP: Effect of estrogen and calcium carbonate on bone loss in postmenopausal women. Ann Intern Med 87:649, 1977.

138. Heaney RP, Recker RR, and Saville PD: Menopausal changes in calcium balance performance. J Lab Clin Med 92:953, 1978.

139. Riis B, Thomsen K, and Christiansen C: Does calcium supplementation prevent post-

menopausal bone loss? A double-blind, controlled clinical study. N Engl J Med 316:173, 1987.

140. Marston RM, and Welsh SO: Nutrient content of the U.S. food supply. Nat Food Rev 25:7, 1984.

141. Advice on limiting intake of bonemeal. FDA Drug Bull 12:5, 1982.

142. Roberts NJ: Potential toxicity due to dolomite and bonemeal. South Med J 76:556, 1983.

143. Lane HW, Roessler GS, Nelson EW, et al: Effect of physical activity on human potassium metabolism in a hot and humid environment. Am J Clin Nutr 31:838, 1978.

144. Talbot NB, Richie RH, and Crawford JD: Metabolic Homeostasis: A Syllabus for Those Concerned with the Care of Patients. Harvard University Press, Cambridge, 1959, p 32.

145. Costill D: Muscle water and electrolytes during acute and repeated bouts of dehydration. In Panzkova J, and Rogozkin VA (eds): Nutrition, Physical Fitness and Health. University Park Press, Baltimore, 1978, p 106.

146. Prasad AS, Oberleas D, Lei KY, et al: Effect of oral contraceptive agents on nutrients: I. Minerals. Am J Clin Nutr 28:377, 1975.

147. Schenker JG, Hellerstein S, Jungreis E, et al: Serum copper and zinc levels in patients taking oral contraceptives. Fertil Steril 22:229, 1971.

148. Carruthers ME, Hobbs CE, and Warren RL: Raised serum copper and caeruloplasmin levels in subjects taking oral contraceptives. J Clin Pathol 19:498, 1966.

149. Prasad AS, Moghissi KS, Lei KY, et al: Effect of oral contraceptives on micronutrients and changes in trace elements due to pregnancy. In Moghissi KS, and Evans TN (eds): Nutritional Impacts on Women Throughout Life with Emphasis on Reproduction. Harper and Row, New York, 1977, p 160.

150. Kosich D, Conlee R, Fisher AG, et al: The effects of exercise and a low-fat diet or a moderate-fat diet on selected coronary risk factors. In Dotson C, and Humphrey J (eds): Exercise Physiology: Current Selected Research, Vol 2. AMS Press, New York, 1986, p 173.

II

Developmental
Phases

CHAPTER 7

The Prepubescent Female

ODED BAR-OR, M.D.

PHYSIOLOGIC RESPONSE TO
  SHORT-TERM EXERCISE
Submaximal Oxygen Uptake
Maximal Aerobic Power
Anaerobic Power and Muscle
  Endurance
Muscle Strength

TRAINABILITY

THERMOREGULATORY CAPACITY
Response to Hot Climate

Response to Cold Climate
High-Risk Groups for Heat- or Cold-
  Related Disorders

GROWTH, PUBERTAL CHANGES,
  AND ATHLETIC TRAINING

COEDUCATIONAL PARTICIPATION
  IN CONTACT AND COLLISION
  SPORTS

Recent years have seen an increasing interest in the physiologic responses of children to exercise. Such interest reflects the greater participation and success of prepubescents and adolescents in elite sports, as well as the recognition that physical exercise is relevant to the health of the nonathletic child.

Although prepubescent athletes of both sexes engage in elite sports, it is primarily the females who have become extremely successful at the national and international levels. Such success is particularly apparent in gymnastics, figure skating, and swimming, in which prepubescents have been performing at levels that, a decade or two ago, were not considered feasible even for adults.

To achieve such excellence, many female athletes have to practice as much as 4 to 6 hours per day and at high intensity. Such involvement and dedication has educational, psychosocial, medical, gynecologic, orthopedic, and physiologic consequences. These have become a focus of research for sports scientists of various disciplines.

Exercise-related research is oriented also toward the young nonathlete, healthy or ill. Study of the healthy child has been of interest, for example, to kinanthropometrists, who are interested in growth patterns and the interrelationships between morphologic and functional changes; to epidemiologists, who assess the possible relationships between habitual activity during childhood and the risk of chronic disease in later years; to motor behaviorists, who study motor learning and skill acquisition; and to physiologists, who seek answers to such maturation-related issues as strength development, energy expenditure of locomotion, trainability, and thermoregulation.

The relevance of exercise to the ill child has also generated growing interest.

129

Pediatric cardiologists and respirologists, for example, are using exercise for the assessment of children with such diseases as congenital heart defects, bronchial asthma, and cystic fibrosis; an exercise prescription is incorporated into the management of the child with diabetes mellitus, obesity, muscular dystrophy, cerebral palsy, and cystic fibrosis; and detrimental effects of exercise are studied in such conditions as aortic stenosis, dysrhythmia, primary amenorrhea, and epilepsy.

This chapter is meant to focus on the physiologic responses to exercise of the healthy prepubescent girl. Emphasis will be given to differences among prepubescents, adolescents, and young adults. Differences will also be pointed out between the responses to exercise of girls and boys. Whenever relevant, the implications to health of such differences will be pointed out.

It is assumed that the reader has some basic knowledge of exercise physiology. Additional information on pediatric exercise physiology can be found in monographs,[1-6] edited books,[7-10] and proceedings of the Pediatric Work Physiology Group.[11-20] Furthermore, a journal (*Pediatric Exercise Sciences,* Human Kinetics, Champaign, IL) is available which is fully dedicated to the effects of exercise in children. A recent monograph[21] includes a comprehensive, longitudinal analysis of relationships between fitness and growth in girls.

PHYSIOLOGIC RESPONSE TO SHORT-TERM EXERCISE

Differences in the response to short-term exercise (less than a 15-minute duration) of prepubescent and older females are summarized in Table 7-1. Table 7-2 is a summary of gender-related differences in the response of prepubescents to short-term exercise. The following discussion will highlight those characteristics of the prepubescent girl that have a direct relevance to her physical performance.

Submaximal Oxygen Uptake

Typically for young girls, oxygen uptake (calculated per body mass unit) while running or walking at any given speed is higher than in adolescent or adult females.[1,22-24] A 5.5-year-old girl, for example, who runs at 10 km/h, consumes about 46 mL of oxygen per kilogram of body weight per minute, compared with 37 $mL \cdot kg^{-1} \cdot min^{-1}$ in a 16-year-old adolescent. Calculated per body surface area, however, such differences disappear.[25]

The implication of such a high metabolic cost is that, at any walking or running speed,

Table 7-1. SOME PHYSIOLOGIC RESPONSES TO ACUTE EXERCISE: COMPARISON BETWEEN PREPUBESCENT GIRLS AND OLDER FEMALES

Physiologic Function	Typical for Girls (Compared with Older Females)
O_2 cost of walking/running	Higher
O_2 uptake max, $L \cdot min^{-1}$	Lower
O_2 uptake max, $mL \cdot kg^{-1} \cdot min^{-1}$	Higher
Heart rate submax	Higher
Stroke volume submax	Lower
Cardiac output submax	Lower
Minute ventilation submax	Higher
Ventilatory equivalent submax and max	Higher
Peak anaerobic power, watt	Lower
Peak anaerobic power, $watt \cdot kg^{-1}$	Lower
Mean anaerobic power, watt	Lower
Mean anaerobic power, $watt \cdot kg^{-1}$	Lower

Table 7-2. GENDER-RELATED COMPARISON OF THE RESPONSE OF PREPUBESCENTS TO ACUTE EXERCISE

Physiologic Function	Girls' Response (Compared with Boys)
O_2 cost of walking/running	Similar
O_2 uptake max, $L \cdot min^{-1}$	Somewhat lower
O_2 uptake max per kg body weight	Somewhat lower
O_2 uptake max per kg lean mass	Similar
Heart rate submax	Higher
Heart rate max	Similar
Stroke volume submax and max	Lower
Minute ventilation submax	Similar
Minute ventilation max	Somewhat lower
Peak anaerobic power, watt	Somewhat lower
Peak anaerobic power, watt $\cdot$ kg^{-1}	Lower
Mean anaerobic power, watt	Somewhat lower
Mean anaerobic power, watt $\cdot$ kg^{-1}	Lower

a young girl operates at a higher percentage of her maximal aerobic power and will fatigue earlier than an older girl or a woman. This may be the main reason why young girls cannot compete on a par with their older counterparts in middle- and long-distance running. Such a difference is virtually nonexistent during cycling.[26-28] This suggests that the biochemical-to-mechanical energy transfer efficiency in muscles is not lower at a young age, but young girls have a more "wasteful" gait, which increases their mechanical output and metabolic demands during the gait cycle. No data are available on the age-related differences in the metabolic cost of swimming. The success of young girls in elite swimming would suggest, however, that a proficient young swimmer is not less economical in her style than her older counterpart.

Maximal Aerobic Power

Throughout childhood and adolescence, maximal aerobic power, as reflected by maximal oxygen uptake ($\dot{V}O_2max$), increases with age. The $\dot{V}O_2max$ of 5-year-old preschoolers is 0.80 to 0.90 $L \cdot min^{-1}$, compared with 1.1 to 1.5 $L \cdot min^{-1}$ and 1.6 to 2.2 $L \cdot min^{-1}$ for 10- and 16-year-old girls, respectively.[1,2] Calculated per kilogram of body weight,

however, there is little change in the $\dot{V}O_2max$ of girls up to the age of 10 to 11 years. During the second decade of life, $\dot{V}O_2max$ per kilogram decreases with age, such that it is approximately 4 to 6 $mL \cdot kg^{-1} \cdot min^{-1}$ lower at age 17 to 18 than at age 10 to 11.[1,2,29,30] It has been suggested that the lower $\dot{V}O_2max$ per kilogram in the pubertal girl is due to the decrease in blood hemoglobin concentration, secondary to menstrual blood loss. This, however, does not explain the drop in $\dot{V}O_2max$ per kilogram of body weight even before menarche. One reason could be the increasing adiposity of many girls who approach puberty.[31-33] Decreasing aerobic power could also result from an age-related decrease in spontaneous habitual activity in the second decade of life.[33-37]

Although gender-related differences in maximal aerobic power are apparent primarily after age 12 to 13 years, boys seem to have a somewhat higher $\dot{V}O_2max$ even at earlier ages.[1,2,33,38-40] In a study comparing the maximal aerobic power of 6- to 16-year-old girls and boys who were tested on the cycle ergometer, such gender-related differences were eliminated when $\dot{V}O_2max$ ($L \cdot min^{-1}$) was plotted against lean leg volume rather than against age.[39] A similar pattern was apparent among 8- to 16-year-old girls and boys when $\dot{W}_{170}$ (i.e., the mechanical power at which they cycle when their heart rate is 170 beats per minute) was plotted against body cell mass.[41] It should be realized, however, that when $\dot{V}O_2max$ is divided by lean leg volume or lean body mass, preadolescent boys still have higher values than preadolescent girls.[33] A more precise determination of body composition is needed to tell whether gender-related differences in maximal aerobic power of prepubescents are fully explained by the mass of their exercising muscles.

Anaerobic Power and Muscle Endurance

High-intensity muscle contractions that cannot be sustained for more than 20 to 30 seconds are dependent primarily on anaerobic energy pathways. Examples of "anaerobic" activities are short and long sprints in running, skating, and cycling, as well as short slalom in downhill skiing. Until recent years, this component of fitness received little attention, compared with maximal aerobic power and muscle strength. This reflected the paucity of reliable and valid laboratory tests for peak muscle power and local muscle endurance. Such tests are currently available, using cycle ergometers or isokinetic machines. These have been added to the Margaria step-running test,[42] which assesses peak muscle power but not muscle endurance. The following information has been obtained using the Margaria test and the Wingate anaerobic test.[43]

The ability of prepubertal girls and boys to perform anaerobic tasks is distinctly lower than that of adolescents and young adults. This was first shown for 8- to 73-year-old sedentary Italians: even when divided by body weight, the peak muscle power of the 8- to 10-year-old girls was only about 60% that of the 20-year-old women.[42] Similar results have been shown for Nilo-Hamitic and Bantu African,[44] British,[39] American,[45] and Israeli[2] populations. In the last, peak muscle power and muscle endurance of the arms and the legs were both lower in the young girls, even when corrected for differences in body weight.

The aforementioned pattern is in contrast to maximal aerobic power which, when calculated per kilogram body weight, is *higher* in the prepubescent girl than in the adolescent or adult female.

The mechanism for the low anaerobic performance of prepubescent girls is not known. In a recent study performed in my laboratory on adolescent girls and boys,[46] lean muscle mass of the upper limb explained much of the variance in arm peak power and muscle endurance of the boys but not of the girls. Performance of both prepubescent girls and boys in the Margaria test, even when corrected for fat-free mass, is lower than that of adolescents and adults.[44] It is quite likely, therefore, that *qualitative* characteristics of the muscles, and possibly their neural control, would explain the rela-

tive deficiency of anaerobic power in the prepubescent. Children of both sexes have lower maximal blood lactate concentration than do adolescents and adults. It has been reported for boys, but not for girls, that creatine phosphate and glycogen concentrations in the resting muscle and, in particular, the rate of glycolysis in the contracting muscle are low before puberty. (For more details, see reference 2.) Based on animal studies, a relationship has been suggested between muscle lactate production and circulating testosterone. Whether this applies also to humans—females or males—has yet to be shown. It can be assumed, however, that a low glycolytic capacity in prepubescents of both sexes is the main cause of their low anaerobic performance.

Muscle Strength

Muscle strength, defined as the maximal force that can be exerted by a muscle or a group of muscles, is similar in girls and boys during their first decade of life.[33,47] Strength is growth-dependent.[33,47–49] However, it does not increase linearly with the growth in body mass or stature. In girls, the main increase in strength occurs during, a few months following, or even just before the "growth spurt" (i.e., the year during which body height velocity is at its peak). In contrast, the increase of strength in boys reaches its peak about 1 year *after* the growth spurt.[50,51] This difference, coupled with the earlier growth spurt in girls (about a 2-year difference), may explain why the greater muscle strength of boys is usually not evident before age 11 or 12 years.

TRAINABILITY

Does a prepubescent girl respond to training in the same manner as an adolescent or an adult female? This question is of utmost relevance to the theory and practice of coaching, but should be of interest also to the pediatric physiotherapist and the physiatrist who wish to apply physiologic principles to rehabilitation.

To obtain definitive answers about trainability (i.e., the ability of body systems to adapt to repeated exercise stimuli) of different age groups, one must conduct a longitudinal training study on these groups. Such a design must satisfy two conditions: (1) the *initial fitness level* of all groups must be similar and (2) the *training dosage* must be equated among the groups.

Unfortunately, neither condition can be adequately satisfied. First, one cannot assume that a 6-year-old girl who, for example, sprints 50 m in 11.0 seconds has the same sprinting ability as a 16-year-old adolescent who runs at the same speed. A better approach might be to use a physiologic criterion for equating the initial fitness level. One cannot be sure, however, that a maximal aerobic power of 40 mL$\cdot$kg$^{-1}\cdot$min^{-1} in a 6-year-old girl denotes the same aerobic fitness as an identical value in a 20-year-old woman. It is also fairly difficult to equate training dosages. Can one assume, for example, that weight training at 70% of their maximal voluntary contraction represents the same physiologic strain in a girl and a woman?

Because of such methodologic constraints, conclusions about the trainability of young girls are not definitive. Some patterns, however, seem to emerge. According to several reports, when prepubescent girls take part in aerobic training, they respond with little or no increase in maximal oxygen uptake, even though their athletic ability may improve.[52-55] This is unlike the response to aerobic training of women, who increase their maximal oxygen uptake and improve their athletic performance. Only a few studies have suggested that prepubescent females do improve their maximal oxygen uptake in response to aerobic training.[56]

A major reason for the improvement of running performance in the absence of increased $\dot{V}O_2$max is the training-induced improvement in running economy, which is manifested by a decrease in the O_2 cost of running. During adolescence, both aerobic power and running economy may improve with training.

Few studies are available on the trainability of muscle strength at different ages. Nielsen and co-workers[49] trained 249 Danish girls aged 7 to 19 years for 5 weeks. One subgroup did isometric knee extension, another the "vertical jump," and the third practiced acceleration in sprints. As in adults, there was *specificity* in the responses: each subgroup improved most in the specific strength (but not sprinting) task at which it had been training. While the authors did not report the pubertal stage of the subjects, the younger girls (less than 13.5 years) improved more than the older ones. Likewise, 8-year-old German girls improved their isometric arm strength more than did adults when given a similar training stimulus.[57] Whether trainability of strength is related to the pubertal stage has yet to be shown. Most research on muscle trainability of children is limited to boys. There are indications, however, that trainability during prepuberty is similar in boys and girls.[58] This is indirect evidence that training-induced strength gains can be achieved without the effect of androgens.

THERMOREGULATORY CAPACITY

Most research on the thermoregulatory characteristics of the exercising child is based on studies in boys. (For a review, see reference 59.) Data are available, however, to suggest that girls are at a disadvantage, compared with women, when exposed to either hot or cold climates. Very few data are available to compare the responses to heat and cold of prepubertal girls and boys.

Response to Hot Climate

Table 7–3 is a summary of the morphologic and physiologic characteristics of prepubescent females, as related to their thermoregulatory capability. As discussed earlier, the smaller the girl, the higher her $\dot{V}O_2$ per kilogram of body weight at any given walking or running speed. Because 75% to 80% or more of the chemical energy during

Table 7–3. MORPHOLOGIC AND PHYSIOLOGIC CHARACTERISTICS OF PREPUBESCENT GIRLS AS RELATED TO THERMOREGULATION

Characteristic or Function	Typical for Girls (Compared with Women)	Implication for Thermoregulation
O_2 cost of running/walking	Higher	High metabolic heat
Surface-to-mass ratio	Larger	Greater heat exchange with environment
Onset of sweating	Later	Greater reliance on convective heat loss
Sweating rate	Somewhat lower	Lower evaporative capacity
Blood flow, peripheral vs. central	Higher	1. Higher heat convection
		2. Lower venous return

muscle contraction is converted into heat, the metabolic heat load of the prepubescent girl is higher (by as much as 5% to 20%) than that of the adolescent or the adult, at equivalent walking or running tasks. Such a difference imposes a greater strain on the young, small girl's thermodissipatory system.

Another size-related difference is the larger skin surface-area–per–mass ratio in the smaller individual. The rate of heat exchange between the body and the environment depends on this surface area. Therefore, when the environment is warmer than the skin, the smaller the girl, the greater the heat gain (through conduction, convection, and radiation) per unit body mass. This difference in heat gain becomes particularly important in extreme climatic heat.

Evaporation of sweat is the main avenue for heat dissipation during exercise, especially in hot climates. When ambient temperature exceeds skin temperature, evaporation is the *only* available means of heat dissipation. Compared with women, prepubertal girls have a slow onset of sweating and a somewhat lower sweating rate while exercising in the heat,[60] which limit their capacity for evaporative cooling. This difference between prepubescents and adults seems to be even more apparent among males.

Girls were found to respond to exercise in the heat with a marked shift of blood from the central to the cutaneous vascular bed. Although greater skin blood flow facilitates greater convection of heat from the body core to the periphery (which, under certain climatic conditions, may compensate for a

low sweating capacity), it also decreases the venous return and stroke volume.[60] The resulting decrease in maximal cardiac output is another explanation for the low ability of prepubertal girls to exercise intensively in hot climates. It should be added that, at any given exercise level, even when performed in neutral environments, cardiac output in young girls is somewhat lower than that of women.[61]

In summary, these geometric and physiologic characteristics suggest that a priori young girls would tolerate exercise in hot climates less effectively than adolescent or adult females. It has indeed been shown that, during extreme climatic heat, prepubescent girls had to terminate their prescribed walking task earlier than did young women.[60,62] In thermoneutral environments, on the other hand, there is no evidence that young age or small body size is detrimental to thermoregulation.[63]

As recently shown,[64] the sweat of prepubescent girls has a lower concentration of sodium and chloride, and a higher concentration of potassium, than the sweat of adolescent females or of women. One possible implication of this difference is that the optimal electrolyte concentration of sports beverages may be different for prepubescent girls and for more mature females.

Response to Cold Climate

In most land-based sports, the rate of metabolic heat production exceeds heat loss, even when the environmental temperature is low. Such is the case, for example, in skating and cross-country skiing. In other winter sports, such as downhill skiing or curling, the rate of heat production may not be high, but clothing usually prevents excessive heat loss. Hypothermia occurs not infrequently in such sports as mountain climbing, snowshoeing, and even long-distance running at low intensity. There is, however, no epidemiologic evidence that prepubescent girls are more prone to hypothermia in these events than are older females.

In contrast, small individuals are at a distinct disadvantage during water-based activities. When swimming at a speed of 30 m/min in 20.3°C water, 8-year-old girls (club swimmers) had a drop in core temperature of as much as 2.5 to 3.0°C and had to be taken out of the water within 18 to 20 minutes owing to marked thermal discomfort. Their 16- to 19-year-old clubmates swam for some 30 minutes, with hardly any drop in core temperature and with little or no thermal discomfort.[65] The reason for the cold intolerance of the younger girls was their large surface area per mass, which facilitated conductive heat loss (water having a heat conductivity at least 25 times that of air). The authors also found that the leaner girls had a greater heat loss than those who had a thicker insulative subcutaneous fat layer.

High-Risk Groups for Heat- or Cold-Related Disorders

Some girls are at a potentially high risk for such heat-related disorders as heat exhaustion or heat stroke, while others may be prone to hypothermia.

Evidence is available that girls with anorexia nervosa have a deficient thermoregulatory capability, both in the heat and in the cold.[66,67] Patients with cystic fibrosis are prone to heat-related disorders,[68] possibly because of their abnormal sweating pattern. Undernourished children are prone to both hypothermia and hyperthermia.[69] Obese individuals perform well and feel comfortable in cold climates but are less tolerant to exercise in the heat than their leaner counterparts. Such intolerance has been documented for college-age women, although the findings for prepubertal girls were inconclusive.[62]

Hypohydration may often lead to heat-related disorders. While data are not available regarding the effects of hypohydration on the thermoregulation and health of prepubescent girls, data on boys suggest that, for a given level of hypohydration, children have a greater rise in core temperature than do young adults.[70] Conditions in which exertion may induce heat-related disorders through hypohydration are *diabetes mellitus, diabetes insipidus, diarrhea,* and *vomiting.* Prepubescent boys[70] and girls (unpublished data from my laboratory), like adults, undergo "voluntary hypohydration" when they exercise for long periods (e.g., 1 to 2 hours), even when fluids are available to them ad libitum. One group of young girls who are prone to hypohydration is those who compete in judo and "make weight" prior to competition. In some states where elementary school girls compete in wrestling, the same practice is probably followed.

Lack of acclimatization to exercise in the heat is perhaps the most important factor that predisposes an individual to heat-related disorders. Data suggest that 8- to 10-year-old boys take longer than adults to acclimatize to the heat.[71] No similar studies are available for girls, but it makes good sense to ensure that young female athletes are well acclimatized to the heat before they are expected to train hard and perform well in warm or humid climates.

As for hypothermia, a small, lean girl who is immersed in water is at a greater risk than a larger girl or one with thicker subcutaneous adipose tissue.

GROWTH, PUBERTAL CHANGES, AND ATHLETIC TRAINING

Trained prepubescent and adolescent girls often have different morphologic and maturational characteristics from those of their untrained counterparts. A question often asked by coaches, physicians, and parents is whether training *per se* affects growth, development, and maturation. To obtain a definitive answer, one would need to launch a prospective study in which nonathletic prepubescent girls are randomly assigned to training and control groups and then followed until after puberty. Such a project has yet to be launched. Data available at present are based on cross-sectional comparisons between athletes and nonathletes and among athletes of various specialties, or on retrospective analyses. The few longitudinal studies lack proper controls.[72] The conclusions derived from such studies therefore are tentative at best and cannot prove causality between training and changes in growth, development, and maturation.

The following are general comments, based on such studies. (For detailed reviews, see Malina,[73] Malina and co-workers,[74] and Wells.[75]) Various female athletes, primarily gymnasts, figure skaters, and ballet dancers, mature later and are shorter than the nonathletic female population. Others, notably swimmers, have little or no delay in maturation and are often taller than nonathletes.[72–74,76–78] These data might suggest that the above morphologic and maturational differences are caused by training. Such conclusions, however, ignore preselection and a possible bias in the drop-out pattern. It is likely, for example, that those girls with delayed puberty and short stature become preferentially attracted to such sports as gymnastics and figure skating, while the taller ones are more attracted to competitive swimming. A recent retrospective study[79] has shown that 8- to 14-year-old female gymnasts who were shorter than the nonathletic population had been shorter even prior to having joined the gymnastics program. Similarly, swimmers, who, as a group, were taller than their nonathletic counterparts, had been taller before training. It is also possible that, within a group of gymnasts, those females who mature early—and thus attain broad hips, relatively short legs, and higher body adiposity—drop out because of unfavorable changes in body mechanics.

Based on reports from the late 1970s and early 1980s, delayed menarche (defined as occurring after age 15 years) was particularly common among divers, figure skaters, gymnasts, and volleyball players.[73] Menarche is particularly delayed in those athletes who are engaged in high-dosage training. Delayed menarche in athletes seems also to correspond to delayed skeletal maturity.[73]

Several factors, singly or in combination, have been suggested to link delayed menarche to physical training. Among these are a low percentage of body fat,[80,81] insufficient calorie intake in conjunction with "energy drain,"[72] onset of training prior to menarche,[76] large sibship,[82] and emotional stress of training and competition. It has also been suggested,[83] but has yet to be confirmed, that hormonal changes which are associated with chronic exercise may be a cause for delayed menarche. In one study,[72] low serum gonadotropins—LH, particularly—were found in premenarcheal ballet dancers. Other endocrinologic studies are based on postmenarcheal athletes (see reference 84 for details).

In a comprehensive review on menarche in athletes, Malina[73] presented a two-part hypothesis on the possible relationship between physical activity and delayed menarche. First is the preselection by body characteristics, in which the girl with a linear physique, long legs, and narrow hips (who is often also a late maturer) is attracted to sports and eventually is successful in them. Second is the "socialization" process, in which early-maturing girls tend to interact socially in a nonsport environment with the appearance of pubertal changes. Conversely, the late maturers are more likely to find sports participation socially gratifying.

Indeed, preselection and the bias in dropping out from athletics may explain the late menarche of athletes as found in cross-sectional and retrospective analyses. One cannot ignore, however, the accumulating data on a more direct, possibly cause-and-effect, relationship between intense sports participation and secondary amenorrhea.

Although primary amenorrhea is a "normal" and common occurrence among athletes, one should not overlook the possibility that it might reflect gynecologic or other hormonal abnormalities. (For details of recommended investigations and of therapeutic approach, see Shangold in reference 85, as well as Chapter 8.)

COEDUCATIONAL PARTICIPATION IN CONTACT AND COLLISION SPORTS

Should prepubescent girls compete with boys in contact (e.g., wrestling, basketball, soccer) and collision (e.g., football, ice hockey) sports? This issue has become highly controversial, attracting media attention, because of its medical, educational, and cultural implications. The following comments are not meant to address the psychologic, sociologic, or ethical aspects of this controversy but only some of the physiologic and medical aspects.

A major issue is the added risk to health that participants of either sex group may incur owing to mixed participation. The main potential cause for such added risk is a marked difference in body mass, strength, or skill among the participants. At age 9 to 12 years, body mass of girls is similar to, or even slightly greater than, that of boys. Body height at that age range is quite similar in boys and girls, and the difference in the strength of various muscle groups is only about 1 to 2 kg in favor of the boys.[51] This is to be contrasted with the increasingly greater muscle strength of males—particularly in the upper body—after puberty.[86] The attainment of such motor skills as throwing, kicking, catching, jumping, hopping, and skipping during the first years of life is similar in boys and girls. Throughout the prepubertal years, these and other motor skills seem to develop and improve at a similar pace in both sex groups.[87]

It should be realized that, at any given chronologic age around puberty, differences in body size and strength of early and late maturers *within* a gender group far surpass the *intergender* differences. Nor is there any evidence to suggest that prepubescent girls are less capable of learning sport skills, are less agile, or have less stamina than boys.[87,88] While not addressing specifically the prepubescent girl, a recent review on orthopedic issues in the young female athlete[89] points out the emergence of "overuse injuries" during the teens. It rejects, however, the notion that girls are more prone to injury than boys.

Based on anthropometric and fitness-related considerations alone, therefore, prepubescent girls can compete successfully with boys in contact and collision sports, and with no undue risk to health. An early maturing girl, in point of fact, may have an edge over boys who are average maturers. It seems as though matching of prepubescent and circumpubescent opponents by body size and maturation level has more relevance to health than the separation into gender groups.

SUMMARY

The physiologic responses to exercise in the prepubescent girl are of a similar pattern to those of the more mature female. There are, however, some age- or development-related differences in these responses. The submaximal O_2 cost during walking or running is higher in the young girl, which causes a lower "metabolic reserve" and early fatigability in endurance events. Likewise, anaerobic muscle power and local muscle endurance are markedly lower in prepubescents, who are therefore unlikely to compete successfully with their older counterparts in events such as jumping and sprinting. Girls are less-effective thermoregulators when exercising in the heat and in the cold. This has implications both to their performance and to their health. Girls with obesity and anorexia nervosa are at special risk for heat-related illness. Although more research is needed, it appears that the training-induced improvement in maximal aerobic power is low before puberty.

A causal relationship among training, growth, and maturation has yet to be established. It seems, however, that the delayed menarche in athletes may be in part a result of intense training.

While coeducational participation in contact and collision sports may be objected to on psychologic and societal grounds, there are no physiologic or medical reasons to ban such activities before puberty.

REFERENCES

1. Åstrand PO: Experimental Studies of Physical Working Capacity in Relation to Sex and Age. Munksgaard, Copenhagen, 1952.
2. Bar-Or O: Pediatric Sports Medicine for the Practitioner: From Physiologic Principles to Clinical Applications. Springer Verlag, New York, 1983.
3. Godfrey S: Exercise Testing in Children. Applications in Health and Disease. WB Saunders, Philadelphia, 1974.
4. Shephard RJ: Physical Activity and Growth. Year Book Medical Publishers, Chicago, 1982.
5. Malina RM, and Bouchard C: Growth, Maturation, and Physical Activity. Human Kinetics, Champaign, IL, 1991.
6. Rowland TW: Exercise and Children's Health. Human Kinetics, Champaign, IL, 1990.
7. Smith NJ (ed): Sports Medicine for Young Athletes. American Academy of Pediatrics, Evanston, IL, 1983.
8. Boileau RA (ed): Advances in Pediatric Sport Sciences, Vol 1. Human Kinetics, Champaign, IL, 1984.
9. Bar-Or O (ed): Advances in Pediatric Sport Sciences, Vol 3. Human Kinetics, Champaign, IL, 1989.
10. Gisolfi CV, and Lamb DR (eds): Perspectives in Exercise Science and Sports Medicine, Vol 2. Benchmark Press, Indianapolis, 1989.
11. Bar-Or O (ed): Pediatric Work Physiology. Wingate Institute, Natanya, Israel, 1973.
12. Berg K, and Eriksson BO (eds): Children and Exercise IX. University Park Press, Baltimore, 1980.
13. Binkhorst RA, Kemper HCG, and Saris WHM: Children and Exercise XI. Human Kinetics, Champaign, IL, 1985.
14. Borms J, and Hebbelinck M (eds): Children and Exercise. Acta Paediatr Belg (Suppl 28):1, 1974.
15. Borms J, and Hebbelinck M (eds): Pediatric Work Physiology. Karger, Basel, 1978.
16. Ilmarinen J, and Valimaki I: Pediatric Work Physiology X. Springer Verlag, Berlin, 1983.
17. Lavallee H, and Shephard RJ (eds): Frontiers of Activity and Child Health. Pelican, Quebec, 1977.
18. Rutenfranz J (ed): Pediatric Work Physiology XII. Human Kinetics, Champaign, IL, 1986.
19. Thoren C (ed): Pediatric Work Physiology. Acta Paediatr Scand (Suppl 213):1, 1971.
20. Frenkel R, and Szmodis I (eds): Children and Exercise. Pediatric Work Physiology XV. Signet, Budapest, Hungary, 1991.
21. Simons J, Beunen GP, Renson R, et al (eds): Growth and Fitness of Flemish Girls: The Leuven Growth Study. Human Kinetics, Champaign, IL, 1990.
22. MacDougall JD, Roche PD, Bar-Or O, et al: Maximal aerobic power of Canadian school children: Prediction based on age-related cost of running. Int J Sports Med 4:194, 1983.
23. Robinson S: Experimental studies of physical fitness in relation to age. Int Z Angew Physiol Einschl Arbeitphysiol 10:251, 1938.
24. Skinner JS, Bar-Or O, Bergsteinová V, et al: Comparison of continuous and intermittent test for determining maximal oxygen uptake in children. Acta Paediatr Scand (Suppl 217):24, 1971.
25. Rowland TW, and Green GM: Physiological responses to treadmill exercise in females: Adult-child differences. Med Sci Sports Exerc 20:474, 1988.
26. Bal MER, Thompson EM, McIntosh EH, et al: Mechanical efficiency in cycling of girls six to fourteen years of age. J Appl Physiol 6:185, 1953.
27. Girandola RN, Wiswell RA, Frisch F, et al: Metabolic differences during exercise in pre- and post-pubescent girls (abstract). Med Sci Sports Exerc 13:110, 1981.
28. Wilmore JH, and Sigerset PO: Physical work capacity of young girls 7–13 years of age. J Appl Physiol 22:923, 1967.
29. Chatterjee S, Banerjee PK, Chatterjee P, et al: Aerobic capacity of young girls. Indian J Med Res 69:327, 1979.
30. Drinkwater BL, Horvath SM, and Wells CL: Aerobic power of females, ages 10 to 68. J Gerontol 30:385, 1975.
31. Forbes GB, and Amirhakimi GH: Skinfold thickness and body fat in children. Hum Biol 42:401, 1970.
32. Karlberg P, and Taranger J: The somatic development of children in a Swedish urban community. Acta Paediatr Scand (Suppl):258, 1977.
33. Sunnegardh J: Physical activity in relation to

energy intake, body fat, physical work capacity and muscle strength in 8- and 13-year-old children in Sweden. Doctoral dissertation, University of Uppsala, Uppsala, 1986.

34. Huenemann RL, Shapiro LR, Hampton MC, et al: Teenagers' activities and attitudes toward activity. J Am Diet Assoc 51:433, 1967.

35. Ilmarinen J, and Rutenfranz J: Longitudinal studies of the changes in habitual physical activity of schoolchildren and working adolescents. In Berg K, and Eriksson BO (eds): Children and Exercise IX, University Park Press, Baltimore, 1980, p 149.

36. Telama R: Secondary School Pupils' Physical Activity and Leisure-Time Sports, Vol III (in Finnish). Institute of Educational Research, University of Jyvaskyla, Report No. 107, Jyvaskyla, Finland, 1971.

37. Verschuur R, and Kemper HCG: The pattern of daily physical activity. In Kemper HCG (ed): Growth, Health and Fitness of Teenagers (Medicine and Sport Science, Vol 20). Karger, Basel, 1985, p 169.

38. Cooper DM, Weiler-Ravell D, Whipp BJ, et al: Growth-related changes in oxygen uptake and heart rate during progressive exercise in children. Pediatr Res 18:845, 1984.

39. Davies CTM, Barnes C, and Godfrey S: Body composition and maximal exercise performance in children. Hum Biol 44:195, 1972.

40. Yoshizawa S, Ishizaki T, and Honda H: Physical fitness of children aged 5 and 6 years. J Hum Ergol (Tokyo) 6:41, 1977.

41. Burmeister W, Rutenfranz J, Stresny W, et al: Body cell mass and physical performance capacity (W_{170}) of school children. Int Z Angew Physiol Einschl Arbeitphysiol 31:61, 1972.

42. Margaria R, Aghemo P, and Rovelli E: Measurement of muscular power (anaerobic) in man. J Appl Physiol 21:1662, 1966.

43. Bar-Or O: The Wingate Anaerobic Test. Characteristics and applications (in French). Symbioses 13:157, 1981.

44. DiPrampero PE, and Cerretelli P: Maximal muscular power (aerobic and anaerobic) in African natives. Ergonomics 12:51, 1969.

45. Kuroski TT: Anaerobic power of children from ages 9 through 15 years. M.Sc. Thesis, Florida State University, 1977.

46. Blimkie JR, Roache P, Hay JT, and Bar-Or O: Anaerobic power of arms in teenage boys and girls: Relationship to lean tissue. Eur J Appl Physiol 57:677, 1988.

47. Asmussen E: Growth in muscular strength and power. In Rarick L (ed): Physical Activity, Human Growth and Development. Academic Press, New York, 1973, p 60.

48. Clarke HH: Physical and motor tests in the Medford Boys' Growth Study. Prentice-Hall, Englewood Cliffs, NJ, 1971.

49. Nielsen B, Nielsen K, Behrendt Hansen M,

et al: Training of "functional muscular strength" in girls 7–19 years old. In Ber K and Eriksson B (eds): Pediatric Work Physiology IX. University Park Press, Baltimore, 1980, p 69.

50. Beunen G, Malina RM, Van'Thof MA, et al: Timing of adolescent changes in motor performance. Symposium on Maturation and Growth, ACSM, Nashville, 1985.

51. Malina RM: Growth, strength and physical performance. In Stull GA (ed): Encyclopedia of Physical Education, Fitness and Sports: Training, Environment, Nutrition and Fitness. Brighton Publishing, Salt Lake City, UT, 1980, p 443.

52. Bar-Or O, and Zwiren LD: Physiological effects of increased frequency of physical education classes and of endurance conditioning on 9- to 10-year-old girls and boys. In Bar-Or O (ed): Pediatric Work Physiology. Wingate Institute, Natanya, Israel, 1973, p 183.

53. Gilliam TB, and Freedson PS: Effects of a 12-week school physical education program on peak $\dot{V}O_2$, body composition and blood lipids in 7 to 9 year old children. Int J Sports Med 1:73, 1980.

54. Mocellin R, and Wasmund U: Investigations of the influence of a running-training programme on the cardiovascular and motor performance capacity in 53 boys and girls of a second and third primary school class. In Bar-Or O (ed): Pediatric Work Physiology. Wingate Institute, Natanya, Israel, 1973, p 279.

55. Yoshida T, Ishiko T, and Muraoka I: Effect of endurance training on cardiorespiratory functions of 5-year-old children. Int J Sports Med 1:91, 1980.

56. Brown CH, Harrower Jr, and Deeter MF: The effects of cross-country running on pre-adolescent girls. Med Sci Sports Exerc 4:1, 1972.

57. Rohmert W: Rechts-links-Vergleich bei isometrichem Armmuskeltraining mit verschiedenem Trainingsreiz bei achtjarigen Kindren. Int Z Angew Physiol Einschl Arbeitphysiol 26:363, 1968.

58. Siegel JA, Camaione DN, and Manfredi TG: The effects of upper body resistance training on prepubescent children. Pediatr Exerc Sci, 1:145, 1989.

59. Bar-Or O: Climate and the exercising child— a review. Int J Sports Med 1:53, 1980.

60. Drinkwater BL, Kuppart IC, Denton JE, et al: Response of prepubertal girls and college women to work in the heat. J Appl Physiol 43:1046, 1977.

61. Bar-Or O, Shephard RJ, and Allan CL: Cardiac output of 10- to 13-year-old boys and girls during submaximal exercise. J Appl Physiol 30:219, 1971.

62. Haymes EM, Buskirk ER, Hodgson JL, et al:

Heat tolerance of exercising lean and heavy prepubertal girls. J Appl Physiol 36:566, 1974.

63. Davies CTM: Thermal responses to exercise in children. Ergonomics 24:55, 1981.

64. Meyer F, Bar-Or O, MacDougall JD, and Heigenhauser JF: Sweat electrolyte loss during exercise in the heat: Effects of gender and level of maturity. Med Sci Sports Exerc 24:776, 1992.

65. Sloan REG, and Keatinge WR: Cooling rates of young people swimming in cold water. J Appl Physiol 35:371, 1973.

66. Davies CTM, Fohlin L, and Thoren C: Thermoregulation in anorexia nervosa patients. In Borms J, and Hebbelinck M (eds): Pediatric Work Physiology. Karger, Basel, 1978, p 96.

67. Wakeling A, and Russel GFM: Disturbances in the regulation of body temperature in anorexia nervosa. Psychol Med 1:30, 1970.

68. Kessler WR, and Andersen DH: Heat prostration in fibrocystic disease of the pancreas and other conditions. Pediatrics 8:648, 1951.

69. Brooke OG: Thermal insulation in malnourished Jamaican children. Arch Dis Child 48:901, 1973.

70. Bar-Or O, Dotan R, Inbar O, et al: Voluntary hypohydration in 10- to 12-year-old boys. J Appl Physiol 48:104, 1980.

71. Inbar O: Acclimatization to dry and hot environment in young adults and children 8–10 years old. Ed.D. dissertation. Columbia University, New York, 1978.

72. Warren MP: The effects of exercise on pubertal progression and reproductive function in girls. J Clin Endocrinol Metab 51:1150, 1980.

73. Malina RM: Menarche in athletes: A synthesis and hypothesis. Ann Hum Biol 10:1, 1983.

74. Malina RM, Meleski BW, and Shoup RF: Anthropometric, body composition, and maturity characteristics of selected school-age athletes. Pediatr Clin North Am 29:1305, 1982.

75. Wells CL: Women, Sport and Performance—A Physiological Perspective. Human Kinetics, Champaign, IL, 1985.

76. Frisch RE, Gotz-Welbergen AV, McArthur JW, et al: Delayed menarche and amenorrhea of college athletes in relation to age of onset of training. JAMA 246:1559, 1981.

77. Malina RM, Harper AB, Avent HH, et al: Age at menarche in athletes and non-athletes. Med Sci Sports 5:11, 1973.

78. Malina RM, Spirduso WW, Tate C, et al: Age at menarche and selected menstrual characteristics in athletes at different competitive levels and in different sports. Med Sci Sports 10:218, 1978.

79. Peltenburg AL, Erich WBM, Bernink MJE, et al: Biological maturation, body composition, and growth of female gymnasts and control groups of school girls and girl swimmers, aged 8 to 14 years: A cross-sectional survey of 1064 girls. Int J Sports Med 5:36, 1984.

80. Frisch RE, Wyshak G, and Vincent L: Delayed menarche and amenorrhea in ballet dancers. N Engl J Med 303:17, 1980.

81. Vanderbroucke JP, van Leer A, and Valkenburg HA: Synergy between thinness and intensive sports activity in delaying menarche. Br Med J 284:1907, 1982.

82. Malina RM, Bouchard C, Shoup RF, et al: Age at menarche, family size, and birth order in athletes at the Montreal Olympic Games. Med Sci Sports 11:354, 1979.

83. Brisson GR, Volle MA, DeCarufel D, et al: Exercise-induced dissociation of blood prolactin response in young women according to their sports habits. Horm Metab Res 12:201, 1980.

84. Shangold MM: Exercise and the adult female: Hormonal and endocrine effects. In Terjung RL (ed): Exercise and Sports Sciences Reviews, Vol 12. Collamore Press, Lexington, MA, 1984, p 53.

85. Shangold MM: Gynecological concerns in young and adolescent physically active girls. Pediatrician 13:10, 1986.

86. Montoye HJ, and Lamphier DE: Grip and arm strength in males and females, age 10 to 69. Res Q Am Assoc Health Phys Ed 48:109, 1977.

87. Branta C, Haubenstricker J, and Seefeldt V: Age changes in motor skills during childhood and adolescence. In Terjung RL (ed): Exercise and Sports Sciences Reviews, Vol 12. Collamore Press, Lexington, MA, 1984, p 467.

88. Rarick GL, and Dobbins DA: Basic components in the motor performance of children six to nine years of age. Med Sci Sports 7:105, 1975.

89. Micheli LJ, and LaChabrier L: The young female athlete. In Micheli LJ (ed): Pediatric and Adolescent Sport Medicine. Little, Brown, Boston, 1984, p 167.

CHAPTER 8

Growth, Performance, Activity, and Training during Adolescence

ROBERT M. MALINA, Ph.D.

Adolescence is a period of transition from childhood to adulthood. It includes changes in the biologic, personal, and social domains that prepare the young girl for adulthood in her particular culture. Thus, the biologic changes that occur during puberty, or sexual maturation, do not occur in isolation; rather, they are related to other developmental events so that any consideration of this period of life must be done in a biosocial or biocultural context.

Biologically, adolescence may be viewed as beginning with an acceleration in the rate of growth (i.e., an increase in size) prior to the attainment of sexual maturity, then merging into a decelerative phase, and eventually terminating with the cessation of growth. The latter is most often viewed as the attainment of adult stature. Sexual maturity and growth are thus closely related.

The events that constitute this phase of the life cycle include changes in the nervous and endocrine systems that initiate and coordinate the sexual, physiologic, and somatic changes; growth and maturation of the primary (ovaries, vagina, and uterus) and secondary (breasts and pubic hair) sex characteristics, leading to menarche and reproductive function; changes in size (i.e., the adolescent growth spurt); changes in proportions, physique, and body composition; and changes in the cardiorespiratory system, among others. The two most prominent outward features of adolescence (excluding behavior) are accelerated growth and appearance of secondary sex characteristics, which appear, on the average, during the second decade of life. However, the neuroendocrine and other physiologic events underlying growth and pubertal change have been in progress for some time prior to the appearance of physical changes. The time span accommodating the growth spurt and puberty is thus wide. It can vary from 8 or 9 years through 17 or 18 years of age in girls, and in some cases may continue into the early 20s. There is variation between individuals in the time and rate at which the structural and functional changes occur; that is, the changes do not begin at the same time and do not proceed at the same rate.

THE ADOLESCENT GROWTH SPURT

Body Size

From birth to adulthood, both height and weight follow a four-phased or double-sigmoid growth pattern: rapid gain in infancy and early childhood; slower, relatively constant gain in middle childhood; rapid gain during adolescence; and slow increase and eventual cessation of growth at the attainment of adult size. Most dimensions of the body—sitting height, leg length, shoulder and hip breadths, limb circumferences, muscle mass, and so on—follow a similar growth pattern. What varies is the timing, tempo, and intensity of the adolescent growth spurt in each. For example, maximum growth (peak velocity) in leg length occurs early in the growth spurt, prior to that for sitting height or trunk length, while maximum growth in body weight occurs after peak height velocity (PHV).

The timing of the growth spurt varies considerably among children. Most data are available for stature. According to data from several longitudinal studies, the adolescent growth spurt (i.e., the acceleration in rate of growth that marks the take-off of the spurt)

starts in some girls as early as 7 or 8 years of age and in others as late as 12 or 13 years, while the age at maximum rate of growth in stature (PHV) occurs in some girls as early as 9 or 10 years of age and in others as late as 13 to 15 years.[1]

Body Composition

The fat-free mass (FFM) of girls, estimated from body density, increases from about 25 kg at 10 years to about 45 kg at 18 years of age, whereas muscle mass, estimated from creatinine excretion, increases from about 12 kg at 10 years to 23 kg at 18 years.[1] However, the major portion of change in FFM and muscle mass between 10 and 18 years occurs during the interval of maximal growth (about 11 to 13 years in girls). This interval includes PHV, which occurs, on average, at about 12 years of age in girls. The adolescent gain in FFM and muscle mass during female adolescence is not, however, as intense as that in males, so that by late adolescence, females attain only about two thirds of the estimated mean values reported for males. Peak velocities of growth in arm and calf musculature occur, on average, after PHV.

Fatness also increases during adolescence, but estimates are highly variable. Densitometric estimates increase from 18% body fat at about 10 years of age to 23% at 18 years.[1] These estimates are adjusted for changes in the estimated chemical composition of FFM (i.e., density of FFM, potassium and water content of FFM) that occur during growth and are lower than those based on adult chemical composition figures. At the time of the growth spurt, however, the rate of fat accumulation slows down in girls. This is especially apparent on the extremities during the interval of PHV in girls.

MENARCHE

The age at menarche is perhaps the most commonly reported developmental milestone of female adolescence. It is, however, a rather late maturational event. Menarche occurs after maximum growth in stature; the average difference between menarche and PHV in a number of studies is about 1.2 to 1.3 years.[1]

Menarche in American girls occurs, on average, just before the 13th birthday. However, there is variability within the U.S. population. In the National Health Examination Survey in the 1960s, the median ages at menarche were 12.5 years for black girls and 12.8 years for white girls.[2] The median age at menarche in American girls has not changed, on average, since the 1950s.[3] Estimates for a number of European samples vary between 12.5 and 13.4 years.[1,4]

In contrast to population surveys of menarche, in which the average age for the population is estimated mathematically on the basis of the number of girls in each age group who have attained menarche, many studies of athletes and of the influence of training on the age at menarche use the retrospective method. This approach relies on the memory of the individual and thus has the limitation of error in recall.

PHYSICAL PERFORMANCE AND ACTIVITY DURING ADOLESCENCE

Characteristics of the adolescent growth spurt and sexual maturation, and of interrelationships among indices of sexual, skeletal, and somatic maturity, are reasonably well documented. Changes in physical performance and activity during female adolescence are less well documented. The data are largely cross-sectional, with but few longitudinal observations spanning the immediate prepubertal and pubertal years.

Strength

Muscular strength improves linearly with age from early childhood through about 15 years of age in girls, with no clear evidence of an adolescent spurt. After age 15, strength of an adolescent spurt. After age 15, strength improves more slowly.[1] This pattern is in contrast to the marked acceleration of strength development during male adolescence, so that sex differences in muscular strength are considerable.

The relationship between strength development and the growth spurt and sexual maturation in girls is not as clear as in boys. Maximum strength development occurs, on the average, after peak height and weight velocity in boys, the relationship being better with weight than with height.[1,5] In girls, the available longitudinal data vary. In the Oakland (California) Growth Study, the time of maximum strength development (a composite strength score of right and left grip and pushing and pulling tests) does not closely correspond to the growth spurt in stature, and a significant percentage of girls experience peak strength gains prior to PHV.[6] Peak strength gain precedes peak weight gain in more than half of the girls, and follows peak weight gain in only about one fourth. On the other hand, in the study of Dutch girls (Growth and Health of Teenagers), peak development of strength (arm pull test) occurs, on average, one-half year after PHV (the same time as it occurs in Dutch boys).[7] The maximum gain in strength at this time is about 6.0 kg/y in girls, which contrasts with a maximum gain of 12.0 kg/y in Dutch boys.[7] The data for Dutch girls are not expressed relative to peak gain in body weight.

Early-maturing girls are slightly stronger than late-maturing girls of the same chronologic age during early adolescence, about 11 through 13 years.[1] The differences between girls of contrasting maturity status, however, do not persist and are no longer evident by 14 to 15 years of age. Further, the differences in muscular strength between girls of contrasting maturity status during adolescence are not as marked as those between early- and late-maturing boys. The strength advantage of girls advanced in maturity status between 11 and 13 years reflects the larger body size of early maturers, since strength is positively related to body mass. When strength is expressed per unit body weight, early maturers have less strength per unit body weight than late-maturing girls; this difference persists through adolescence.[1]

Motor Performance

Average performances of girls in a variety of motor tasks (dash, standing long jump, jump and reach, distance throw, and others) improve more or less linearly from childhood through about 13 or 14 years of age, followed by a plateau in the ability to perform some tasks and a decline in others.[1,8,9] In most tasks, the average performances of girls fall within one standard deviation of the boys' averages in early adolescence. After 13 to 14 years of age, however, the average performances of girls are often outside the limits defined by one standard deviation below the boys' mean performance. Overhand throwing performance is an exception; few girls approximate the throwing performances of boys at all ages from late childhood on.

Longitudinal data relating the motor performance of girls to the timing of the adolescent growth spurt are not available. Cross-sectional analysis of longitudinal data does not suggest adolescent spurts in the motor performances of girls. Performances in a variety of motor tasks show no tendency to peak before, at, or after menarche (which occurs, on average, about 1 year after PHV); rather, performances are generally stable across time.[5] Among boys, on the other hand, motor performances show rather clear adolescent spurts. Maximal gains in functional strength and power tests (flexed arm hang and vertical jump) occur, on average, after PHV, whereas maximal gains in speed tests (shuttle run, speed of hand movement) and flexibility (sit and reach) occur before PHV.[10]

Correlations between skeletal and sexual maturity and motor performance in girls are low and, for many tasks, negative. The latter suggests that later maturation is more often associated with better motor performance in girls, whereas the opposite is more often true in boys.[1,11,12] For example, a comparison of high- and low-performing girls indicated that the superior performers were about 0.5 year less mature skeletally and 0.4 year later in menarche.[12] This trend is apparent in elite female athletes (i.e., skilled performers), who tend to be later in age at menarche and delayed in skeletal maturation.[13,14]

Maximal Aerobic Power

Absolute maximal oxygen uptake (mL/min) has a growth pattern in girls similar to that for motor performance: it increases linearly with age from 7 years through 13 to 14 years in untrained girls, and then declines slightly.[15] In contrast, in untrained boys, it increases linearly with age through adolescence, so that by 16 years of age the difference between maximal oxygen uptake in untrained boys and girls is about 56%. When expressed relative to body weight ($mL \cdot kg^{-1} \cdot min^{-1}$), aerobic power declines with age from 6 through 16 years in untrained girls, but is more or less constant in untrained boys. The slope of the regression in girls declines from a value of 52.0 $mL \cdot kg^{-1} \cdot min^{-1}$ at 6 years of age to 40.5 $mL \cdot kg^{-1} \cdot min^{-1}$ at 16 years. Values for untrained boys at corresponding ages are 52.8 and 53.5 $mL \cdot kg^{-1} \cdot min^{-1}$, respectively, yielding a negligible sex difference of 1.5% at 6 years, but a considerable difference of 32% at 16 years.[15]

The sex difference in aerobic power per unit of body weight at 16 years of age is probably related to sex differences in body composition. The aerobic power of girls per unit of body weight is approximately 77% of the value for boys. This percentage is not too different from estimates of lean body and muscle mass in late adolescence; that is, girls attain, on the average, only about two thirds of the values for boys. The increase in relative fatness associated with the sexual maturation of girls probably contributes to the sex difference in aerobic power per unit of body weight.

Absolute aerobic power (mL/min) shows a clear adolescent spurt in both girls and boys, which on average occurs close to that for stature.[16] This reflects the growth of heart and lung functions in proportion to overall body size.[1] Given the size differences between early- and late-maturing girls, the former have a slightly larger absolute aerobic power, especially during early adolescence. When expressed per unit of body weight, however, relative aerobic power is higher in late maturers.[17]

Aerobic power responds positively to training, so that absolute and relative maximal oxygen uptakes are greater in trained than in untrained girls at all ages. The differences between trained and untrained girls are greatest during adolescence. It is also interesting to note that trained girls and boys differ by only 24% for absolute and 18% for relative oxygen uptake at age 16, in contrast to comparable differences of 56% and 32% in untrained boys and girls of the same age.[15]

Studies of aerobic power seldom control for the maturity status of the subjects, and the few studies that do are largely limited to boys. Correlations between skeletal age and aerobic power are generally low,[15] but the association between body mass and skeletal maturity confounds the relationship.[1]

Physical Activity Habits

Physical activity is a major component of the daily energy expenditure. Energy expenditure in free-living children and youth is difficult to measure, and the few available studies are limited to rather small samples with narrow age ranges, and largely to boys.[18] Standardized questionnaires, interviews, and diaries are often used to estimate physical activity habits in large samples of youngsters, usually 10 years of age and older. The data, however, are largely descriptive and do not consider growth and maturity characteristics. Results of several surveys of European, Canadian, and American youth indicate a slight decline in time spent in physical activity by girls during adolescence.[18] In the United States survey,[19] for example, the average weekly time engaged in physical activity outside of school physical education was 11.5 hours in grades 5 and 6 (10 to 11 years), 12.5 hours in grades 7

through 9 (12 to 14 years), and 11.8 hours in grades 11 and 12 (15 to 17 years). Although the data suggest a trend, more specific changes with age cannot be examined. In a mixed-longitudinal sample of Dutch girls,[20] the average number of hours per week spent in physical activity with an average energy expenditure of 4 metabolic equivalents (METs) or more declined from 9.6 hours at 12 to 13 years to 8.1 hours at 17 to 18 years. The earlier adolescent years were not considered.

Intensity is a critical variable when considering physical activity. In the mixed-longitudinal Dutch study, girls aged 12 to 13 participated, on the average, in only 4.0 h/wk of activities of medium intensity (7 to 10 METs), and 0.5/h/wk in activities of heavy intensity (10+ METs). By 17 to 18 years, the corresponding hours per week were 1.5 and 0.3.[20] Clearly, the majority of the activities of these girls were of light intensity.

Given the type of data available, it is difficult to make inferences about activity habits during the adolescent growth spurt and sexual maturation, as well as about possible effects of rapid growth and maturation on activity habits. The figures do suggest, however, that most adolescent girls are not getting sufficient regular physical activity to maintain a high level of aerobic fitness.

Significance of the Adolescent Plateau in Performance

Data relating the physical performance of girls to the timing of the growth spurt and sexual maturation are not extensive. A question that merits more detailed study is the relative flatness of the performance curves of girls during adolescence. That is, their level of performance shows little improvement in many tasks after 13 to 14 years of age, and in some tasks it actually declines. Is this trend related primarily to biologic changes in female adolescence (e.g., sexual maturation, fat accumulation, physique changes), or is it related to cultural factors (e.g., changing social interests and expectations, pressure from peers, lack of motivation, limited opportunities to participate in performance-related physical activities)? Most likely both biologic and cultural factors are reflected in the trend. Thus, the overall age-related pattern of physical performance during female adolescence may change with the recent emphasis on and opportunity for athletic competition for young girls, and the wider acceptability of women in the role of athlete.

INFLUENCE OF TRAINING ON THE TEMPO OF GROWTH AND MATURATION DURING ADOLESCENCE

Under adequate environmental conditions, the timing of the adolescent growth spurt and sexual maturation is genetically determined. However, these processes can be influenced by environmental factors. The delaying effects of chronic undernutrition are well documented. Socioeconomic variation in growth and maturation is evident in some societies but not in others.[1] Criteria of socioeconomic status, of course, vary from country to country, but data from industrialized countries indicate inconsistent trends in ages at PHV and menarche relative to indices of socioeconomic status. Another factor related to age at menarche is the number of children in the family. Girls from larger families tend to experience menarche later than those from smaller families, and this applies to athletes as well as nonathletes. The estimated effect of each additional sibling on the age at menarche ranges from 0.11 to 0.22 years in several samples of athletes and nonathletes.[21]

Stressful life events are also significant. They are especially evident in the growth and maturation of youngsters experiencing disturbed home environments,[22] and in the "unusually 'fractured' curves of growth and pubertal development in girls translated to unfamiliar boarding schools at various times in puberty."[23] Studies of secular change in menarche suggest that the timing of this maturational event may be programmed by conditions early in life and not necessarily by those conditions that may be operating at or about the time of puberty.[24,25]

A question of concern, therefore, is the role of intensive training for sport and perhaps of the stress of competition on the timing and tempo of growth and sexual maturation during adolescence. *It should be obvious that physical activity is only one of the many factors that may influence growth and maturation.*

Stature and Body Composition

Regular physical training has no apparent effect on statural growth. It is, however, a significant factor in the regulation of body weight and composition, specifically fatness. Changes in response to short- or long-term training programs largely reflect fluctuating levels of fatness, with minimal or no change in FFM. The role of regular activity in the development of adipose tissue cellularity and subcutaneous fat distribution is not clearly established.[26]

Regular training is a significant factor in the growth and integrity of skeletal and muscle tissues. Changes in bone tissue include greater mineralization, density, and mass. Training-associated changes in muscle tissue are generally specific to the type of program followed. Strength or resistance training is associated with hypertrophy, whereas endurance training is associated with increases in oxidative enzymes. The direction of responses to training in growing individuals is similar to those observed in adults, but the magnitude of the responses varies.[26]

The persistence of beneficial training effects on adipose and muscular tissues depends upon continued activity. In contrast, evidence is accumulating that excessive training associated with altered menstrual function (see below and Chapter 9) and diet contributes to bone loss in some athletes.[27,28] Thus, there may be a threshold for some adolescent athletes: regular training has a beneficial effect on the integrity of skeletal tissue up to a point, but excessive activity may alter menstrual function and have a negative influence on bone mass.

Sexual Maturation

Longitudinal data on the effects of training on sexual maturation of girls (and boys too) are lacking, and the available cross-sectional data do not indicate a significant effect of training on sexual maturation. Much of the discussion of training and sexual maturation is based on comparisons of later mean ages at menarche of athletes with those of the general population, with the inference that intensive training for sport "delays" menarche.[13] The menarcheal data are generally consistent with observations of breast and pubic-hair development and skeletal maturity of young athletes engaged in figure skating, ballet, gymnastics, and track—that is, they develop later.[14] However, girls training for sport at prepubertal ages are not necessarily representative of those who are successful at later ages, who in turn constitute the samples of athletes upon whom most menarcheal data are based. Also, Title IX legislation has influenced sport opportunity for girls and women, so that many now continue to train and compete through the college years. In the not-too-distant past, on the other hand, many young girls stopped training and competing at 16 or 17 years of age. The opportunity provided by Title IX most likely has influenced the composition of the female athlete population at the college level, particularly in swimming. The age at menarche in college-age swimmers in recent estimates[21,29] is considerably older than that of elite swimmers about 20 years ago,[13] and this is in contrast to the advanced pubertal status and skeletal maturity often observed in age group swimmers.[14]

Although not the first to suggest that training may delay menarche, Frisch and colleagues[30] concluded that for every year a girl trains before menarche, her menarche will be delayed by up to 5 months. This conclusion is based on a correlation of $+0.53$

between years of training before menarche and age at menarche, a moderate correlation that accounts for only about 28% of the sample variance. Correlation does not imply a cause-and-effect sequence, however; the association is more likely an artifact. The older a girl is at menarche, the more likely she would have begun her training prior to menarche, and conversely, the younger a girl is at menarche, the more likely she would have begun training after menarche or would have a shorter period of training prior to menarche.[29] It could also be that later maturation is a factor in a girl's decision to take up sport, rather than the training causing the lateness.[13] Further, athletes as a group tend to be rather select, and other factors known to influence menarche are not considered in the analysis.

It has also been suggested that menarche occurs later specifically in those disciplines that emphasize low body weight, such as ballet and gymnastics.[31] Emphasis on low body weight may involve dietary practices that adversely influence maturation, so that it would be difficult to partition dietary from training effects. In addition, such sports tend to have rather rigorous selection criteria, which are often applied early in childhood and which favor the morphologic characteristics of the late-maturing girl. Finally, data for elite university-level athletes indicate later mean ages at menarche in athletes across several sports that differ considerably in training load and emphasis on body weight: diving, track and field, swimming, tennis, golf, basketball, and volleyball.[21]

Nevertheless, two questions merit consideration. First, are regular, intensive, prepubertal training for sport and regular competition sufficiently stressful to prolong the prepubertal state and in turn delay the adolescent growth spurt and sexual maturation? Second, do intensive training for sport and the stress of competition during the adolescent growth spurt and sexual maturation produce conditions that are sufficiently adverse to influence the progress and thus the timing of these maturational events?

Hormonal Responses

The suggested mechanism for the association between training and later menarche is hormonal. It is suggested that intensive training and perhaps the associated energy drain influence circulating levels of gonadotropic and ovarian hormones, and in turn, menarche.

Exercise is an effective means of stressing the hypothalamic-pituitary-ovarian axis, producing short-term increases in serum levels of all gonadotropic and sex steroid hormones.[32,33] Other factors also influence hormonal levels, including diurnal variation, state of feeding or fasting, emotional states, and so on, and these need to be considered. Further, virtually all hormones are episodically secreted, so that studies of hormonal responses based on single serum samples may not reflect the overall pattern. What is needed are studies in which 24-hour levels of hormones are monitored or in which actual pulses are sampled every 20 minutes or so in response to exercise. Otherwise, the evidence from the available studies on the hormonal response to exercise is inconclusive.

It should be noted that the majority of hormonal data do not deal with chronic changes associated with regular, intensive training. Further, the data are largely derived from samples of postmenarcheal women, both athletes and nonathletes, who are physiologically quite different from the maturing girl. What is specifically relevant for the prepubertal or pubertal girl is the possible cumulative effects of hormonal responses to regular training. The hormonal responses are apparently essential to meet the stress that intensive activity imposes on the body. Do they have an effect on the hypothalamic center, which apparently triggers and coordinates the changes that initiate sexual maturation and eventually menarche? Such data are now lacking.

Hormonal data for prepubertal or pubertal girls involved in regular training are limited, and the results are variable and inconclusive. Low gonadotropin secretion in association with only "mild" growth stunting, for example, has been reported in premenarcheal ballet dancers.[34] The dancers were delayed in breast development, menarche, and skeletal maturation, which would suggest a prolonged prepubertal state. However, they were not delayed in pubic hair development.

Lower plasma levels of estrone, testosterone, and androstenedione have been observed in 11-year-old prepubertal gymnasts than in swimmers of the same age and maturity status, but plasma gonadotropin and dehydroepiandrosterone-sulfate (DHEAS) levels did not differ in the two samples. On the other hand, plasma levels of the seven hormones assayed did not differ between early pubertal (stage 2 of breast development) gymnasts and swimmers, although the latter were an average of 0.5 year older.[35] Both the prepubertal and early pubertal gymnasts had been training regularly for a longer period than the swimmers. The two groups of gymnasts had been training since 4.8 and 5.0 years of age, respectively, whereas the two groups of swimmers had been training since 7.2 and 8.0 years of age. The similar levels of DHEAS in the prepubertal gymnasts and swimmers suggests a similar stage of adrenarche, although the gymnasts had been training for a significantly longer period. This observation thus does not support the suggestion that training delays adrenarche and prolongs the prepubertal state.[36] Moreover, recent evidence does not support the view that secretion of adrenal androgens triggers sexual maturation.[37] Early childhood growth data for the two groups of athletes suggest physique differences. Since 3 years of age, the gymnasts had been shorter and lighter than Dutch reference data, whereas the swimmers had been taller and heavier. Midparental heights (height of mother and height of father, divided by 2) and weights were also less in the gymnasts than in the swimmers, and the groups did not differ in socioeconomic status.[35]

Changes in basal levels of hormones in association with training in young athletes may be significant. Similar basal levels of ACTH, cortisol, prolactin, and testosterone have been reported during a 24-week training season in small samples of premenarcheal and postmenarcheal competitive swimmers 13 to 18 years of age.[38] During the season, ACTH levels gradually increased, prolactin levels tended to increase, and testosterone levels decreased, whereas cortisol levels showed a variable pattern in the combined sample. As expected, basal estradiol levels differed between the premenarcheal and postmenarcheal swimmers, but both groups experienced a decrease in basal levels during the first 12 weeks of training, followed by a rise at 24 weeks. Basal levels of estradiol at the start of training and after 24 weeks of training did not differ in the premenarcheal swimmers, whereas the basal level after 24 weeks was lower than at the start of training in the postmenarcheal swimmers.[38]

A role for β-endorphins in the amenorrhea of runners and, in turn, in later menarche in athletes has been postulated. Administration of naloxone, an opiate receptor antagonist, to amenorrheic athletes, for example, results in a marked increase in luteinizing hormone (LH).[39] Responses of normal prepubertal girls and boys to naloxone under basal conditions are different from those of adults, however.[40] Naloxone apparently does not have an effect on LH secretion in children. A study of the effects of naloxone during exercise conditions in children might be enlightening, but ethical concerns make collection of such data difficult.

Fatness and Menarche

A corollary of the suggestion that training delays menarche is that changes in weight or body composition associated with intensive training may function to delay menarche; that is, training may delay maturation in young girls by keeping them lean. This idea is related to the critical weight or critical fatness hypothesis, which suggests that a certain level of weight (about 48 kg) or fatness (about 17%) is necessary for menarche to

occur.[41] Accordingly, intensive, regular training functions to reduce and maintain fatness below the hypothesized minimal level, thereby delaying menarche. The critical weight or fatness hypothesis has been discussed at length by many authors,[21,42] and the evidence does not support the specificity of weight or fatness, or of a threshold level, as the critical variable for menarche to occur.

Other Maturity Indicators

Since indicators of sexual maturity are reasonably well related to indicators of skeletal and somatic maturity during adolescence,[1] it seems logical to consider the effects of training on other maturity indicators. If the hormonal responses to regular training are viewed as important influences on sexual maturation, one might expect them to influence the growth spurt, which occurs a year or so before menarche, and skeletal maturation around the time of menarche. (For example, epiphyseal capping and fusion are influenced by gonadal hormones, among others.)

Regular physical activity, including training for sport, has no apparent effect on other indices of biologic maturation used in growth studies. Age at PHV is not affected by training, while skeletal maturation is neither accelerated nor delayed by regular training for sport during childhood and adolescence.[1,2,26]

Overtraining

The issue of overtraining—that is, excessive training without adequate time for recovery—must be considered, since a significant number of adolescent girls (and boys) are involved in intensive training for sport. Overtraining can be short-term or chronic, and when it is chronic, it results in an array of behavioral, emotional, and physiologic symptoms.[43] Data for adults indicate weight loss, decreased performance, and slow recovery after training. Reduction in both FFM and fat mass probably accompany weight loss, and a reduction in efficiency and maximal working capacity accompany the decrease in performance. Implications for growing girls should be obvious. The behavioral, emotional, and physiologic complications of overtraining have the potential to negatively influence growth and maturation.

SUMMARY

Variation in the timing, tempo, and magnitude of the adolescent growth spurt is considerable. Although on the average girls enter and complete the growth spurt earlier than boys, adolescent gains in FFM and muscle mass in girls are not as great as in boys. Thus, young adult women attain about two thirds of the estimated FFM and muscle mass levels of young adult men. In contrast, absolute and relative fatness increase more in adolescent girls.

Menarche is a relatively late pubertal event that usually occurs a year or so after maximum growth in stature during the adolescent spurt. In American girls, menarche occurs, on average, near the 13th birthday.

Strength, motor performance, and absolute aerobic power improve during adolescence, but the average performance levels tend to reach a plateau between 13 and 15 years of age. Well-defined growth spurts in the strength and motor performances of adolescent girls are not clearly apparent. However, maximal aerobic power shows a definite spurt near the time of PHV. Trained girls have higher performance levels than do untrained girls, and girls who are later in sexual and skeletal maturity tend to be better performers.

Under adequate environmental circumstances, the timing of the growth spurt and sexual maturation is genetically determined. The evidence that regular training before sexual maturity may delay maturation of girls is not convincing.

The stress of training and competition as a factor that influences growth and biologic maturation needs more systematic and controlled study. Prospective studies are needed in which youngsters of both sexes are followed from prepubescence through puberty, in which several indicators of growth and maturity are observed, and in which both training and other factors known to influence growth and maturation are monitored.

REFERENCES

1. Malina RM, and Bouchard C: Growth, Maturation, and Physical Activity. Human Kinetics Publishers, Champaign, IL, 1991.
2. MacMahon B: Age at menarche, United States. Vital and Health Statistics, Series 11, No. 133, 1973.
3. Malina RM: Research on secular trends in auxology. Anthropol Anz 48:209, 1990.
4. Danker-Hopfe H: Menarcheal age in Europe. Yrbk Phys Anthropol 29:81, 1986.
5. Beunen G, and Malina RM: Growth and physical performance relative to the timing of the adolescent spurt. Exerc Sport Sci Rev 16:503, 1988.
6. Faust MS: Somatic development of adolescent girls. Mon Soc Res Child Dev 42(1), 1977.
7. Kemper HCG, and Verschuur R: Motor performance fitness tests. In Kemper HCG (ed): Growth, Health and Fitness of Teenagers. S Karger, Basel, 1985, p 107.
8. Branta C, Haubenstricker J, and Seefeldt V: Age changes in motor skills during childhood and adolescence. Exerc Sport Sci Rev 12:467, 1984.
9. Haubenstricker JL, and Seefeldt VD: Acquisition of motor skills during childhood. In Seefeldt V (ed): Physical Activity and Well-Being. American Alliance for Health, Physical Education, Recreation and Dance, Reston, VA, 1986, p 41.
10. Beunen GP, Malina RM, Van't Hof MA, et al: Adolescent Growth and Motor Performance: A Longitudinal Study of Belgian Boys. Human Kinetics Publishers, Champaign, IL, 1988.
11. Beunen G, Ostyn M, Renson R, et al: Skeletal maturation and physical fitness of girls aged 12 through 16. Hermes (Leuven) 19:445, 1976.
12. Espenschade A: Motor performance in adolescence. Monogr Soc Res Child Dev 5(1):1940.
13. Malina RM: Menarche in athletes: A synthesis and hypothesis. Ann Hum Biol 10:1, 1983.
14. Malina RM: Biological maturity status of young athletes. In Malina RM (ed): Young Athletes: Biological, Psychological, and Educational Perspectives. Human Kinetics Publishers, Champaign, IL, 1988, p 121.

15. Krahenbuhl GS, Skinner JS, and Kohrt WM: Developmental aspects of maximal aerobic power in children. Exerc Sport Sci Rev 13:503, 1985.
16. Mirwald RL, and Bailey DA: Maximal Aerobic Power. Sport Dynamics, London, Ontario, 1986.
17. Kemper HCG, Verschuur R, and Ritmeester JW: Maximal aerobic power in early and late maturing teenagers. In Rutenfranz J, Mocellin R, and Klimt F (eds): Children and Exercise XII. Human Kinetics Publishers, Champaign, IL, 1986, p 213.
18. Malina RM: Energy expenditure and physical activity during childhood and youth. In Demirjian A (ed): Human Growth: A Multidisciplinary Review. Taylor and Francis, London, 1986, p 215.
19. Ross JG, Dotson CO, Gilbert GG, et al: The National Children and Youth Fitness Survey: After school physical education . . . Physical activity outside of school physical education programs. J Phys Educ Rec Dance 56:77, 1985.
20. Kemper HCG, Dekker HJP, Ootjers MG, et al: Growth and health of teenagers in the Netherlands: Survey of multidisciplinary longitudinal studies and comparison to recent results of a Dutch study. Int J Sports Med 4:202, 1983.
21. Malina RM: Darwinian fitness, physical fitness and physical activity. In Mascie-Taylor CGN, and Lasker GW (eds): Applications of Biological Anthropology to Human Affairs. Cambridge University Press, Cambridge, 1991, p 143.
22. Patton RG: Growth and psychological factors. In Mechanisms of Regulation of Growth, Report of the 40th Ross Conference on Pediatric Research. Ross Laboratories, Columbus, OH, 1962, p 58.
23. Tanner JM: Fetus into Man. Harvard University Press, Cambridge, MA, 1989.
24. Ellison PT: Morbidity, mortality, and menarche. Hum Biol 53:635, 1982.
25. Leistol K: Social conditions and menarcheal age: The importance of early years of life. Ann Hum Biol 9:521, 1982.
26. Malina RM: Growth and maturation: Normal variation and effect of training. In Gisolfi CV and Lamb DR (eds): Perspectives in Exercise Science and Sports Medicine, Vol 2. Youth, Exercise, and Sport. Benchmark Press, Indianapolis, IN, 1989, p 223.
27. Drinkwater BL, Nilson K, Chestnut ÇH, et al: Bone mineral of amenorrheic and eumenorrheic athletes. N Engl J Med 311:277, 1984.
28. Warren MP, Brooks-Gunn J, Hamilton LH, et al: Scoliosis and fractures in young ballet dancers. N Engl J Med 314:1348, 1986.
29. Stager JM, Robertshaw D, and Miescher E: Delayed menarche in swimmers in relation to age at onset of training and athletic performance. Med Sci Sports Exerc 16:550, 1984.
30. Frisch RE, Gotz-Welbergen AV, McArthur JW, et al: Delayed menarche and amenorrhea of college athletes in relation to age of onset of training. JAMA 246:1559, 1981.
31. Warren MP, and Brooks-Gunn J: Delayed menarche in athletes: The role of low energy intake and eating disorders and their relation to bone density. In Laron Z, and Rogol AD (eds): Hormones and Sport. Raven Press, New York, 1989, p 41.
32. Shangold MM: Exercise and the adult female: Hormonal and endocrine effects. Exerc Sport Sci Rev 12:53, 1984.
33. Keizer HA, and Rogol AD: Physical exercise and menstrual cycle alterations: What are the mechanisms: Sports Med 10:218, 1990.
34. Warren MP: The effects of exercise on pubertal progression and reproductive function in girls. J Clin Endocrinol Metab 51:1150, 1980.
35. Peltenburg AL, Erich WBM, Thijssen JJH, et al: Sex hormone profiles of premenarcheal athletes. Eur J Appl Physiol 52:385, 1984.
36. Brisson GR, Dulac S, Peronnet F, et al: The onset of menarche: A late event in pubertal progression to be affected by physical training. Can J Appl Sport Sci 7:61, 1982.
37. Wierman ME, and Crowley WR Jr: Neuroendocrine control of the onset of puberty. In Falkner F, and Tanner JM (eds): Human Growth, Vol 2. Plenum, New York, 1986, p 225.
38. Carli G, Martelli G, Viti A, et al: The effect of swimming training on hormone levels in girls. J Sports Med Phys Fit 23:45, 1983.
39. McArthur JW, Bullen BA, Beitins IZ, et al: Hypothalamic amenorrhea in runners of normal body composition. Endocr Res Commun 7:13, 1980.
40. Fraioli F, Cappa M, Fabbri A, et al: Lack of endogenous opioid inhibitory tone on LH secretion in early puberty. Clin Endocrinol 20:299, 1984.
41. Frisch RE: Fatness of girls from menarche to age 18 years, with a nomogram. Hum Biol 48:353, 1976.
42. Bronson FH, and Manning JM: The energetic regulation of ovulation: a realistic role for body fat. Biol Reprod 44:945, 1991.
43. Kuipers H, and Keizer HA: Overtraining in elite athletes: Review and directions for the future. Sports Med 6:79, 1988.

CHAPTER 9

Menstruation and Menstrual Disorders

MONA M. SHANGOLD, M.D.

Increased participation of women in sports has led to greater awareness of the menstrual cycle alterations that frequently accompany exercise and training. This raised consciousness has inspired more scientists to investigate the etiologic mechanisms responsible for such changes and has led many athletes to seek medical attention. Unfortunately, many other athletes still avoid physician consultation, usually because they fear they will be told to stop exercising. It is the responsibility of all physicians and other health professionals to advise exercising women about what is known regarding reproductive effects of exercise and to assist them in formulating therapeutic plans.

PREVALENCE OF MENSTRUAL DYSFUNCTION AMONG ATHLETES

Oligomenorrhea (infrequent menses) and amenorrhea (absent menses) are more prevalent among athletes (10% to 20%)[1,2] than among the general population (5%) and are found more often in runners than in swimmers or cyclists[3] (Fig.

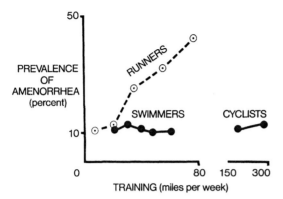

Figure 9-1. The prevalence of amenorrhea in runners, swimmers, and cyclists, relative to training mileage. (From Sanborn,[3] with permission.)

9-1). Among competitive athletes, the prevalence of amenorrhea has been reported to be as high as 50%.[3] However, the prevalence of menstrual dysfunction does not correlate with average weekly mileage, running pace, or number of years of training.[2,4] Bachmann and Kemmann[5] have reported that the prevalences of oligomenorrhea and amenorrhea among college students are 11% and 3%, respectively. However, this population includes some athletes, for whom exercise and training contribute to the problem. The prevalence of menstrual dysfunction among college students is higher than that among the rest of the population because college students tend to experience more emotional stress than the general population and because many college students have not undergone full maturation of the hypothalamic-pituitary-ovarian axis, making them more susceptible to menstrual disorders. It is worth mentioning that the general population has previously been considered to be sedentary, but the rising numbers of exercising women will undoubtedly increase the percentage of exercising women in the gen-

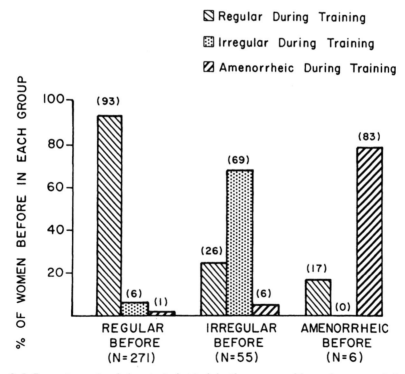

Figure 9-2. Percent menstrual change during training for women with regular menses before training, irregular menses before training, and amenorrhea before training. Of those women who had regular menses before training, 93% continued to have regular menses during training. (From Shangold,[2] with permission.)

eral population and may raise the prevalence of menstrual dysfunction in this
group.

Although it is tempting to presume that
exercise itself is responsible for the higher
prevalence of amenorrhea associated with
it, many factors change simultaneously during the course of an athletic training program, making it difficult to isolate causal factors. The fact that amenorrheic runners
have a higher incidence of prior menstrual
irregularity[1,2] suggests that exercise alone
may not be responsible for menstrual dysfunction in many cases (Fig. 9–2).

REVIEW OF MENSTRUAL PHYSIOLOGY

A brief review of menstrual physiology
follows, to facilitate the understanding of
readers from diverse backgrounds. It is necessary to be familiar with the basic hormonal events of the menstrual cycle, in
order to appreciate both the hormonal and
menstrual alterations that accompany exercise and training. For more comprehensive
reviews, the reader is referred to other publications.[6–8]

A normal menstrual cycle (counting from
the beginning of one period to the beginning
of the next period) lasts from 23 to 35 days.
An ovarian **follicle** is the structure that contains an egg; a **corpus luteum** is what develops from a follicle after the egg has been ex-
pelled. The **follicular phase** is the portion of
the ovarian cycle that extends from the first
day of menstruation until ovulation; this
corresponds temporally with the **prolifera-
tive phase** of the endometrial cycle. The **luteal phase** of the ovarian cycle extends from
ovulation until the onset of the next menstrual period; this corresponds temporally
with the **secretory phase** of the endometrial
cycle. A normal luteal phase should approach 14 days, while a normal follicular
phase may vary considerably in length.
Thus, fluctuations in the length of the menstrual cycle of a woman who ovulates usually

result from variations in the length of the follicular phase, or the time required for a follicle to enlarge and mature enough to undergo ovulation.

Throughout the menstrual cycle, the hypothalamus secretes **gonadotropin-releasing hormone (GnRH),** which is also referred to as luteinizing hormone-releasing
hormone (LH-RH) or luteinizing hormone-
releasing factor (LRF). This decapeptide is
produced by cells in the arcuate nucleus of
the hypothalamus; it promotes synthesis,
storage, releasability, and secretion of both
pituitary gonadotropins: **follicle-stimulating hormone (FSH)** and **luteinizing hormone (LH).** FSH promotes growth of the
ovarian follicle and synthesis of estrogen
from androgen precursors. LH stimulates
ovarian androgen production, maintaining a
supply of androgens available for conversion to estrogens.

In a normal menstrual cycle, a woman produces estrogen all the time and produces
significant progesterone only after ovulation. Blood estrogen levels vary greatly
throughout the cycle, being quite low during
the early follicular phase and quite high during the late follicular phase. It is the high estrogen level in the late follicular phase that
triggers ovulation. During the luteal phase,
levels of both estrogen and progesterone
are high.

Estrogen stimulates the endometrium
(the inner lining of the uterus) to proliferate;
progesterone promotes maturation and stabilization of an estrogen-stimulated endometrium. It is the decline in the concentrations of estrogen and progesterone near the
end of the menstrual cycle that results in
menstruation, which is the desquamation of
the endometrium (Fig. 9–3).

TYPES OF MENSTRUAL DYSFUNCTION

With any insult to a woman's reproductive
system, menstrual disturbance probably follows an orderly sequence of increasing

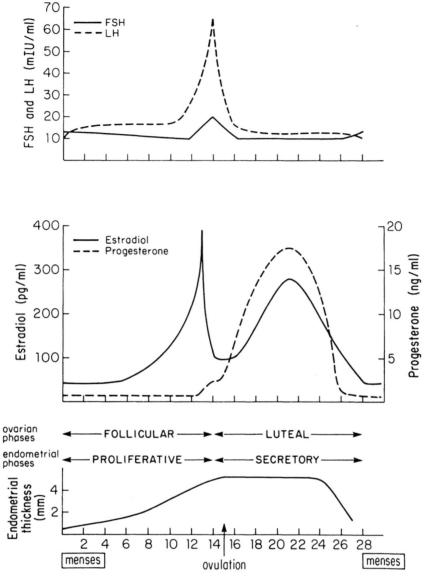

Figure 9-3. Hormonal events of the menstrual cycle, phases of the ovarian and endometrial cycles, and endometrial height throughout the menstrual cycle.

severity: (1) luteal phase deficiency, (2) euestrogenic anovulation, and (3) hypoestrogenic amenorrhea. Thus, any condition that disturbs the delicate balance of carefully timed hormonal events needed for regular ovulation and menstruation usually produces luteal phase deficiency first. If the condition continues, euestrogenic anovulation will probably follow. If the condition continues even longer, hypoestrogenic

amenorrhea is likely to ensue. Many women do not seek attention when menstrual dysfunction is mild or of recent onset and may have hypoestrogenic amenorrhea by the time they first seek attention. Although progression of this sequence has not been documented in prospective studies, it is likely, nevertheless, and provides a useful model for understanding menstrual dysfunction.

MENSTRUAL CYCLE CHANGES WITH EXERCISE AND TRAINING

The data collected from the surveys reported are derived from records of women who recorded only their menstrual patterns. Most, but not all, women who bleed at regular intervals have normal ovulatory and luteal function. More accurate information about menstrual cyclicity can be derived from basal body temperature records and hormonal measurements. By having 14 subjects record their basal body temperatures to indicate that and when ovulation had occurred, Prior and co-workers[9] have shown in 48 menstrual cycles that even among athletic women with apparently regular menses, approximately one third have anovulation, one third have luteal phase deficiency, and one third have normal luteal function. This suggests that menstrual disturbance among exercising women may be more pervasive than has been appreciated.

In addition to the epidemiologic studies that demonstrate a higher prevalence of oligomenorrhea/amenorrhea among athletes than among sedentary women, several prospective investigations have demonstrated changes in menstrual cyclicity in individual women who trained. Each of these has studied a number of factors that vary during training, any of which may contribute to menstrual cycle alteration. It is usually very difficult to separate the many contributory variables that change simultaneously during training, including body composition, physical and emotional stress, diet, and certain hormone levels (Table 9–1).

Weight Loss and Thinness

Many women lose both weight and body fat when they begin to exercise regularly. Some attain and maintain very low levels of weight and fat. Simple weight loss and thinness may lead to amenorrhea, even in the absence of exercise. Shangold and Levine[2] have reported that amenorrheic runners are lighter than eumenorrheic (regularly menstruating) runners. Schwartz and associates[1]

Table 9–1. FACTORS TO WHICH AN ATHLETE IS OFTEN SUBJECTED DURING TRAINING

1. Weight loss
2. Low weight
3. Low body fat
4. Dietary alterations
5. Nutritional inadequacy
6. Physical stress
7. Emotional stress
8. Acute hormone alterations
9. Chronic hormone alterations

have demonstrated that amenorrheic runners were thinner and had lost more weight after initiating regular running.

Despite claims that women need a minimum amount of body fat in order to maintain regular menstrual cyclicity, this hypothesis remains unproven and suspect. If such a minimum amount of fat must be exceeded, the mechanism by which this functions also remains unproven. Adipose tissue produces and retains estrogen, but the amount of estrogen contributed by adipose tissue is negligible compared with the very large quantity produced by normal ovaries. Since muscle tissue contains aromatizing enzymes too, and since athletic women tend to have more muscle and less fat than sedentary women, aromatizing capability should be comparable in both groups. Thus, the mechanism by which thinness promotes menstrual dysfunction remains to be shown.

Following the original suggestion by Frisch and McArthur[10] that thinness caused amenorrhea, many investigators have probed the relationships between thinness and hormone production and metabolism. Previously it was shown that thin women metabolize most of their estradiol by 2-hydroxylation, while obese women excrete most estradiol after 16-hydroxylation.[11] Recently, Snow and her associates[12] have shown that elite oarswomen who develop menstrual dysfunction during training metabolize a greater fraction of administered [2-³H]estradiol by 2-hydroxylation than do sedentary controls or elite oarswomen who remain eumenorrheic during training. How the resultant catecholestrogens affect menstrual function remains to be shown.

Physical and Emotional Stress

Schwartz and colleagues[1] have shown that amenorrheic runners associate more stress with their exercise than do eumenorrheic runners. This supports the concept that the physical and emotional stress of both training and competition may be substantially greater than appreciated. Although regular exercise tends to relieve stress and anxiety, this action may be outweighed in busy women who are determined to incorporate a specific quantity of exercise into their daily schedules.

Warren[13] has demonstrated the complexity and interrelationship of the factors contributing to the development of menstrual dysfunction in two ballet dancers (Fig. 9–4). The dancer in the upper graph experienced no change in weight or body composition throughout the year in which she had three menstrual periods, each during an interval of inactivity. The dancer in the lower graph developed regular menses when she gained both weight and body fat, although she maintained her customary level of activity. She continued menstruating regularly, despite a loss of both weight and body fat that occurred during an inactive vacation interval. With no further loss of weight, she ceased menstruating altogether when she resumed her customary level of activity. It is likely that stress levels are higher during intervals of intensive dancing, compared with vacation intervals. Thus, activity, fat, weight, and stress must be considered variables in the changes observed.

Dietary Factors

Many women who begin to exercise regularly alter their dietary patterns because they become more concerned about healthful living. Those who have been exercising regularly for a long time often eat differently from nonathletes. Schwartz and co-workers[1] reported that protein constituted a smaller percentage of the total caloric intake of amenorrheic runners compared with that of eumenorrheic runners and eumenorrheic nonrunners. These amenorrheic runners consumed more total calories than the other groups, however, so that equal quantities of protein were consumed by all three groups. Calabrese and colleagues[14] have demonstrated that professional and student ballet dancers consume fewer calories (1358 calories) than the recommended dietary allowance (RDA) (2030 calories) established by the National Research Council,[15] a figure intended for an "average" woman, weighing 58 kg and exercising very little or not at all. Although the mean daily protein intake by these dancers (47.4 g) fell slightly below the RDA for "average-sized women" (50 g), this protein intake was adequate when based on the RDA of 0.8 g/kg[15] and the subjects' mean weight of 53.1 kg. Frisch and associates[16] have reported that a group of collegiate women who began athletic training prior to menarche consumed less fat (65 g) and protein (71 g) than a group who began training after menarche (95 g of fat and 92 g of protein), and that the former group also had higher incidences of oligomenorrhea and amenorrhea. Very low levels of fat intake are difficult to attain, and such diets have been associated with insidious negative calcium balance.[17] Deficiencies of the fat-soluble vitamins, which require fat for absorption, have never been reported in people consuming low-fat diets, but such deficiencies remain a theoretical hazard. Deuster and her co-workers[18] have described differences between the dietary intakes of eumenorrheic and amenorrheic runners, and they have reported that many amenorrheic runners consume less than the recommended dietary allowances of some nutrients. Pirke and associates[19] have described menstrual dysfunction that developed in association with caloric restriction, especially in association with a vegetarian diet. These investigators have demonstrated impairment of episodic LH secretion during dieting.[20]

Despite the suggestion that amenorrheic runners may consume inadequate choles-

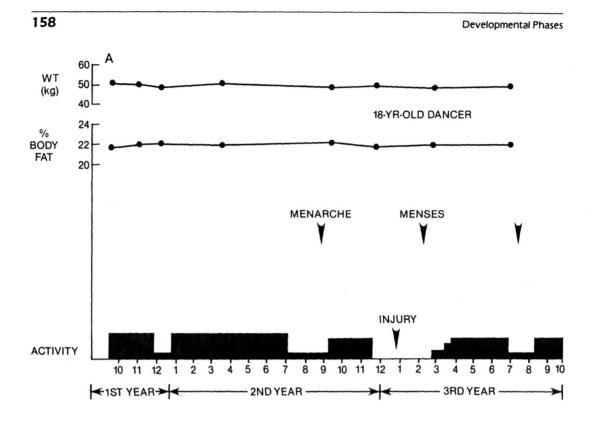

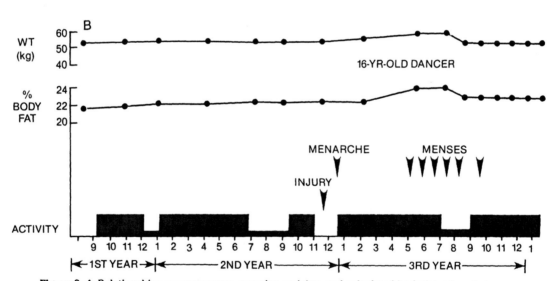

Figure 9–4. Relationships among menses, exercise, weights, and calculated body fat values in two young ballet dancers. (From Warren,[13] with permission.)

terol to produce sufficient estrogen, there remains no evidence that dietary cholesterol is necessary for hormone synthesis. The corpus luteum cannot make enough cholesterol de novo to synthesize adequate

progesterone during a normal luteal phase, but the rest of the body can provide enough cholesterol to serve as precursor for adequate luteal progesterone production.

Although there is little to prove that estrogen production is affected by these dietary differences, there is evidence that estrogen metabolism is altered. Longcope and co-workers[21] have shown that the ingestion of a low-fat diet promotes the same pattern of estrogen metabolism observed in thin women: increased production of catecholestrogens (the result of 2-hydroxylation) and reduced production of estriol (the result of 16-hydroxylation).

Myerson and her associates[22] have shown that the resting metabolic rate (RMR) of amenorrheic runners is significantly less than that of eumenorrheic runners, which is significantly less than that of eumenorrheic sedentary controls. The RMR of the amenorrheic runners remained lower than that of each of the other two groups after adjustment for body weight or for fat-free mass. Although the absolute caloric intake of the amenorrheic runners was less than that of the eumenorrheic runners and was similar to that of the sedentary controls, the differences were not significant, probably due to large intragroup variability and small sample size. The amenorrheic runners also had higher scores on the eating attitudes test (EAT-26, modified), including two subscales and total score; this reflected a higher level of aberrant dietary patterns in the amenorrheic group. Thus, a growing body of information has brought our attention to the role of dietary intake as a contributing cause of menstrual dysfunction among athletes.

HORMONAL CHANGES WITH EXERCISE AND TRAINING

Acute Hormone Alterations with Exercise

Blood levels of several protein and steroid hormones increase transiently during continuous, aerobic exercise. The long-term effects of such repetitive, but brief, alterations remains unknown. Reported exercise-induced changes in gonadotropin levels are inconsistent and have been confused by the pulsatile nature of gonadotropin release. Circulating concentrations of prolactin,[23] estradiol,[24] progesterone,[24] and testosterone[23] rise during exercise and return to normal within an hour or two after cessation of exercise. Exercise-associated increments in ACTH, opioid peptides, melatonin, and cortisol are facilitated by training.[25,26] Since testosterone[27] and cortisol[28] increase also in anticipation of exercise, it is probable that psychologic factors contribute to the reported changes as well. Rebar and co-workers[29] have shown that dexamethasone suppression abolishes all effects of exercise on adrenal and gonadal hormones, including those in anticipation of exercise. Detailed review of the many studies of hormonal changes during exercise sessions, ranging in duration from a few minutes to the time required to complete a marathon, is beyond the scope of this chapter. For a more comprehensive review, readers are referred elsewhere.[30-32]

Factors Influencing Hormone Levels

Plasma hormone levels represent a balance among production, metabolism, utilization, clearance, and plasma volume, all of which may change simultaneously during exercise. Levels of many hormones also are affected by episodic secretion, diurnal variation, state of sleep or wakefulness, state of feeding or fasting, dietary composition and caloric adequacy, temperature, body weight and composition, emotional factors, and body position. The hormonal response to exercise in any person is often influenced by the person's fitness, which affects the relative workload of any given activity and, in some cases, alters hormonal responsiveness during exercise. Difficulty in controlling these many variables during any specific investigation makes it even harder to interpret the observed exercise-induced changes in hormone levels.

Chronic Hormone Alterations with Training

Shangold and associates[33] have observed one runner during 18 menstrual cycles in which she varied her weekly mileage. This woman had shortening of the luteal phase and lower progesterone levels in cycles of greater mileage (Figs. 9–5 and 9–6). Prior and colleagues[34] have also reported luteal phase deficiency in two runners during several menstrual cycles of varying mileage. One of these two runners had a normal pregnancy when she stopped running, suggesting that exercise-induced luteal phase deficiency is a reversible phenomenon.

Similarly, Frisch and associates[35] observed a long-distance swimmer prior to, during, and after intensive training, with monitoring of basal body temperature records, as well as blood and urine hormone measurements. She developed a luteal phase defect, followed by an anovulatory cycle, during intensive training. Three months after completion of a long-distance swim (the English Channel), she regained a normal, biphasic basal body temperature pattern. This confirms that the menstrual cycle alterations associated with intensive training occur in swimming as well as in running.

Menstrual and hormonal changes in two groups of untrained women have been studied prospectively.[36] One group lost weight during a running program of increasing mileage, and the other group maintained weight during the same program. The prev-

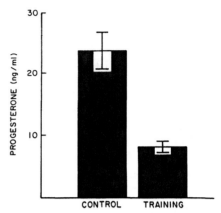

Figure 9–6. Midluteal phase plasma progesterone concentrations obtained 3 to 7 days after change in cervical mucus (presumptive evidence of ovulation), comparing seven samples from three control cycles and seven samples from three training cycles. Bars indicate means plus or minus standard errors ($p < 0.001$). (From Shangold,[33] reproduced with permission of The American Fertility Society.)

alence of menstrual dysfunction was high in both groups during intensive training, but was much higher in the weight-loss group; 94% of them experienced menstrual disturbances, compared with 75% of the weight-maintenance group. Of those who lost weight, 63% experienced abnormal luteal function, as did 66% of the weight-maintenance group. All subjects regained normal menstrual cyclicity within 6 months of termination of the study (and presumably of training). As has been shown by Warren,[13] weight loss and exercise act synergistically in promoting menstrual dysfunction. However, these data[36] suggest that a compensatory increase in caloric intake cannot prevent exercise-induced menstrual dysfunction in most cases.

In the same investigation of training-induced menstrual dysfunction,[37] two types of luteal dysfunction were described: a short luteal phase and an inadequate luteal phase. The short luteal phase was marked by decreased luteal phase length, while the inadequate luteal phase was characterized by insufficient progesterone secretion, measured by the concentration in overnight urine collections. The significance of these differences remains to be shown, but these

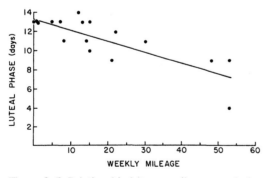

Figure 9–5. Relationship between mileage run during the first 6 days of the follicular phase and the length of the luteal phase, defined as the interval between the day of change in cervical mucus and onset of the next menses, in 18 cycles. ($y = 13.3 - 0.11x$; $r = -0.81$; $p < 0.001$). Point (1,13) represents three values. (From Shangold,[33] reproduced with permission of The American Fertility Society.)

investigators have shown that menstrual dysfunction can be induced in normal women with intense training. It remains to be shown, however, whether a critical level of exertion must be exceeded, and why some women are predisposed to this type of dysfunction in response to training. If a critical level exists, the level undoubtedly differs among various women.

Russell and associates[38,39] found similar weights and body fat levels among athletic and inactive women, but found a correlation among strenuous exercise, anovulatory oligomenorrhea, and elevated levels of β-endorphins and catechol estrogens. Although endogenous opiates are known to modulate pulsatile luteinizing hormone release in humans,[40] it is unlikely that circulating levels of these peptides correspond to the brain levels influencing hypothalamic secretion.

The fact that a generalized increase in "stress" hormones occurs with exercise and endurance training has been confirmed by Villanueva and colleagues,[41] who demonstrated increased cortisol production in both eumenorrheic and amenorrheic runners. Although the amenorrheic runners had higher levels of both serum cortisol and urinary cortisol, the differences between these two groups of runners were not statistically significant.

Loucks and her associates[42] have demonstrated that both eumenorrheic and amenorrheic athletes have higher morning serum cortisol levels than do eumenorrheic sedentary women, and that the serum cortisol levels in the amenorrheic athletes remained higher throughout the day compared to those in the eumenorrheic sedentary women. However, these three groups did not differ in plasma ACTH pulse frequency, pulse amplitude, or mean level during any time interval, and also did not differ in serum cortisol pulse frequency. The eumenorrheic athletes had reduced serum cortisol pulse amplitude during the day. Other investigators have also described mild hypercortisolism in amenorrheic runners.[43] Loucks and co-workers[42] have also shown a blunted response of plasma ACTH and

serum cortisol to bolus administration of human corticotropin-releasing hormone (CRH), and to meals, among both eumenorrheic and amenorrheic athletes compared to eumenorrheic sedentary controls. These data suggest that the hypothalamic-pituitary-adrenal axes of athletic women are characterized by increased CRH stimulation, increased cortisol negative feedback, normal ACTH secretion, normal corticotroph responsiveness to cortisol-induced negative feedback, and decreased responsiveness to ACTH. In an excellent review, DeSouza and Metzger[44] have suggested that the adrenal response may be blunted because the adrenal is functioning near capacity at rest, unable to mount a greater response to stimulation.

Boyden and associates[45] have provided an important clue toward understanding the alterations in menstrual function associated with intensive exercise. They have shown that GnRH-stimulated LH levels in eumenorrheic women decrease with endurance training (distance running).

Cumming and co-workers[46] further enhanced our understanding of these changes when they reported that eumenorrheic runners (at rest) have lower LH pulse frequency, LH pulse amplitude, and area under the LH curve over 6 hours, compared with eumenorrheic sedentary women (Figs. 9-7 and 9-8). These investigators[47] then found that acute exercise reduces LH pulse frequency but does not change pulse amplitude or area under the 6-hour curve. These important findings suggest that acute exercise has an inhibitory effect on LH pulsatile release at the hypothalamic level in eumenorrheic runners, perhaps contributing to the observed alterations with training.

Several recent studies have provided even more information about LH pulsatile patterns in athletes. Veldhuis and co-workers[48] demonstrated reduced LH pulse frequency and normal LH pulse amplitude in amenorrheic or severely oligomenorrheic runners compared to eumenorrheic sedentary controls. These investigators also reported normal or accen-

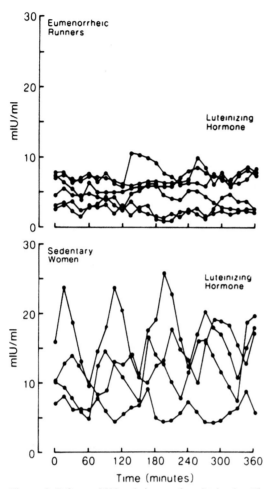

Figure 9–7. Serum LH levels in samples obtained at 15-minute intervals over 6 hours in six eumenorrheic runners *(upper)* and four sedentary controls *(lower)*. The studies were performed in the early follicular phase of the menstrual cycle (days 3 to 6). (From Cumming,[46] with permission.)

tuated LH release and normal estradiol release in response to exogenous GnRH pulses.

Loucks and co-workers[42] have shown reduced LH pulse frequency and increased LH pulse amplitude in eumenorrheic athletes compared to eumenorrheic sedentary controls; both the LH pulse frequency and amplitude of the amenorrheic athletes were lower than those of the eumenorrheic athletes. An exogenous GnRH bolus caused blunted FSH release in the eumenorrheic athletes and augmented FSH and LH release

in the amenorrheic athletes, compared to the eumenorrheic sedentary controls. These data suggest that exercise-induced menstrual dysfunction results from inhibition of hypothalamic release of GnRH at the level of the hypothalamus or higher brain centers influencing hypothalamic function.

CONSEQUENCES OF MENSTRUAL DYSFUNCTION

Luteal Phase Deficiency

The major adverse condition associated with luteal phase deficiency is infertility, and this association remains controversial. Preliminary findings suggesting that progesterone deficiency may be linked to an increased breast cancer risk[49] have not been confirmed. Prior and her associates[50] have recently demonstrated that shortening the luteal phase correlates with loss of bone density.

Anovulatory Oligomenorrhea

Chronic anovulation is associated with chronic, unopposed estrogen production, which leads to continuous endometrial stimulation and, as a consequence, an increased risk of endometrial hyperplasia and adenocarcinoma. Although this association has been documented in women with polycystic ovary syndrome,[51–54] it has never been reported in athletes. It remains unknown whether anovulatory athletes carry the same, increased risk of developing endometrial hyperplasia and adenocarcinoma as nonathletes with chronic anovulation. Perhaps inadequate reporting or history-taking, or both, has led to the absence of such reports (i.e., gynecologists may not routinely elicit athletic histories, particularly when diagnosing cancer), or perhaps anovulatory athletic women do not maintain high enough estrogen levels long enough to induce hyperplasia or cancer. Until this question is answered, it seems reasonable to assume that the endometrium of the athlete

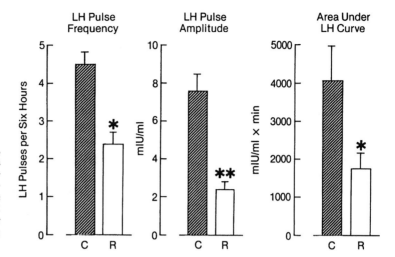

Figure 9–8. LH pulse frequency, pulse amplitude, and the area under the LH curve in eumenorrheic runners and sedentary controls in the early follicular phase of the menstrual cycle. (*p < 0.05, **p < 0.01 on Mann-Whitney U test.) (From Cumming,[46] with permission.)

responds the same as that of the nonathlete to estrogen stimulation. Thus, an increased risk of endometrial hyperplasia and adenocarcinoma should be presumed until it is disproved.

Recent studies have suggested that anovulatory women may also be at increased risk of developing breast cancer.[55] This preliminary report requires further confirmation. This suggestion, too, has not described the athletic habits of subjects. Thus, if chronic anovulation leads to an increased risk of breast carcinoma, it remains to be shown whether this increased risk includes anovulatory athletes.

Although Frisch and associates[56] have reported a lower prevalence of breast cancer among former college athletes compared with former college nonathletes, this report did not relate breast cancer prevalence to recent athletic participation. Thus, it remains to be demonstrated whether regular exercise has any effect on breast cancer risk. Prior and her colleagues[50] have shown that anovulatory cycles are also associated with loss of bone density.

Chronic anovulation usually leads to infrequent, heavy bleeding at unpredictable times. At best, this is an inconvenience, particularly to competitive athletes, and at worst, it may require hospitalization to control blood loss. Between these extremes, women with chronic, unopposed estrogen

production may be iron-deficient or anemic. Either of these conditions can impair athletic performance, as can heavy bleeding during training or competition. The prevalence of heavy bleeding among athletes remains to be shown. As suggested earlier, it is possible that anovulatory athletic women do not maintain high enough estrogen levels long enough to induce sufficient thickening of the endometrial lining and consequent profuse bleeding. However, heavy, infrequent bleeding episodes are common among adolescents, even those who are athletes; it is probable that more mature athletes are subject to the same risk.

Hypoestrogenic Amenorrhea

Estrogen promotes beneficial effects on calcium metabolism, lipid metabolism, and urogenital epithelial maturation. Hypoestrogenic women lack these favorable effects. Many reports have demonstrated that athletes with hypoestrogenic amenorrhea have reduced bone density and increased risk of musculoskeletal injury, compared with eumenorrheic athletes.[57–63]

Cann and co-workers[57] were the first to bring this finding to our attention. They reported that women with hypothalamic amenorrhea, in many cases associated with exercise, had lower vertebral bone density than several other groups of eumenorrheic and amenorrheic women, including those with hyperprolactinemia and premature ovarian failure. This surprising, incidental finding led several other investigators to the same issue. It had been shown by others that exercise has a beneficial effect on bone density, as discussed in Chapter 5. In view of the higher prevalence of hypoestrogenic amenorrhea among athletes, it became important to resolve whether exercise is beneficial enough to compensate for an estrogen deficiency.

Rigotti and colleagues[58] reported that amenorrheic women with anorexia nervosa had lower radial bone density than eumenorrheic controls and that those anorectics who reported a high physical activity level had a greater bone density than those who were less active. This suggested that physical activity offers some protection against bone loss induced by estrogen deficiency.

In a study by Drinkwater and co-workers,[59] lower vertebral bone density was found in amenorrheic athletes than in eumenorrheic athletes. However, these groups differed not only in their estrogen status but also in their calcium intake. Although the absolute values of calcium ingested by the groups were not significantly different, the amenorrheic group, but not the eumenorrheic group, consumed much less calcium than the amount recommended for hypoestrogenic women. Since estrogen enhances calcium absorption, hypoestrogenic women require an additional 500 mg of calcium daily, compared with that required by euestrogenic women. (It is recommended that euestrogenic women consume 1000 mg of calcium daily and that hypoestrogenic women consume 1500 mg daily.[64]) Thus, it is unclear whether the lower bone density of these amenorrheic athletes was caused by estrogen deficiency, calcium deficiency, or both.

Marcus and colleagues[60] also reported that eumenorrheic runners had greater vertebral bone density than eumenorrheic sedentary women, who had greater bone density than amenorrheic runners, who had greater bone density than amenorrheic sed-

entary women. This suggested that exercise is beneficial in increasing bone density, but not as beneficial as a normal estrogen level. Unfortunately, differences in calcium intake between some of these groups introduced another variable, as occurred in the Drinkwater study.[59] It remains difficult to separate estrogen, exercise, and calcium intake as variables in pinpointing causality in such studies.

It was demonstrated by Jones and associates[61] that radial bone density regresses in a linear fashion with increasing duration of amenorrhea, regardless of etiology, confirming that hypoestrogenic young women lose bone density in the same pattern as that observed for postmenopausal women.[65]

Warren and co-workers[62] have reported that ballet dancers have a higher prevalence of scoliosis and a greater incidence of fractures with increasing menarcheal age. They also found a higher incidence and longer duration of secondary amenorrhea among dancers with stress fractures. These findings suggest that menarcheal delay and prolonged intervals of hypoestrogenic amenorrhea may predispose ballerinas to scoliosis and stress fractures.

The suggestion of increased susceptibility to musculoskeletal injuries among amenorrheic athletes has been supported by the work of Lloyd and colleagues.[63] These authors reported that women who were injured during their running program were more likely to have had absent or irregular menses, were less likely to have used oral contraceptives, and had been running for more years than those running women who were not injured.

The increased risk of cardiovascular disease that occurs after menopause results mostly from adverse changes in lipids, induced by estrogen deficiency. Most of the adverse effects of the hypoestrogenic state on low-density lipoprotein cholesterol concentrations tend to be offset by endurance training. In addition, most athletes have a reduced risk of cardiovascular disease, compared with the general population. On the other hand, exercise-induced hypoestrogenic amenorrhea can reverse the beneficial effects of strenuous exercise on plasma apolipoprotein concentrations.[66]

Because estrogen leads to maturation of the urogenital epithelium, a deficiency causes thinning of the vaginal epithelium and increased susceptibility to atrophic urethritis and vaginitis. These uncomfortable conditions are most common after menopause, probably because development of urogenital atrophy requires several years in the hypoestrogenic state. Since few athletes remain severely hypoestrogenic long enough to develop atrophic vaginitis, this condition is relatively uncommon among athletes and can usually be treated easily when it occurs.

DIAGNOSTIC EVALUATION OF MENSTRUAL DYSFUNCTION IN ATHLETES

I believe that all oligomenorrheic and amenorrheic athletes deserve the following: (1) a thorough history, including detailed dietary intake; (2) a physical examination, including a pelvic examination; and (3) some blood tests (Table 9-2). The dietary record should be reviewed by a trained nutritionist. Although most athletes with menstrual disturbances will be found to have no serious conditions, it is impossible to determine, without this assessment, whether the menstrual dysfunction is related to exercise or to some serious pathologic condition. A complete blood count, measurement of electrolytes and liver enzymes, and urinalysis are useful screening tests for the general

Table 9-2. INITIAL DIAGNOSTIC EVALUATION OF OLIGOMENORRHEA OR AMENORRHEA

1. History, including dietary intake
2. Physical examination, including pelvic examination
3. Prolactin, free thyroxine, TSH, FSH, LH, DHEAS, testosterone, β-HCG, estradiol
4. Progestin challenge test

population. However, because these tests have not proved cost-effective for patients in my practice who have only menstrual dysfunction, I no longer perform these tests routinely.

Menstrual disturbances may be caused by hyperprolactinemia, hypothyroidism, ovarian failure, hyperandrogenism, and pregnancy. To detect these conditions, it is necessary to measure the following: serum prolactin, thyrotropin (TSH), free thyroxine, follicle-stimulating hormone (FSH), luteinizing hormone (LH), dehydroepiandrosterone sulfate (DHEAS), testosterone, and β-human chorionic gonadotropin (β-HCG). I also measure serum estradiol, in order to determine whether the patient is hypoestrogenic. Hyperprolactinemia may result from a pituitary adenoma or microadenoma; it requires further evaluation and specific treatment. If both FSH and LH are very low, the sella turcica should be assessed (probably by a lateral cone-down film), to detect a large hypothalamic or pituitary lesion. An elevated TSH level or a low free-thyroxine level indicates hypothyroidism, which also requires further evaluation and specific treatment. Hyperandrogenism may result from any of several etiologies, including polycystic ovarian syndrome, adrenal hyperplasia, an ovarian tumor, an adrenal tumor, or drug abuse; hyperandrogenism requires further evaluation and treatment. Although many women with hyperandrogenism will also have peripheral signs of androgen excess, not all women do. Some hyperandrogenic women develop menstrual dysfunction before acne, hirsutism, or other symptoms of androgen excess. Therefore, I believe it is worthwhile to measure DHEAS and testosterone in all women with menstrual dysfunction, regardless of whether other symptoms are present. Pregnancy, of course, requires further care. Ovarian failure requires at least counseling and possibly also further evaluation and treatment. In a patient younger than age 30, ovarian failure warrants a blood karyotype to detect the presence of a Y chromosome, which confers an increased risk of gonadal malignancy. In a patient older than age 30, no further evaluation is required. At the time of the initial evaluation, and after blood has been drawn for the above determinations, the patient may be given a prescription for a 5- or 10-day course of medroxyprogesterone acetate, to assess whether her endometrium has been stimulated by endogenous estrogen. If she has no withdrawal bleeding, her endometrium had not been stimulated and the rest of her body probably also lacks sufficient estrogen. Direct measurement of serum estradiol gives more accurate information, however, and is more useful in planning treatment.

After evaluating an athlete with oligomenorrhea or amenorrhea in this manner, and upon finding that all of these tests except the estradiol concentration are within normal limits, the athlete can be reassured that serious causes of menstrual dysfunction have been ruled out. She should be counseled about potential risks that may result from the condition. Her serum estradiol concentration may be helpful in planning treatment.

TREATMENT OF MENSTRUAL DYSFUNCTION IN ATHLETES

Even if no serious causative pathology is detected during the hormonal evaluation for menstrual dysfunction, treatment usually is indicated to prevent serious resultant pathology.

The association between luteal phase deficiency and infertility is generally accepted, but the links between luteal phase inadequacy and breast cancer and bone loss seem preliminary at the present time. Until confirming studies for the latter two conditions are available, treatment for only infertility is recommended. Thus, at the present time, luteal phase deficiency requires no treatment unless and until pregnancy is desired.

As discussed, euestrogenic anovulatory women are at increased risk of developing endometrial hyperplasia and should be treated with monthly progestin administra-

tion to protect the endometrium adequately. This can be effected by one of the following regimens: (1) medroxyprogesterone acetate 5 to 10 mg daily for 10 to 14 consecutive days of every month; (2) oral contraceptive pills, each containing 30 to 35 μg of ethinyl estradiol and 0.15 to 1.0 mg of progestin; or (3) clomiphene citrate to induce ovulation (Table 9–3). Ovulation induction should be reserved for those women desiring pregnancy at the time of evaluation. The first two choices are acceptable for women who do not seek pregnancy now, regardless of whether they are sexually active. Although oral contraceptive pills obviously provide contraception, medroxyprogesterone acetate does not, and this regimen requires individuals to use barrier contraceptive methods if they are sexually active.

Hypoestrogenic amenorrheic women require hormone replacement, primarily for skeletal protection, but also for urogenital protection. Such athletes should be treated with one of the following treatment protocols: (1) conjugated estrogens 0.625 to 0.9 mg daily and medroxyprogesterone acetate 5 to 10 mg daily on days 1 to 12 of every calendar month; (2) transdermal estradiol 0.05 to 0.10 mg daily and medroxyprogesterone acetate 5 to 10 mg daily on days 1 to 12 of every calendar month; (3) oral contraceptive pills, each containing 30 to 35 μg of ethinyl estradiol and 0.15 to 1.0 mg of progestin; or (4) clomiphene citrate or human menopausal gonadotropins to induce ovulation (Table 9–4). Ovulation induction should be reserved for women desiring pregnancy at the time of evaluation.

Oral contraceptive pills may be recommended to any hypoestrogenic amenorrheic athlete who does not desire pregnancy

Table 9–3. TREATMENT OF EUESTROGENIC OLIGOMENORRHEA

1. If not sexually active or using barrier contraception: monthly progestin therapy
2. If contraception needed or preferred: oral contraceptives
3. If fertility desired: clomiphene citrate

Table 9-4. TREATMENT OF
HYPOESTROGENIC AMENORRHEA

1. If fertility desired: clomiphene citrate
2. If contraception needed or preferred: oral contraceptives
3. If contraception and fertility not of concern: cyclic estrogen and progestin therapy
4. If diet inadequate: correct deficiencies
5. If very thin: weight gain?
6. If exercising very heavily: less exercise?

Table 9-5. ABSOLUTE
CONTRAINDICATIONS TO ESTROGEN
THERAPY

1. Abnormal liver function
2. History of thromboembolic or vascular disease
3. Breast or endometrial carcinoma
4. Undiagnosed vaginal bleeding

at the time of evaluation, regardless of whether she is sexually active; no additional contraceptive method is needed by athletes selecting this form of hormone replacement therapy. Those who select the more physiologic regimen of conjugated estrogens or transdermal estradiol and medroxyprogesterone acetate, separately, should be advised to use mechanical methods of contraception if they are sexually active. The major advantages of taking oral contraceptive agents are convenience and contraception; the major disadvantages are their two most common side effects: breakthrough bleeding (bleeding on the days of pill ingestion) and amenorrhea (lack of withdrawal bleeding at the end of the hormone-containing pills in each package). These side effects are inconvenient but not serious; both can be alleviated by hormone manipulation. The low-dose oral contraceptive pills recommended are associated with much lesser side effects and complications than the higher doses prescribed commonly more than a decade ago; the low-dose preparations are also associated with a reduction in many disease risks, compared with the risk to the general population.

Another advantage of oral contraceptives for athletes with menstrual dysfunction is predictable bleeding and continued endometrial and skeletal protection. Many athletes may produce enough endogenous estrogen to have withdrawal bleeding following progestin administration for several months and then produce too little estrogen to do so during the next few months. It is disturbing to many athletes to experience such

fluctuations in their observed responses, and many experience psychologic benefit from the regularity and predictability of oral contraceptive therapy.

The major advantages of taking either progestin alone or estrogen and progestin as separate pills are the ingestion of more physiologic doses of medication and the likelihood of having predictable bleeding. Although the risks of exogenous hormone administration are much less than the risks of hormone deficiency, in my view, certain women should probably avoid estrogen and others should definitely avoid it. Absolute contraindications to estrogen therapy are listed in Table 9-5; relative contraindications are listed in Table 9-6.

Many athletes have an aversion to exogenous hormone ingestion and do not comprehend the difference between physiologic replacement and pharmacologic therapy. It requires careful and concerned counseling to convince many of these women that hormone replacement therapy is advisable.

If the dietary intake record reveals caloric or other nutritional inadequacy, the athlete should be evaluated and counseled by a nutritionist and possibly a psychologist or psychiatrist, if an eating disorder is suspected

Table 9-6. RELATIVE
CONTRAINDICATIONS TO ESTROGEN
THERAPY

1. Hypertension
2. Diabetes mellitus
3. Fibrocystic disease of the breast
4. Uterine leiomyomata
5. Familial hyperlipidemia
6. Migraine headaches
7. Gallbladder disease

(see Chapter 17). Many athletes will be willing to increase their food intake when they understand that dietary inadequacy may be contributing to the problem. Those who are unwilling to change their diets should be referred for such counseling by a specialist.

Although some of them may prefer to gain weight or to reduce training intensity or quantity, to see if menses return without hormone therapy, it is not recommended that these measures postpone for longer than 6 months the initiation of hormone replacement. A shorter trial is reasonable, particularly if the athlete herself makes this suggestion. I believe that the benefits of regular exercise far outweigh these potential reproductive hazards, which can and should be evaluated and treated if they develop.

Despite the demonstration by several investigators that exercise-associated menstrual dysfunction is often a reversible phenomenon, there is no evidence that it is reversible in *all* cases, nor is there any method of predicting when normal function will return, if ever. It seems unlikely that chronic, unopposed estrogen stimulation of the uterus will cause hyperplasia or adenocarcinoma in an athlete in less than one year. However, endometrial hyperplasia can develop within 6 months in postmenopausal women being treated with unopposed estrogen.[67,68] This raises my concerns about permitting any women with euestrogenic, anovulatory oligomenorrhea to remain untreated. Similarly, bone loss takes place at an accelerated rate as soon as a woman becomes hypoestrogenic, and a significant amount of bone will be lost within the first 3 years of hypoestrogenism. I believe that it is best to initiate hormone replacement therapy by the time 6 months have passed, for both oligomenorrheic and amenorrheic athletes. I also believe that pelvic examination and blood evaluation should be repeated annually in all athletes with menstrual dysfunction, regardless of whether they are receiving hormone replacement (Table 9-7).

Many athletes claim that they prefer to be amenorrheic. However, there is an obvious difference between not wanting to menstru-

Table 9-7. RECOMMENDATIONS FOR FOLLOW-UP OF ATHLETES WITH OLIGOMENORRHEA OR AMENORRHEA

1. Annual history and physical examination
2. Annual prolactin, TSH, free thyroxine, FSH, LH, DHEAS, testosterone, β-HCG, estradiol
3. Annual progestin challenge test
4. Hormone replacement therapy

ate on the day of an important competitive event and *never* wanting to menstruate at all. It is likely that most would prefer to have normal reproductive function, rather than amenorrhea, even if many are unwilling to admit this to themselves.

EVALUATION AND TREATMENT OF PRIMARY AMENORRHEA

Primary amenorrhea refers to the condition in which menstruation has never occurred. *Secondary amenorrhea,* to which we have referred until now, refers to the condition in which menstruation had occurred in the past but subsequently has ceased. Because menarche is often delayed in athletic girls, as discussed thoroughly in Chapters 7 and 8, it is tempting to assume that menarcheal delay is related to exercise. However, this assumption is as dangerous as that for secondary amenorrhea. Serious pathologic conditions can easily be missed if they are not sought.

Any girl who has not developed any secondary sexual characteristics by the age of 13 should be examined and possibly evaluated further. The same should be done for any girl who has not begun to menstruate by age 16. Physical findings will direct appropriate testing for these problems. As shown in Table 9-8, the diagnostic evaluation of primary amenorrhea is similar to that for secondary amenorrhea, except for the greater emphasis in primary amenorrhea upon detection of a uterus.

Müllerian agenesis (which includes the absence of the uterus) is the second most

Table 9–8. DIAGNOSTIC EVALUATION OF ATHLETES WITH PRIMARY AMENORRHEA

1. History, including dietary intake
2. Physical examination, including pelvic examination
3. Prolactin, free thyroxine, TSH, FSH, LH, DHEAS, testosterone, β-HCG, estradiol
4. Progestin challenge test
5. If uterus not palpable on pelvic examination: sonogram
6. If uterus absent: testosterone, karyotype
7. If FSH high: karyotype

common pathologic cause of primary amenorrhea, second only to gonadal dysgenesis. If the presence of a uterus cannot be determined with certainty by pelvic examination, a pelvic sonogram should be performed. The third most common pathologic cause of primary amenorrhea is androgen insensitivity syndrome (testicular feminization). Thus, the absence of a uterus requires further testing to distinguish between these two entities. The blood testosterone concentration should be measured, and a blood karyotype performed. Abnormal findings should be followed with appropriate testing, as indicated.

However, the most common cause of primary amenorrhea, particularly among athletes, is constitutional delay. If examination indicates good estrogen effect, the girl can be reassured that menarche is likely to occur soon spontaneously. Copious estrogenic cervical mucus usually indicates that spontaneous menarche will occur within 6 to 12 months. Hormone replacement therapy for euestrogenic or hypoestrogenic athletes is optional between the ages of 16 and 18, in my view, but should not be postponed beyond the age of 18 because of the risk of osteopenia.

SUMMARY

The tremendous increase in research in this field has enhanced our understanding of the pathophysiology of exercise-associated menstrual dysfunction. We now realize that, in many cases, dietary factors, weight loss, and exercise act synergistically to promote hormone alterations in both women with regular menses and those without.

Athletes are more likely than sedentary women and girls to experience menstrual dysfunction and menarcheal delay. However, this greater susceptibility should not discourage any athletes from exercising intensely or frequently. The benefits of regular exercise far outweigh this potential hazard.

The increased susceptibility of athletes to menstrual dysfunction also should not lead to the presumptive diagnosis of "exercise-induced" until completion of a comprehensive hormonal evaluation to rule out all other pathologic causes. It must be emphasized that the diagnosis of "exercise-related menstrual dysfunction" can be made only by excluding all other etiologies. Any woman or girl experiencing one of these problems should be evaluated and treated.

REFERENCES

1. Schwartz B, Cumming DC, Riordan E, et al: Exercise-associated amenorrhea: A distinct entity? Am J Obstet Gynecol 141:662, 1981.
2. Shangold MM, and Levine HS: The effect of marathon training upon menstrual function. Am J Obstet Gynecol 143:862, 1982.
3. Sanborn CF, Martin BJ, and Wagner WW: Is athletic amenorrhea specific to runners? Am J Obstet Gynecol 143:859, 1982.
4. Wakat DK, Sweeney KA, and Rogol AD: Reproductive system function in women cross-country runners. Med Sci Sports Exerc 14:263, 1982.
5. Bachmann GA, and Kemmann E: Prevalence of oligomenorrhea and amenorrhea in a college population. Am J Obstet Gynecol 144:98, 1982.
6. Judd HL (guest ed): Reproductive endocrinology. Clin Obstet Gynecol 21:15, 1978.
7. Shangold MM: Menstrual irregularity in athletes: Basic principles, evaluation, and treatment. Can J Appl Sport Sci 7:68, 1982.
8. Speroff L, Glass RH, and Kase NG: Clinical Gynecologic Endocrinology and Infertility, 4th Ed. Williams and Wilkins, Baltimore, 1989.
9. Prior JC, Cameron K, Ho Yuen B, et al: Menstrual cycle changes with marathon training: Anovulation and short luteal phase. Can J Appl Sports Sci 7:173, 1982.
10. Frisch RE, and McArthur JW: Menstrual cy-

cles: Fatness as a determinant of minimum weight for height necessary for their maintenance or onset. Science 185:949, 1974.

11. Fishman J, Boyar RM, and Hellman L: Influence of body weight on estradiol metabolism in young women. J Clin Endocrinol Metab 41:989, 1975.

12. Snow RC, Barbieri RL, and Frisch RE: Estrogen 2-hydroxylase oxidation and menstrual function among the oarswomen. J Clin Endocrinol Metab 69:369, 1989.

13. Warren MP: The effects of exercise on pubertal progression and reproductive function in girls. J Clin Endocrinol Metab 51:1150, 1980.

14. Calabrese LH, Kirkendall DT, Floyd M, et al: Menstrual abnormalities, nutritional patterns, and body composition in female classical ballet dancers. Phys Sportsmed 11(2):86, 1983.

15. Recommended Dietary Allowances, 9th Ed. Washington, DC, National Research Council, Food and Nutrition Board, National Academy of Sciences, 1980.

16. Frisch RE, Botz-Welbergen AV, McArthur JW, et al: Delayed menarche and amenorrhea of college athletes in relation to age of onset of training. JAMA 246:1559, 1981.

17. Godara R, Kaur AP, and Bhat CM: Effect of cellulose incorporation in a low fiber diet on fecal excretion and serum levels of calcium, phosphorus, and iron in adolescent girls. Am J Clin Nutr 34:1083, 1981.

18. Deuster PA, Kyle SB, Moser PB, et al: Nutritional intakes and status of highly trained amenorrheic and eumenorrheic women runners. Fertil Steril 46:636, 1986.

19. Pirke KM, Schweiger U, Laessle R, et al: Dieting influences the menstrual cycle: Vegetarian versus nonvegetarian diet. Fertil Steril 46:1083, 1986.

20. Pirke KM, Schweiger U, Strowitzki T, et al: Dieting causes menstrual irregularities in normal weight young women through impairment of episodic luteinizing hormone secretion. Fertil Steril 51:263, 1989.

21. Longcope C, Gorbach S, Goldin B, et al: The effect of a low fat diet on estrogen metabolism. J Clin Endocrinol Metab 64:1246, 1987.

22. Myerson M, Gutin B, Warren MP, et al: Resting metabolic rate and energy balance in amenorrheic and eumenorrheic runners. Med Sci Sports Exerc 23:15, 1991.

23. Shangold MM, Gatz ML, and Thysen B: Acute effects of exercise on plasma concentrations of prolactin and testosterone in recreational women runners. Fertil Steril 35:699, 1981.

24. Bonen A, Ling W, MacIntyre K, et al: Effects of exercise on the serum concentrations of FSH, LH, progesterone and estradiol. Eur J Appl Physiol 42:15, 1979.

25. Carr DB, Bullen BA, Skrinar GS, et al: Physical conditioning facilitates the exercise-induced secretion of beta-endorphin and beta-lipotropin in women. N Engl J Med 305:560, 1981.

26. Carr DB, Reppert SM, Bullen B, et al: Plasma melatonin increases during exercise in women. J Clin Endocrinol Metab 53:224, 1981.

27. Cumming DC, and Rebar RW: Exercise and reproductive function in women. Am J Ind Med 4:113, 1983.

28. Hartley LH, Mason JW, Hogan RP, et al: Multiple hormonal responses to prolonged exercise in relation to physical training. J Appl Physiol 33:607, 1972.

29. Rebar RW, Bulow S, Stern B, et al: Patterns of endocrine response to exercise in normal and dexamethasone suppressed women. Sixty-fifth annual meeting, Endocrine Society, 1983, Abstract 464.

30. Shangold MM: Exercise and the adult female: Hormonal and endocrine effects. Exerc Sport Sci Rev 12:53, 1984.

31. Cumming DC, and Rebar RW: Hormonal changes with acute exercise and with training in women. Sem Reprod Endocrinol 3:55, 1985.

32. Loucks AB, and Horvath SM: Athletic amenorrhea: A review. Med Sci Sports Exerc 17:56, 1985.

33. Shangold MM, Freeman R, Thysen B, and Gatz M: The relationship between long-distance running, plasma progesterone and luteal phase length. Fertil Steril 31:130, 1979.

34. Prior JC, Ho Yuen B, Clement P, et al: Reversible luteal phase changes and infertility associated with marathon training. Lancet 2:269, 1982.

35. Frisch RE, Hall GM, Aoki TT, et al: Metabolic, endocrine, and reproductive changes of a woman channel swimmer. Metabolism 33:1106, 1984.

36. Bullen BA, Skrinar GS, Beitins IZ, et al: Induction of menstrual disorders by strenuous exercise in untrained women. N Engl J Med 312:1349, 1985.

37. Beitins IZ, McArthur JW, Turnbull BA, et al: Exercise induces two types of human luteal dysfunction: Confirmation by urinary free progesterone. J Clin Endocrinol Metab 72:1350, 1991.

38. Russell JB, Mitchell D, Musey PI, and Collins DC: The relationship of exercise to anovulatory cycles in female athletes: Hormonal and physical characteristics. Obstet Gynecol 63:452, 1984.

39. Russell JB, Mitchell DE, Musey PI, and Collins DC: The role of beta-endorphins and catechol estrogens on the hypothalamic-pituitary axis in female athletes. Fertil Steril 42:690, 1984.

40. Ropert JF, Quigley ME, and Yen SSC: Endogenous opiates modulate pulsatile luteinizing hormone release in humans. J Clin Endocrinol Metab 52:583, 1981.

41. Villanueva AL, Schlosser C, Hopper B, et al: Increased cortisol production in women runners. J Clin Endocrinol Metab 63:133, 1986.

42. Loucks AB, Mortola JF, Girton L, and Yen SSC: Alterations in the hypothalamic-pituitary-ovarian and the hypothalamic-pituitary-adrenal axes in athletic women. J Clin Endocrinol Metab 68:402, 1989.

43. Ding J-H, Sheckter CB, Drinkwater BL, et al: High serum cortisol levels in exercise-associated amenorrhea. Ann Int Med 108:530, 1988.

44. DeSouza MJ, and Metzger DA: Reproductive dysfunction in amenorrheic athletes and anorexic patients: A review. Med Sci Sports Exerc 23:995, 1991.

45. Boyden TW, Pamenter RW, Stanforth PR, et al: Impaired gonadotropin responses to gonadotropin-releasing hormone stimulation in endurance-trained women. Fertil Steril 41:359, 1984.

46. Cumming DC, Vickovic MM, Wall SR, and Fluker MR: Defects in pulsatile LH release in normally menstruating runners. J Clin Endocrinol Metabol 60:810, 1985.

47. Cumming DC, Vickovic MM, Wall SR, et al: The effect of acute exercise on pulsatile release of luteinizing hormone in women runners. Am J Obstet Gynecol 153:482, 1985.

48. Veldhuis JD, Evans WS, Demers LM, et al: Altered neuroendocrine regulation of gonadotropin secretion in women distance runners. J Clin Endocrinol Metab 61:557, 1985.

49. Cowan LD, Gordis L, Tonascia JA, and Jones GS: Breast cancer incidence in women with history of progesterone deficiency. Am J Epidemiol 114:209, 1981.

50. Prior JC, Vigna YM, Schechter MT, and Burgess AE: Spinal bone loss and ovulatory disturbances. N Engl J Med 323:1221, 1990.

51. Fechner RE and Kaufman RH: Endometrial adenocarcinoma in Stein-Leventhal syndrome. Cancer 34:444, 1974.

52. Jafari K, Ghodratollah I, and Ruiz G: Endometrial adenocarcinoma and the Stein-Leventhal syndrome. Obstet Gynecol 51:97, 1978.

53. Coulam CB, Annegers JF, and Kranz JS: Chronic anovulation syndrome and associated neoplasia. Obstet Gynecol 61:403, 1983.

54. Dennefors BL, Knutson F, Janson PO, et al: Ovarian steroid production in a woman with polycystic ovary syndrome associated with endometrial cancer. Acta Obstet Gynecol Scand 64:387, 1985.

55. Gonzales ER: Chronic anovulation may increase post-menopausal breast cancer risk. (Medical News), JAMA 249:445, 1983.

56. Frisch RE, Wyshak G, Albright NL, et al: Lower prevalence of breast cancer and cancers of the reproductive system among former college athletes compared to nonathletes. Br J Cancer 52:885, 1985.

57. Cann CE, Martin MC, Genant HK, and Jaffe RB: Decreased spinal mineral content in amenorrheic women. JAMA 251:626, 1984.

58. Rigotti NA, Nussbaum SR, Herzog DB, and Neer RM: Osteoporosis in women with anorexia nervosa. N Engl J Med 311:1601, 1984.

59. Drinkwater BL, Nilson K, Chesnut CH, et al: Bone mineral content of amenorrheic and eumenorrheic athletes. N Engl J Med 311:277, 1984.

60. Marcus R, Cann C, Madvig P, et al: Menstrual function and bone mass in elite women distance runners. Ann Int Med 102:158, 1985.

61. Jones KP, Ravnikar VA, Tulchinsky D, and Schiff I: Comparison of bone density in amenorrheic women due to athletics, weight loss, and premature menopause. Obstet Gynecol 66:5, 1985.

62. Warren MP, Brooks-Gunn J, Hamilton LH, et al: Scoliosis and fractures in young ballet dancers. N Engl J Med 314:1348, 1986.

63. Lloyd T, Triantafyllou SJ, Baker ER, et al: Women athletes with menstrual irregularity have increased musculoskeletal injuries. Med Sci Sports Exerc 18:374, 1986.

64. Heaney RP, Recker RR, and Saville PD: Menopausal changes in calcium balance performance. J Lab Clin Med 92:953, 1978.

65. Meema S and Meema HE: Menopausal bone loss and estrogen replacement. Isr J Med Sci 12:601, 1976.

66. Lamon-Fava S, Fisher EC, Nelson ME, et al: Effect of exercise and menstrual cycle status on plasma lipids, low density lipoprotein particle size, and apolipoproteins. J Clin Endocrinol Metab 68:17, 1989.

67. Schiff I, Sela HK, Cramer D, et al: Endometrial hyperplasia in women on cyclic or continuous estrogen regimens. Fertil Steril 39:79, 1982.

68. Gelfand M, and Ferenczy A: A prospective 1-year study of estrogen and progestin in postmenopausal women: Effects on the endometrium. Obstet Gynecol 74:398, 1989.

CHAPTER 10

Pregnancy

MARSHALL W. CARPENTER, M.D.

Exertion and pregnancy are the two most profound normal alterations in mammalian physiology. Exertion causes acute changes in cardiac output, blood flow distribution, oxygen uptake, fuel mobilization, and the endocrine responses that facilitate these changes. Chronic exercise stress (exertional training) alters resting cardiovascular and metabolic homeostasis, the circulatory response to exertion, and aerobic capacity. Pregnancy appears to induce a primary vasodilatation with associated increases in cardiac output, oxygen carrying capacity, oxygen uptake, and pulmonary changes. Whereas many of the cardiovascular changes that characterize pregnancy at rest are similar to those seen in acute exertion, the endocrine and metabolic changes of pregnancy differ considerably from those seen with acute exertion. Acute maternal adaptation to exertion and to exercise training has recently received increased investigational attention. The effect of maternal acute and chronic exercise stress on fetal homeostasis and growth and the role of maternal nutrition remain only superficially understood in humans, based primarily on animal investigation. The limited physiologic and epidemiologic investigation available, however, form the foundation for the guidelines and counsel that can be offered to pregnant women.

This chapter examines the effects of pregnancy on resting physiology, and its interaction with the effects of acute exertion. The impact of acute exertion on fetal homeostasis and the effect of exercise training on pregnancy outcome are also explored. These observations will be related to recommendations which may be offered to pregnant women in clinical circumstances.

PHYSIOLOGIC CHANGES OF PREGNANCY

Cardiovascular changes begin early in pregnancy and are well established by the midtrimester, thereby anticipating later fetal/placental requirements for oxygen and nutrition. Plasma volume increases 45% by 30 to 34 weeks,[1,2] with measurable changes by 8 weeks. Despite a dilutional anemia, red cell volume increases by 20% to 30% by mid-pregnancy.[2]

Cardiac output may increase secondary to a primary increase in circulating plasma volume or decreased systemic vascular resistance,[3] though the relationship of these factors remains speculative.[4] By 8 weeks, cardiac output increases by 23% and stroke volume by 20%.[5-7] The maximal increment in cardiac output (34%) exceeds the 13% increase in body weight during pregnancy. This is due, partly, to the 13% to 30% increase in resting oxygen uptake observed in pregnancy[8-10] and also to the decreased arteriovenous oxygen difference in pregnancy.

End diastolic volume[6,7] and stroke volume[11] appear to increase through midpregnancy. Venous compliance increases by the second trimester and is greater in the lower extremities.[12,13] These vascular changes and the expanding uterus may impede vena caval blood flow, so that maternal position increasingly alters measurements of hemodynamic function as pregnancy progresses. The further increase in resting cardiac output later in pregnancy seems to be heart-rate dependent but variable, due to differences in maternal stature and position.

Respiratory changes in pregnancy involve respiratory control and pulmonary function. Changes in respiratory control are reflected in a 17% increase in minute ventilation relative to oxygen uptake (the ventilatory equivalent).[14] This results in a fall in arterial P_{CO_2} from 39 to 31 torr, which produces a mild respiratory alkalosis, increasing pH to 7.44. Increased total lung capacity and increased tidal volume account for most of the increase in minute ventilation, rather than changes in respiratory frequency. The increased resting oxygen uptake observed in pregnancy is an early phenomenon, half of which occurs by 8 weeks and three quarters by 15 weeks' gestation. However, resting oxygen uptake remains proportional to body weight, not changing from the antepartum to postpartum state.[15,16]

ACUTE PHYSIOLOGIC RESPONSE TO EXERTION IN THE NONPREGNANCY STATE

The cardiovascular and respiratory systems act in concert during acute exertion to ensure adequate oxygen delivery to exercising muscle while maintaining function in other tissues. Oxygen consumption is the product of oxygen delivery (heart rate, stroke volume) and oxygen extraction (arteriovenous O_2 difference), as expressed in the modified Fick equation:[17]

$$\dot{V}_{O_2} = HR \cdot SV \cdot avD_{O_2}$$

During incremental exercise to maximal intensity, $\dot{V}_{O_2}$ increases linearly to values typically 10 to 20 times that at rest. Near the peak intensity of exertion, a plateau of oxygen uptake ($\dot{V}_{O_2}$) occurs, which persists despite greater exercise intensity. This upper limit of oxygen uptake ($\dot{V}_{O_2}max$) occurs as maximal aerobic power is reached and is the most important indicator of cardiovascular fitness. The percentage of $\dot{V}_{O_2}max$ may be used, therefore, to describe relative intensity of exertion among individuals with different aerobic capacities when comparing physiologic responses that are related to exertional intensity. $\dot{V}_{O_2}max$ is usually limited by cardiac output. (See Chapters 1 and 4.)

Cardiac output typically increases four-tofivefold from rest to maximum exertion. Cardiac output increases with $\dot{V}_{O_2}$ in normal individuals in a ratio ranging from 5:1 to 6:1.

Heart rate increases linearly with $\dot{V}_{O_2}$. Initial increases during mild exertion result from release from vagal tone, and increases at higher exercise intensities are caused by increases in sympathetic tone. Up to 40% $\dot{V}_{O_2}$ max, stroke volume increases with increased venous return to 1.5 to 2.0 times that at rest. Above a heart rate of 100, however, further increases in cardiac output are pulse-dependent.[18]

Peripheral as well as central hemodynamic changes are necessary to effectively deliver required oxygen and fuel to exercising muscle. Blood flow is redistributed by sympathetic nerve activity, which is reflected in increased plasma norepinephrine concentrations.[19] Norepinephrine concentration is closely related to intensity of exertion and to heart rate above 100.[17] This redistribution results in an early and sustained linear reduction in splanchnic and renal blood flow and, at high exertional intensity, causes decreased cutaneous perfusion.

The proportion of total cardiac output perfusing exercising muscle increases with the relative intensity of exertion regardless of individual aerobic fitness. However, this proportion is higher at maximal aerobic power among individuals with high levels of aerobic fitness. Therefore, the increment in $\dot{V}_{O_2}$max obtained with exercise training is attributable to increased oxygen uptake of exercising muscle, while nonexercising vascular beds receive the same low absolute blood flow.

Oxygen uptake during exertion is also enhanced by increased oxygen extraction from each volume of blood perfusing exercising muscle. This is reflected in a three- or fourfold increase in arteriovenous oxygen difference at maximal exertion compared to rest.[17,20]

Ventilation increases linearly with oxygen uptake (at 20 to 25 L per liter of O_2 uptake) to about 50% $\dot{V}_{O_2}$max, above which the increase in ventilation is greater, relative to oxygen uptake, approaching a ratio of 40 L of air per liter of O_2 uptake. This change in ventilatory pattern has been referred to as the "ventilatory threshold"[21,22] but has uncertain physiologic significance. It is loosely associated with elevated levels of plasma lactate, found at high exertional intensity. Exercise training results in a greater increase in $\dot{V}_{O_2}$ at ventilatory threshold than in $\dot{V}_{O_2}$max. Maximal voluntary ventilation does not limit $\dot{V}_{O_2}$max in normal individuals.

ACUTE METABOLIC RESPONSE TO EXERTION

The profound increase in the energy requirements of muscle during exercise necessitates the mobilization and distribution of fuel from other tissues to sustain exertion beyond the first seconds of movement. Energy consumption may increase over 10-fold above resting values during intense exertion.[21,23,24] Muscle can oxidize glucose, free fatty acids, glycerol and ketones to produce energy. The proportion of fuel types available to muscle is a function of exercise intensity, duration, nutritional state, and the physical fitness of the individual, and is determined largely by the acute hormonal response to exertion.

Carbohydrate stores in the body are found in muscle glycogen (300 to 400 g, $5 \cdot 10^3$ kJ), hepatic glycogen (80 to 90 g, $1.5 \cdot 10^3$ kJ), and blood glucose (20 g, 30 kJ). This is dwarfed by the energy stored as fat (about 15 kg, $6 \cdot 10^5$ kJ). Protein is not significantly available as fuel during acute exercise. At rest, free fatty acids provide the primary fuel for muscle in the fasting state.

As exertional intensity increases beyond 60% $\dot{V}_{O_2}$max, carbohydrate is oxidized in higher proportions, so that at $\dot{V}_{O_2}$max, all the energy expended by muscle is derived from carbohydrate oxidation. At this intense level of exertion, adenosine triphosphate (ATP) is provided increasingly by anaerobic glycolysis, which is reflected in rising plasma lactate concentrations above 60% $\dot{V}_{O_2}$max. Elevated plasma lactate may act to suppress lipolysis,[25] thereby increasing demands on carbohydrate as fuel. Consequently, exercise at $\dot{V}O_2$max can only be sustained for a short duration, being limited by the modest stores of carbohydrate available to sustain exertion at this intensity. Most investigators employ some criterion for a "plateau" of oxygen uptake with increasing workload to establish that $\dot{V}O_2$max has been achieved. The uncertainty about criteria to establish a maximum $\dot{V}O_2$ plateau and the subject's difficulty in maintenance of this level of exertion make observations under this condition problematic, especially in pregnancy. Data from such studies thereby require some judgment in their interpretation.

Exercise duration also influences fuel metabolism. The immediate, local sources of energy (ATP and phosphocreatine) provide energy for the first 6 to 8 seconds of muscle contraction. Glycogenolysis and local lactate production provide carbohydrate for 1 to 3 minutes of exertion at maximal aerobic exertion. Exercise beyond 5 to 10 minutes becomes increasingly dependent on free fatty acids. Moderate-intensity exertion for 40 minutes results in a fourfold rise in glucose production by glycogenolysis and gluconeogenesis to maintain plasma glucose concentration for tissue with obligate glucose needs. This response is reduced 15% to 60% by glucose infusion, and 67% by glucose and insulin infusion.[26]

Diet antecedent to exercise may alter exercise capacity at $\dot{V}O_2$max. A high carbohydrate diet following intense exercise increases muscle glycogen stores. Low carbohydrate diets decrease muscle and hepatic glycogen. Exercise capacity is increased when muscle glycogen stores are augmented.[21,23,24,27] Carbohydrate ingestion during exertion increases exercise endurance.[21,23,24,27]

The neuroendocrine response to exertion facilitates the mobilization of fuels for muscle contraction. Norepinephrine, released from synaptic nerve endings, stimulates hepatic glycogenolysis and peripheral lipolysis. It also stimulates islet α-adrenergic receptors to inhibit insulin release and stimulate glucagon release, which, in turn, augment hepatic glycogenolysis and peripheral lipolysis.[28,29] Both norepinephrine and epinephrine increase with percent $\dot{V}O_2$max and pulmonary artery oxygen saturation. Epinephrine concentration is increased with intense exertion, is produced by the adrenal medulla, and correlates positively with norepinephrine and negatively with glucose concentrations.[30,31] Therefore, the net effect of these changes is to augment and sustain the release of glucose.

Exertion also alters the metabolic effects of insulin. The drop in insulin concentration during acute exertion does not impede the marked rise in peripheral glucose uptake during exercise.[32] Under these conditions, only an absolute lack of insulin causes a reduction in glucose uptake (in the pancreatectomized dog), suggesting that insulin may only have a permissive role in peripheral uptake during intense exertion.[32] Isolated exertion increases insulin-mediated glucose uptake (insulin sensitivity) and glucose uptake at maximal effective insulin concentration (insulin responsiveness) up to 48 hours after exercise.[33]

Intense or prolonged moderate exertion is required to produce a rise in circulating levels of glucagon,[29,34] growth hormone,[35] and cortisol. Growth hormone response correlates with $\dot{V}O_2$ and plasma lactate concentration.[35]

EFFECT OF PREGNANCY ON THE ACUTE PHYSIOLOGIC RESPONSE TO EXERTION

The impact of pregnancy on exercise response to submaximal and maximal exercise differs. During pregnancy, we found that absolute oxygen consumption (L·min^{-1}) was 14% higher at rest, 9% higher during identical workloads during submaximal, weight-supported cycle ergometry, and 12% higher during identical submaximal treadmill exertion[16] compared to postpartum values. Similar investigations by others have not consistently shown an increased oxygen uptake during submaximal cycle exercise in pregnancy compared to nonpregnant controls.[8–11,37,38] However, identical submaximal treadmill exertion has been found to result in increased $\dot{V}O_2$ during pregnancy.[8,16] When oxygen consumption is expressed relative to body weight ($mL \cdot kg^{-2} \cdot min^{-1}$), however, there are no differences in submaximal oxygen uptake with either mode of exercise. Of the increased oxygen uptake of submaximal exertion, 75% can be accounted for when the contribution of increased maternal weight is controlled for experimentally during pregnancy. This was accomplished by comparing non–weight-bearing and weight-bearing exercise during pregnancy and postpartum, and by using weight belts during postpartum weight-bearing exertion to mimic pregnancy weight.[16] These data suggest that gravid women have an increased resting and exertional percent $\dot{V}O_2max$ due, largely, to the increased metabolic demands of the conceptus as well as the increased work of moving a heavier body.

Pregnancy may alter the relative contribution of stroke volume and heart rate to increased cardiac output during incremental workloads at high levels of exercise intensity. In the nonpregnant state, stroke volume does not increase with incremental exertion above 60% $\dot{V}O_2max$; further increases in cardiac output are due to increased heart rate. In contrast, limited data in pregnancy suggest that further increases in stroke volume are still possible above this level of exertional intensity.[10] This change in the relative contribution of stroke volume to incremental cardiac output with increased workload alters the regression equation of $\dot{V}O_2$ on heart rate during pregnancy. Consequently, the mathematic model for predicting $\dot{V}O_2max$ from submaximal $\dot{V}O_2$/heart-rate data in pregnant women is altered.[39]

In contrast to submaximal exertion, the limited studies performed on pregnant women at maximal aerobic exertion show little, if any, change in maternal cardiovascular response under this condition. Pregnancy is not associated with any change in the usual coupling of $\dot{V}O_2$ to cardiac output.[10]

Likewise, peak age-specific heart rate appears to be unchanged by pregnancy at maximal aerobic exertion. Also, we and others have found no difference in maximal aerobic power in pregnancy when compared with postpartum values.[10]

Recovery from exertion in the upright position may differ in pregnancy. Stroke volume recorded within 3 minutes of exercise cessation has been observed to fall 26% during the third trimester, compared to only 11% postpartum.[40] Cardiac output did not differ, being maintained by a compensatory increase in heart rate. This change in post-exertional recovery may be related to increased venous compliance and capacity and possible vena caval obstruction that may characterize late pregnancy, though this remains to be documented.

EFFECT OF PREGNANCY ON THE ACUTE METABOLIC RESPONSE TO EXERTION

Pregnancy produces alterations in hormonal and metabolic homeostasis, which distinguish it from the nonpregnant resting and exercising state. Pregnancy produces insulin resistance, which is reflected in an elevated fasting insulin-glucose ratio. This may be observed more quantitatively by inducing hyperinsulinemia by intravenous infusion and measuring the rate of glucose infusion required to maintain steady-state euglycemia. This euglycemia, hyperinsulinemic clamp technique demonstrates a reduced requirement for infused glucose during pregnancy in order to maintain euglycemia compared to that required in the nonpregnant state under the same hyperinsulinemic conditions.[41] Insulin binding on red cells is unaffected by pregnancy, but binding is reduced on adipocytes during pregnancy.[42] Pregnancy is characterized by postprandial hyperglycemia and by fasting hypoglycemia. Free fatty acid and triglyceride concentrations are increased in pregnancy.

Acute hormonal responses to exercise

stress support internal homeostasis in two ways. First, release of catecholamines by peripheral nerves serves to increase and redirect cardiac output to exercising muscle while maintaining "adequate" perfusion to nonexercising vascular beds. Second, the medullary release of catecholamines, and the release of glucagon, cortisol, and growth hormone result in providing the peripheral circulation with fuel to maintain both intense and sustained exertion.

Little has been published about alterations in the hormonal response to exertion induced by pregnancy. Resting plasma norepinephrine and epinephrine levels are unchanged in pregnancy, though standing is associated with a reduced rise in norepinephrine concentration in pregnancy.[43] Exertion appears to produce a similar norepinephrine response in pregnancy as in the nonpregnant state.[44,45] Insulin concentration does not appear to fall during mild exertion during pregnancy[46] but has not been examined at more vigorous exercise. Glucagon, which is increased in pregnancy, has been observed to rise twofold with maternal exertion to a pulse of only 104,[46] but this was not confirmed in later studies.[44] In the nonpregnant state, increased glucagon concentrations are observed after only intense or prolonged exertion.[29] The effect of pregnancy

on glucagon, growth hormone, and cortisol response to moderate or intense exertion has not been examined.

Consequently, the nature and degree of pregnancy-induced alterations of acute hormonal response to exertion are largely unexamined. Possible direct or indirect effects of these changes on fetal homeostasis during maternal exertion are likewise unknown.

MATERNAL THERMOREGULATION DURING EXERCISE

Published studies of maternal thermoregulation have examined gravidae only during submaximal exertion lasting 20 to 30 minutes in a controlled laboratory environment of 19 to 21°C with a relative humidity of 30% to 55%. Two studies examined stationary cycle exercise at approximately 60% $\dot{V}O_2$max,[47,48] and one[49] had subjects perform treadmill exercise at a maternal heart rate of approximately 158 beats per minute (bpm) (approximately 60% $\dot{V}O_2$max). Under these conditions, the range of mean rectal temperature rise was 0.3 to 0.8°C during exercise, inversely related to gestational age (Fig. 10–1). Pregnant women appear to maintain

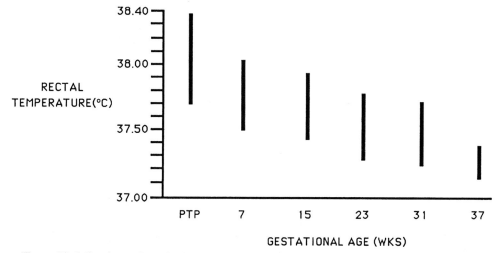

Figure 10–1. Resting and maximal rectal temperatures (at the bottom and top of each column, respectively) during, and 10 minutes after, a 20-minute cycle exercise period at 61%–64% maximal oxygen uptake. (Adapted from Clapp[48]).

their core temperature within narrow limits, though maternal thermoregulatory capacity during exertion under more stressful ambient conditions has not been examined. Associated fetal effects also have not been examined.

ACUTE EFFECTS OF MATERAL EXERTION ON THE FETUS

Splanchnic perfusion falls linearly with the percentage of $\dot{V}O_2$max, as blood flow is redistributed to exercising muscle. A similar reduction in uterine blood flow with moderate and extreme maternal exertion during pregnancy has been demonstrated in sheep[50-52] and goats[53] and suggested in humans (Fig. 10-2).[54-56] In sheep, this exercise-induced reduction of uterine perfusion was found to be associated with a fall in fetal PO_2 of 11% with moderate maternal exertion, and 30% with exhausting exertion.[51] However, no measurable net lactate production by the conceptus has been observed under these conditions. This suggests that oxygen delivery is, in most fetal tissues, adequate for aerobic metabolism during these short-term experiments.

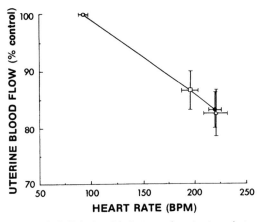

Figure 10–2. Relationship between heart rate and uterine blood flow as percent of control in near-term pregnant sheep: ○ = rest, □ = 10-minute exercise at 70% $\dot{V}O_2$max; ● = 10-minute exercise at 100% $\dot{V}O_2$max; △ = 40-minute exercise at 70% $\dot{V}O_2$max. (From Lotgering,[51] with permission).

Early studies in human pregnancy examined fetal heart-rate response to maternal exertion using the same Doppler fetal monitors used clinically on quiet, recumbent women during labor. These reports described frequent fetal bradycardia with only brief and mild maternal exertion,[57,58] but the findings may have been confounded by motion artifact during maternal activity.

Subsequent investigation has employed two-dimensional sonographic fetal heart-rate documentation. In one such study, 85 submaximal and 79 maximal exercise bouts[59] produced no unexplained fetal bradycardia (<110 bpm) during exertion. However, postexertional fetal bradycardia was noted within 3 minutes of cessation of maximal aerobic effort in 19% (15 out of 79) of cases (Fig. 10-3). This bradycardia was not associated with the duration of maximal aerobic exertion, changes in maternal blood pressure during and after exertion, or with gestational age. It was more likely to occur in women with higher $\dot{V}O_2$max values, suggesting that maternal cardiovascular fitness does not protect against this event. All fetuses had normal fetal heart-rate patterns and fetal activity within 30 minutes of maternal exercise, and the birth outcome in the pregnancies with fetal bradycardia was uncomplicated.

These data suggest that fetal homeostatic reserve is not compromised by even extreme levels of maternal exertion in the human. The possible adverse impact of maternal upright posture on fetal homeostasis during maternal recovery remains to be explored. The observed postexertional fall in stroke volume in exercising gravid women may indicate that visceral perfusion may be compromised in pregnancy under these conditions.

Observations of baseline fetal heart rate before, during, and after maternal exertion has generally shown a 10 to 15 bpm increase in fetal heart rate with moderate exertion lasting 30 minutes or more. Generally maternal exertion at 60% $\dot{V}O_2$max which lasts less than 20 minutes will not produce fetal tachycardia. Exertion at this level which lasts 20 to 30 minutes will produce a rise in fetal heart rate which correlates with gestational age over 20 to 36 weeks. This response does not correlate with the minor changes in maternal core temperature (0.3°C) observed in these subjects, however.[47]

MATERNAL EXERCISE TRAINING EFFECTS ON FETAL GROWTH AND PERINATAL OUTCOME

The epidemiology of the workplace environment and activity and maternal and perinatal outcome occupies a large body of literature. Discussion here will be limited to studies examining the association of recreational exercise with maternal and perinatal outcome. Prospective studies of recreational exertion can be divided into nonrandomized and randomized, controlled comparisons of exercising and sedentary pregnant women. Nonrandomized studies have shown both no effect on maternal weight gain[60] and significantly reduced maternal weight gain caused by chronic maternal exercise.[61] Likewise, nonrandomized observations have documented either no effect of chronic maternal exercise on birth weight and duration of pregnancy[60,62] or a significant reduction in birth weight, percentile birth weight, percentage body fat,[63] and earlier gestational age at birth.[61,64] Exercising mothers were found to have either a lower rate of labor complications[60,64] or no significant difference from their nonrandomized controls.[62] It should be noted that most of these nonrandomized studies[63–65] examine the effect of the cessation of maternal recreational exertion before or early in pregnancy among women who are exercise enthusiasts. The remainder are simply comparisons of

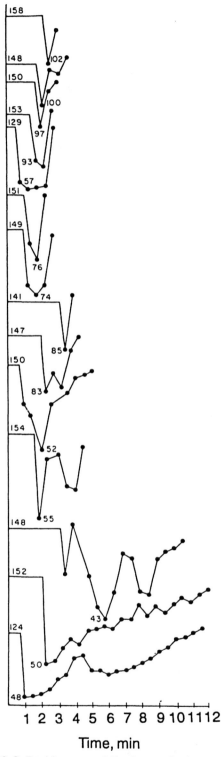

Figure 10–3. Fetal heart rate following maximal exertion during 14 episodes of fetal bradycardia. Fetal heart rate was averaged over 10 cardiac cycles every 30 seconds during the postexercise period, using videotaped recordings of two-dimensional fetal imaging. Predeceleration baseline fetal heart rate and nadir fetal heart rate are noted for each deceleration. Zero time is time of cessation of maximal effort. (From Carpenter,[59] with permission).

women who have self-selected exercise programs or sedentary activity.

Two randomized, controlled trials[66,67] examined the effect of instituting exercise training during pregnancy in sedentary pregnant women. Only one provided observed exercise training in a laboratory environment.[67] Both studies documented objective signs of cardiovascular training effect in the groups randomized to exercise training; however, in contrast to the nonrandomized investigations, neither randomized trial showed any effect of maternal exercise training on maternal weight gain, length of gestation, birth weight, Apgar scores, or mode of delivery. One study[66] suggested that primigravid trainers had a shorter second stage of labor.

Differences between the results of nonrandomized and randomized prospective studies suggest that self-selected women may differ in daily activity, percentage body fat, caloric intake or food type, or other factors that affect fetal growth, medical treatment during labor, and maternal and perinatal outcome. Some of the nonrandomized studies are detraining studies rather than investigations of training effects in sedentary women, and thereby present problems in applying findings in atheletes to the more common, inactive pregnant woman. Women who enter pregnancy with a history of frequent vigorous exertion may differ metabolically from those who are relatively sedentary.

Transabdominal pressure transducer monitoring of pregnant women during exercise has shown, in one study,[68] that uterine contractions are associated with nonrecumbent types of exercise. Another investigation,[69] however, examined uterine contractions by the same method immediately after the cessation of maternal exertion and found no increased uterine activity. These studies and practical experience in the use of these transducers in laboring women suggest that the uterine activity detected in up to 50% of gravidae during exercise is likely to represent artifact due to maternal motion.

Available data suggest that maternal exertion does not predispose to preterm labor.

RECOMMENDATIONS ABOUT RECREATIONAL EXERCISE

The limited scope of applied research regarding the effects of pregnancy on acute exercise and training and the effects of exertion on pregnancy limit the advice that can be confidently given to the pregnant patient. In 1985, the American College of Obstetricians and Gynecologists published two prescriptive articles,[70,71] which commented on exercise during pregnancy. These recommendations preceded much of the clinical research performed in this area. As such, they were an attempt to form a consensus opinion about principles of maternal and fetal safety during maternal exertion, and they reflected a necessarily conservative approach to exercise in pregnancy that could be used, practically, in a clinical setting. Some later studies have addressed some of these issues.

The principles documented in these published guidelines are listed below. In italics, the uncertainty attending these guidelines or modifying data available from subsequently published research are discussed.

1 Maternal joints become more unstable during pregnancy and may be more prone to injury during exertion. Exercises should avoid "ballistic" movement and extreme extension and flexion of joints. *No observational or experimental studies have quantified the risk of joint injury during pregnancy. These proscriptions may reduce injury, however.*

2 More physically fit individuals will perform a given task at a relatively lower percentage of maximal aerobic capacity. It is therefore desirable for women to become aerobically trained before pregnancy and thereby reduce fetal risk of asphyxia and bradycardia during maternal exertion during pregnancy. *Di-*

rect observation of fetal heart-rate response during maternal exertion has shown no fetal heart rate decelerations during exertion of any relative intensity, and none following maternal exertion up to a maternal pulse of 150 bpm in the maternal age range of 21 to 37 years of age. The occasional fetal bradycardia that follows maximal maternal exertion is more common in the more aerobically fit mother. Maternal exertion may increase the baseline fetal heart rate.[72] However, exercise-associated fetal tachycardia and episodic bradycardia are unassociated with any measurable fetal or neonatal morbidity.[59] The usually recommended warm-up and slow cool-down periods with exercise should probably be used during pregnancy.

3 Pregnant women may develop a high maternal core temperature during exercise exceeding 15 minutes, especially in hot and humid environments. High maternal core temperature may be associated with teratogenesis or respiratory compromise in animals, suggesting risk in the exercising mother. Human experiments describe only a 0.3 to 0.8°C rise in maternal core temperature with moderate to severe maternal exertion of 30 minutes' duration,[47,48,73] an increase of little physiologic consequence. The effect of maternal exertion under conditions of high ambient temperature and humidity on fetal homeostasis and core temperature has not been examined.

4 Maternal fasting glucose levels are significantly lower than in the nonpregnant state. Since pregnant women use more carbohydrate during exertion, hypoglycemia may occur during exertion. Little human experimental evidence is available about maternal glycemic response to exertion. Animal experiments performed in the nonpregnant state indicate that both sympathetic and glucagon response to exertion must be ablated to cause exertional hypoglycemia. Gravidae consume a relatively higher proportion of carbohydrates during exertion if exercise is carried out at a higher percentage of aerobic capacity, so it may be desirable during pregnancy to exercise at levels that elicit maternal heart rates of less than 150 bpm.

5 Exercise during pregnancy may result in premature labor due to release of norepinephrine. Experimental data show no consistent evidence of increased uterine contractions immediately following exertion. Preterm labor among exercisers does not appear to be increased in either detraining or training studies.

6 Previously sedentary women should engage in activity of very low intensity and avoid exertional intensity known to increase exertional cardiovascular fitness. Limited human experimental data show no increased maternal or fetal compromise during and after acute exertion. Pregnant women with lower $\dot{V}o_2$max values had a lower rate of fetal bradycardia after maximal exertion,[59] suggesting that prior sedentary lifestyle is not a contraindication to vigorous exertion during pregnancy.

7 Pregnant women should practice good nutritional principles (see below) and avoid cigarettes and alcohol. The vasodilatory effects of alcohol and vasoconstrictive and hypoxemic effects of cigarette smoking may compromise the homeostatic reserve of the mother and the fetoplacental unit during maternal exertion. Women who smoke and drink during pregnancy should probably avoid exertion at times when exposed to these drugs. No human observational studies or experiments have been performed examining these interactions directly.

8 Women whose pregnancies are compromised by any maternal diseases or any untoward symptoms should contact their physician for consultation. The importance of consultation of a patient with her physician should be emphasized. Though data are not available, caution regarding exertion in many con-

ditions complicating pregnancy should be counseled by physicians.

We use several principles when counseling pregnant women regarding exercise:

1 We recognize the value of continued recreation during pregnancy, which for many women includes vigorous exertion. Unless prior observational or experimental data or the individual circumstances of the patient's pregnancy appear to contradict a proposed exercise activity during pregnancy, we do not proscribe exertion for the patient.

2 Relative exertional intensity, as described in terms of percentage of $\dot{V}o_2$max, produces similar cardiovascular, respiratory, and hormonal responses. Likewise, fetal homeostasis is similarly maintained at a given relative exertional intensity, regardless of the exertional fitness of the experimental animal. We infer that this is also true for pregnant patients and allow physical exertion in all healthy patients up to a heart rate of 150 bpm. Since heart rate is difficult to monitor during competitive sports and levels of peak exertion tend to be high, we discourage competitive exertion for pregnant women.

3 Exercise studies during pregnancy have been limited to short bouts of exertion under "comfortable" ambient conditions. Since exertion for prolonged periods or with high heat and humidity has not been examined in human pregnancy, we discourage exercise under these conditions in pregnant patients.

4 Pregnant patients are probably more prone to trauma because of changes in weight distribution and resulting "clumsiness." Consequently, we caution patients about potentially traumatic sports, especially in the last half of pregnancy, when the uterus is more exposed to frontal trauma.

5 Fetal homeostasis during pregnancy compromised by uteroplacental insufficiency, cardiac or respiratory disease, or significant anemia may be adversely

affected by maternal exercise. The significance of these interactions is impossible to estimate; thus, we remain cautious in our counseling of potentially affected pregnant patients.

6 Patients with a history of poor pregnancy outcome due to repeated abortion, abruptio placenta, preterm labor, or preterm rupture of membranes are probably not compromised by exercise in pregnancy, based on limited studies in normal women. Appropriate investigation of exercise effects on patients with these histories have not been performed, however. We counsel patients with such histories who desire to exercise about our lack of knowledge, and about their potential sense of responsibility should another mishap occur in the present pregnancy. In this circumstance, however, we are nondirective in our counseling. Patients with histories of incompetent cervix, DES exposure, or with uterocervical abnormalities are counseled to avoid exertion during pregnancy.

NUTRITIONAL REQUIREMENTS OF PREGNANT EXERCISERS

It seems appropriate to advise pregnant exercisers also about possible changes in nutritional requirements to support the energy demands of exercise and the increased caloric costs of accretion of maternal and fetal tissues. Pregnancy, but not exercise, substantially increases dietary protein requirements. Other than fetal demands for essential free fatty acids, neither exercise nor pregnancy requires a net increase in dietary fat.

Estimates of increased caloric needs of pregnancy were originally based on cross-sectional data of increased maternal and fetal mass in pregnancy.[73,74] The fetal mass of 3.5 kg, the placental mass of 0.6 kg, the increase in uterine and breast mass of 5 kg, of maternal fat of 4 kg, and the estimated increase in metabolic rate were used to estimate the total caloric cost of pregnancy to be approximately 83,000 kcal. This estimate suggests that an increase of ~250 kcal in daily caloric intake is needed in pregnancy, consistent with the FAO/WHO/UNU,[75] the United Kingdom Department of Health and Social Security,[76] and the National Research Council.[77] Longitudinal investigations of pregnancy begun prior to conception provide different data, however. A cohort of 162 women from Scotland and the Netherlands underwent prospective measurements of weight, body fat, dietary intake, metabolic rate at rest, and daily activity pattern.[78] The estimated increased energy cost of pregnancy was ~69,000 kcal. The increase in dietary intake during pregnancy was estimated based on fairly rigorous weighed-inventory 5-day measurements performed every 2 to 4 weeks during pregnancy. These estimates suggested that the average increment in dietary intake during pregnancy was only ~22,000 kcal. The 47,000-kcal discrepancy suggests either that the estimates of caloric intake are in error or that there is a reduction in physical activity and an increase in mechanical efficiency during pregnancy. Nevertheless, during normal pregnancy with documented sedentary lifestyle, daily incremental caloric intake appears to be 80 to 100 kcal/d in the first half of pregnancy, and approximately 150 to 200 kcal/d during the second half. Since chronic exercise may increase basal metabolic rate and the character, duration, frequency, and intensity of exercise will otherwise affect the increased caloric cost of exertion, these estimates are complex and need to be individualized. Since maternal weight gain probably offers a reproducible correlate with fetal growth in the second half of uncomplicated, sedentary pregnancy, weekly weight gain may provide a practical measure of the adequacy of caloric support in exercising women. The utility of maternal weight gain as a measure of fetal nutritional adequacy in pregnancy in exercising women has not been adequately tested, however.

Requirements for most vitamins are increased during pregnancy, but adequate amounts will be provided by a balanced diet with sufficient increased calories. The exercise-related requirements for thiamine, niacin, riboflavin, and pantothenic acid likewise are probably supported by a calorically adequate diet.

Mineral needs, in the form of iron and calcium, are probably not increased in exercising individuals. Pregnancy results in a fetal accretion of 300 mg of elemental iron and a maternal erythropoietic requirement of 500 mg. Exercise training will produce an increase in plasma volume and erythrocyte mass which requires a transient increase in iron utilization. Recommendations for the daily intake of iron (30 to 60 mg of elemental iron) and calcium (1200 to 1500 mg of elemental calcium) during pregnancy will meet the needs of exercising as well as sedentary pregnant women.

SUMMARY

Both pregnancy and exercise produce profound adaptive cardiovascular and endocrine responses which affect fetal homeostasis. The early cardiovascular and hematologic changes of pregnancy include increased stroke volume, increased cardiac output, decreased peripheral vascular resistance, increased venous compliance, increased minute respiration, and increased plasma and red cell volume. These "adaptations" occur well before the fetoplacental unit develops the increased gas and nutrient transport that is supported by these changes.

Exercise in pregnancy is associated with many of the same physiologic responses associated with exertion in the nonpregnant state. Vasoconstriction occurs in vascular beds, except those serving exercising muscle. Mild exertion induces increases in pulse and stroke volume, which both contribute to increased cardiac output. Limited data suggest that the neuroendocrine response and insulin and glucagon response to exertion during pregnancy are similar to those found in the nonpregnant state. However, pregnancy is associated with a decreased arteriovenous O_2 difference and an increased stroke volume, which may impact on response to intense physical exertion. For example, during cycle exercise, increases in stroke volume appear to contribute to incremental cardiac output at extreme exertional intensity, which does not occur in nonpregnant humans.

The increased weight in pregnancy and the increase in metabolically active fetoplacental tissue results in higher pulse, cardiac output, and oxygen uptake at rest and at similar external workloads during pregnancy, compared to postpartum values. Similar external exertional power thereby requires exertion at a higher percentage of $\dot{V}o_2max$ during pregnancy. Pregnancy does not affect the weight-specific oxygen uptake at rest and during weight-supported exertion, however.

Maternal thermoregulation maintains the core maternal temperature within 0.3 to 0.8°C in human pregnancy, when exercise is limited to 20 to 30 minutes. The effect of more prolonged exertion under conditions of high ambient heat or humidity have not been examined.

Fetal response to maternal exertion has been examined most directly in the ungulate model. Uterine perfusion falls in proportion to duration and intensity of maternal exertion, but even under conditions of extreme exertion, fetoplacental oxygen uptake is maintained. Human studies using two-dimensional fetal imaging have shown no fetal heart-rate decelerations during even maximal maternal exertion, nor following submaximal maternal exercise. Frequent fetal heart-rate decelerations observed following maximal maternal exertion suggest that fetoplacental perfusion or blood pressure may be disturbed by this maneuver.

Studies of maternal and perinatal outcome following chronic maternal exercise are largely flawed by nonrandom assignment of subjects to comparison groups. The few randomized trials suggest that exercise training can be instituted during pregnancy without morbid effect. Continued exercise training by athletes after conception may reduce fetal birth weight, though this thesis requires further investigation.

Clinical recommendations for patients desirous of engaging in recreational exercise are limited by the small number of clinical studies available. Consequently, current published recommendations are conservative, recognizing that the benefits of maternal recreational exercise for the fetus are probably miminal and the potential risks unknown.

REFERENCES

1. Hytten FE, and Paintin DB: Increase in plasma volume during normal pregnancy. J Obstet Gynaecol Br Com 70:402, 1963.
2. Lund CJ, and Donovan JC: Blood volume during pregnancy. Am J Obstet Gynecol 98:393, 1967.
3. Phippard AF, Horvath JS, Glynn EM, et al: Circulatory adaptation to pregnancy—serial studies of haemodynamics, blood volume, renin and aldosterone in the baboon. J Hypertens 4:773, 1986.
4. Longo LD: Maternal blood volume and cardiac output during pregnancy: a hypothesis of endocrinologic control. Am J Physiol 245:R720, 1983.
5. Capeless EL, and Clapp JF: Cardiovascular changes in early phase of pregnancy. Am J Obstet Gynecol 161:1449, 1989.
6. Laird-Meeter K, van de Ley G, Bom TH, et al: Cardiocirculatory adjustments during pregnancy—an echocardiographic study. Clin Cardiol 2:328, 1979.
7. Rubler S, Damani PM, and Pinto ER: Cardiac size and performance during pregnancy estimated with echocardiography. Am J Cardiol 40:534, 1977.
8. Knuttgen HG, and Emerson K: Physiological response to pregnancy at rest and during exercise. J Appl Physiol 36:549, 1974.
9. Pernoll ML, et al: Oxygen consumption at rest and during exercise in pregnancy. Respir Physiol 25:285, 1975.
10. Sady SA, et al: Cardiovascular response to cycle exercise during and after pregnancy. J Appl Physiol 65:336, 1989.
11. Ueland K, et al: Maternal cardiovascular dynamics. Am J Obstet Gynecol 104:856, 1969.
12. Fawer R, et al: Effect of the menstrual cycle, oral contraception and pregnancy on forearm blood flow, venous distensibility and

clotting factors. Eur J Clin Pharmacol 13:251, 1978.

13. Barwin BN, and Roddie IC: Venous distensibility during pregnancy determined by graded venous congestion. Am J Obstet Gynecol 125:921, 1976.

14. Boutourline-Young H, and Boutourline-Young E: Alveolar carbon dioxide levels in pregnant parturient and lactating subjects. J Obstet Gynaecol Br Com 63:509, 1956.

15. Clapp JF: Cardiac output and uterine blood flow in the pregnant ewe. Am J Obstet Gynecol 130:419, 1978.

16. Carpenter MW, et al: Effect of maternal weight gain during pregnancy on exercise performance. J Appl Physiol 68:1173, 1990.

17. Rowell LB: Circulatory adjustments to dynamic exercise. In Rowell (ed): Human Circulation. Regulation during Physical Stress. Oxford University Press, New York, 1986, p 226.

18. Karpman VL: Cardiovascular System in Physical Exercise. CRC Press, Boca Raton, FL, p 140.

19. Christensen NJ, and Galbo H: Sympathetic nervous activity during exercise. Annu Rev Physiol 45:139, 1983.

20. Dempsey JA: Is the lung built for exercise? Med Sci Sports Exerc 18:143, 1986.

21. Brooks GA, and Fahey TD: Metabolic response to exercise In Brooks GA, and Fahey TD (eds): Exercise Physiology: Human Bioenergetics and its Applications. John Wiley & Sons, New York, 1985, p 189.

22. Jones NL, and Ehrsam, RE: The anaerobic threshold. Exerc Sport Sci Rev 10:49, 1982.

23. McArdle WD, Katch FI, and Katch VL: Exercise Physiology, Energy, Nutrition, and Human Performance. Lea & Febiger, Philadelphia, 1986.

24. Åstrand PO, and Rodahl K: Physical performance. In Åstrand PO, and Rodahl K (eds): Textbook of Work Physiology. Physiological Bases of Exercise. New York, 1986, p 295.

25. Fredholm B: Inhibition of fatty acid release from adipose tissue by high arterial lactate concentrations. Acta Physiol Scand (Suppl 330):77, abstract #106, 1969.

26. Felig P, and Wahren J: Role of insulin and glucagon in the regulation of hepatic glucose production during exercise. Diabetes 28 (Suppl 1):7175, 1979.

27. Horton ES: Exercise and diabetes mellitus. Med Clin North Am 72:1301, 1988.

28. Hoelzer DR, et al: Glucoregulation during exercise: Hypoglycemia is prevented by redundant glucoregulatory systems, sympathochromaffin activation and changes in islet hormone secretion. J Clin Invest 77:212, 1986.

29. Galbo H, Holst J, and Christensen NJ: Glucagon and plasma catecholamine responses to graded and prolonged exercise in man. J Appl Physiol 38:70, 1975.

30. Christensen NJ, et al: Catecholamines and exercise. Diabetes 28(Suppl 1):58, 1979.

31. Scheurink AJW, et al: Adrenal and sympathetic catecholamines in exercising rates. J Appl Physiol 66:R155, 1989.

32. Pruett EDR: Plasma insulin during prolonged work at near maximal oxygen uptake. J Appl Physiol 29:155, 1970.

33. Mikines KJ, Sonne B, and Farrell PA: Effect of physical exercise on sensitivity and responsiveness to insulin in humans. Am J Physiol 254:E248, 1988.

34. Bottger I, et al: The effect of exercise on glucagon secretion. J Clin Endocrinol Metab 35:117, 1972.

35. VanHelder WP, Casey K, and Radomski MW: Regulation of growth hormone during exercise by oxygen demand and availability. Eur J Appl Physiol 56:628, 1987.

36. Ueland K, Novy MJ, and Metcalfe J: Cardiorespiratory responses to pregnancy and exercise in normal women and patients with heart disease. Am J Obstet Gynecol 115:4, 1973.

37. Lehmann V, and Regnat K: Untersuchung sur korperlichen belastungsfahigkeit schwangeren frauen. Der einfluss standardisierter arbeit auf herzkreislaufsystem, ventilation, gasaustausch, kohlenhydratstoffwechsel und saure-basen-haushalt. Z Beburtshilfe Perinato 180:279, 1976.

38. Blackburn MW, and Calloway DH: Heart rate and energy expenditure of pregnancy and lactating women. Am J Clin Nutr 42:1161, 1985.

39. Sady SA, et al: Prediction of VO_2max during cycle exercise in pregnant women. J Appl Physiol 65:657, 1988.

40. Morton MJ, et al: Exercise dynamics in late gestation: Effects of physical training. Am J Obstet Gynecol 152:91, 1985.

41. Ryan ED, O'Sullivan MJ, and Skyler JS: Insulin action during pregnancy: Studies with the euglycemic clamp technique. Diabetes 34:380, 1985.

42. Hjollund E, et al: Impaired insulin receptor binding and postbinding defects of adipocytes from normal and diabetic pregnant women. Diabetes 35:598, 1986.

43. Barron WM, et al: Plasma catecholamine responses to physiologic stimuli in normal human pregnancy. Am J Obstet Gynecol 154:80, 1986.

44. Artal R, Wiswell R, and Romeo Y: Hormonal responses to exercise in diabetic and nondiabetic pregnant patients. Diabetes 34(Suppl 2):7880, 1985.

45. Airaksinen KEJ, et al: Effect of pregnancy on autonomic nervous function and heart rate in diabetic and nondiabetic women. Diabetes Care 10:748, 1987.

46. Artal R, et al: Exercise in pregnancy I. Maternal cardiovascular and metabolic responses in normal pregnancy. Am J Obstet Gynecol 140:123, 1981.

47. Carpenter MW, et al: Maternal exercise duration and intensity affect fetal heart rate. 1989 American College of Sports Medicine Annual Meeting.

48. Clapp JF: The changing thermal response to endurance exercise during pregnancy. Am J Obstet Gynecol 165:1684, 1991.

49. Jones RL, et al: Thermoregulation during aerobic exercise in pregnancy. Obstet Gynecol 65:340, 1985.

50. Clapp JF: Acute exercise stress in the pregnant ewe. Am J Obstet Gynecol 136:489, 1980.

51. Lotgering FK, Gilbert RD, and Longo LD: Exercise responses in pregnant sheep: Blood gases, temperatures and fetal cardiovascular system. J Appl Physiol 55:842, 1983.

52. Chandler KD, and Bell AW: Effects of maternal exercise on fetal and maternal respiration and nutrient metabolism in the pregnant ewe. J Dev Physiol 3:161, 1981.

53. Hohimer AR, et al: Maternal exercise reduced myoendometrial blood flow in the pregnant goat. Fed Proc 41:1490, 1982.

54. Morris N, Osborn SB, and Payling Wright H: Effect on uterine blood-flow during exercise in normal and pre-eclamptic pregnancies. Lancet 2:481, 1956.

55. Morrow RJ, Knox Ritchie JW, and Bull SB: Fetal and maternal hemodynamic responses to exercise in pregnancy assessed by Doppler ultrasonography. Am J Obstet Gynecol 160:138, 1989.

56. Rauramo I, and Forss M: Effect of exercise on placental blood flow in pregnancies complicated by hypertension, diabetes or intrahepatic cholestasis. Acta Obstet Gynecol Scand 67:15, 1988.

57. Artal R, Paul RH, Romeo Y, and Wiswell R: Fetal bradycardia induced by maternal exercise. Lancet 2:258, 1984.

58. Jovanovic L, Kessler A, and Peterson CM: Human maternal and fetal response to graded exercise. J Appl Physiol 58:1719, 1985.

59. Carpenter MW, et al: Fetal heart rate response to maternal exertion. JAMA 259:3006, 1988.

60. Dale E, Mullinax KM, and Bryan DH: Exercise during pregnancy: Effects on the fetus. Can J Appl Sport Sci 7:98, 1982.

61. Clapp JF, and Dickstein S: Endurance exercise and pregnancy outcome. Med Sci Sports Exerc 16:556, 1984.

62. Hall DC, and Kaufmann DA: Effects of aerobic and strength conditioning on pregnancy outcomes. Am J Obstet Gynecol 157:1199, 1987.

63. Clapp JF, and Capeless EL: Neonatal morphometrics after endurance exercise during pregnancy. Am J Obstet Gynecol 163:1805, 1990.

64. Clapp JF: The course of labor after endurance exercise during pregnancy. Am J Obstet Gynecol 163:1799, 1990.

65. Clapp JF: The effects of maternal exercise on early pregnancy outcome. Am J Obstet Gynecol 161:1453, 1989.

66. Kulpa PJ, White BM, and Visscher R: Aerobic exercise in pregnancy. Am J Obstet Gynecol 156:1395, 1987.

67. Carr SR, et al: Obstetrical outcome in aerobically trained women. Am J Obstet Gynecol SPO Abstracts 166:1(pt 2):380 (abstr 376), 1992.

68. Durak EP, Jovanovic-Peterson L, and Peterson CM: Comparative evaluation of uterine response to exercise on five aerobic machines. Am J Obstet Gynecol 162:754, 1990.

69. Veille JC, et al: The effect of exercise on uterine activity in the last eight weeks of pregnancy. Am J Obstet Gynecol 151:727, 1985.

70. ACOG Technical Bulletin: Women and Exercise. ACOG Technical Bulletin Number 87, September, Washington DC, 1985.

71. ACOG Home Exercise Programs: Exercise during pregnancy and the postnatal period. May, Washington DC, 1985.

72. Collings C, and Curet LB: Fetal heart rate response to maternal exercise. Am J Obstet Gynecol 151:498, 1985.

73. Hytten FE, and Leitch I: The Physiology of Human Pregnancy, ed 2. Blackwell, Oxford, 1971.

74. Hytten FE, and Chamberlain GVP: Clinical Physiology in Obstetrics. Blackwell, Oxford, 1980.

75. FAO/WHO/UNU: Energy and protein requirements. WHO Tech Rep Ser No 724. World Health Organization, Geneva, 1985.

76. Department of Health and Social Security: Recommended daily amounts of food energy and nutrients for groups of people in the United Kingdom. Rep Health Soc Subj 15, 1979.

77. National Research Council, Food and Nutrition Board: Recommended dietary allowances. National Academy, Washington DC, 1989.

78. Durnin JV: Energy requirements of pregnancy. Diabetes 40(Suppl 2):152, 1991.

CHAPTER 11

Menopause*†

MORRIS NOTELOVITZ, M.D., Ph.D., and MONA M. SHANGOLD, M.D.

MENOPAUSE IN PERSPECTIVE

Menopause is a natural phenomenon that usually lasts about 1 week—the duration of the last menstrual period. It is the biologic marker of the gradual but persistent decrease in ovarian steroidogenesis that precedes the cessation of menstruation by about 15 years and that postdates that event by a similar duration. This period of reproductive senescence is known as the climacteric. The differentiation between "menopause" and the "climacteric" involves more than semantics, since it serves to illustrate that the midlife physical and psychologic needs of women extend over a 30-year continuum. There are two additional features of note: (1) the attenuation in endocrine function of the ovarian follicle affects many systems remote from the reproductive tract; and (2) the climacteric occurs at a time when certain age-related changes become apparent, so that one must differentiate between biologically induced and chronologically induced pathophysiology.

*Supported by grants from the National Institute on Aging R01 AG 00976, Nautilus Sports/Medical Industries, Inc.

†Although, as discussed at the beginning of this chapter, the period is more properly called the "climacteric," "menopause" is certainly the more commonly used term.

The date of menopause can be accurately pinpointed, but it is a retrospective diagnosis: a year of amenorrhea has to pass before the clinical diagnosis can be confirmed. The mean age of onset of menopause in western societies is 51 years.[1] The climacteric may be empirically but pragmatically categorized into three decades of clinical presentation and need (Fig. 11–1): the early climacteric (age 35 to 45), premenopausal and postmenopausal periods (age 46 to 55), and the late climacteric (56 to 65).[2] Contrary to the theory that follicular depletion is the cause of menopause, primordial follicles are frequently found in the ovaries of postmenopausal women, but they are unable to respond to stimulation of the pituitary gonadotropins—FSH and LH. The resultant alteration in ovarian function brings about the dysfunctional uterine bleeding patterns that characterize this phase. As the climacteric progresses, the decrease in estradiol production results in menopause and in a number of so-called hormone-dependent symptoms such as hot flushes and changes in temperament, mood, and sleeping patterns. The late climacteric is often associated with conditions resulting from chronic estrogen deprivation—chronic atrophic vaginitis, the urethral syndrome, and urinary incontinence.

Although the conditions just listed have an impact on an individual's quality of life, none is life-threatening. There are, however, two asymptomatic potential complications of the late climacteric that may have a serious adverse effect and that are responsible for much of the morbidity and mortality associated with older age in women: osteoporosis and atherogenic disease. In the United States, the total number of hip fractures among white women was 158,000 in 1986, and this number is expected to increase to 252,000 in the year 2020 and to 367,000 by the year 2040.[3] Of this figure, approximately 12% to 20% will die as a result of factors directly attributable to their hip fracture.[4] Only a third of the survivors will regain normal activity.[5] Of all hip fractures, 70% to 80% affect women. The total annual cost of hip fractures was approximately $7.2 billion in 1984, and this cost, adjusted for 5% inflation,

THREE DECADES OF HEALTH NEEDS

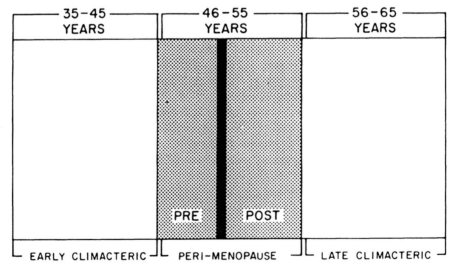

Figure 11–1. Diagrammatic representation of the menopause as a single event in the larger context of the climacteric. (From Notelovitz[2] with permission.)

is expected to increase to $240 billion by 2040.[3] This cost, of course, does not take into account the physical and psychologic pain suffered by these women.

In 1989, approximately 500,000 persons died from ischemic heart disease, the leading cause of death in the United States.[6] Annual health-care costs for cardiovascular disease alone exceed $135 billion, while the added costs of related injury and disability exceed $170 billion.[7] Cardiovascular disease has a significant influence on the well-being of the fastest-growing age group in the United States: an estimated 1000 individuals join the ranks of the elderly every day.[8] A woman aged 65 can now expect to live an additional 18.8 years (14.5 years for men).[9]

Exercise can play an important role in ensuring an appropriate quality of life in middle age and later, but to be maximally effective, it needs to be introduced as a premenopausal lifestyle—hence the emphasis on recognizing the climacteric as an important transitional phase in the pathogenesis of potentially preventable disease.

OSTEOPOROSIS AND BONE HEALTH

Osteoporosis is preventable. It is a condition that is relatively uncommon in men and in black women, owing in part to their having a greater bone mass. Cohn and co-workers[10] examined the skeletal and muscle mass of normal black women and found that their total body calcium was 16.7% higher than that of age-matched white women. More than half of this difference (9.7%) was calculated to be due to a greater muscle mass in the black women. Thus, despite the complexity of bone physiology, two practical issues need to be addressed: (1) women need to acquire as much bone as possible before menopause, and (2) the rate at which bone is lost thereafter needs to be modulated. Exercise plays a pivotal role, in that it is one of the few known means of stimulating new bone formation. Central to the entire

issue is the fact that bone is a living tissue and needs to be treated as such.

Osteogenesis: A Brief Overview

Bone formation depends upon a five-stage cycle that results in "old" bone being removed and replaced with "new" bone. Normally, this process is coupled; the amount of old bone removed is replaced with an equal amount of freshly formed bone. Initiation of the cycle is dependent upon the recruitment and activation of osteoclasts. This activity usually takes place on the inner aspect of the bone's surface—the endosteal layer—and results in the dissolution of bone mineral and collagen, and the formation of a cavity. Resorption ceases when the mean depth of the cavity reaches 60 μm (trabecular bone) and 100 μm (cortical bone) from the surface.[11] At this point, mononuclear cells lay down a highly mineralized, collagen-poor bone matrix known as cement substance. It is from this surface that new bone is laid down by osteoblasts. These cells probably originate from bone marrow stromal cells (preosteoblasts), thereby sharing the ability of another cell type, the fibroblasts, to synthesize collagen.[11] The stimulus for osteoblast recruitment may be mechanical owing to humoral and/or locally produced substances (for example, human skeletal growth and other bone growth factors).[12]

The osteoblasts are responsible for the synthesis of collagen, which is the main component of newly formed bone matrix, or osteoid. The latter matures and is later mineralized by a process that largely depends on an adequate supply of calcium and phosphate and the formation of hydroxyapatite crystals.[10] At a microstructural level, numerous small crystallites of hydroxyapatite may be seen in intimate juxtaposition and in highly organized geometric arrangements with collagen fibrils.[11]

The elastic and tensile strength of bone depends in large measure on this interrelationship. Another very important determinant of the mechanical strength of bone is the orientation of the collagen fibrils in the bone matrix and the three-dimensional network of plates and bars found especially in trabecular bone (such as vertebrae), and to a lesser extent in cortical bone (for example, the radius), resulting in a scaffoldlike arrangement of vertical and horizontal trabeculae (Fig. 11–2). Interruption of this support system—for example, loss of horizontal trabeculae as a result of aging—can impair the structural integrity of the bone and result in

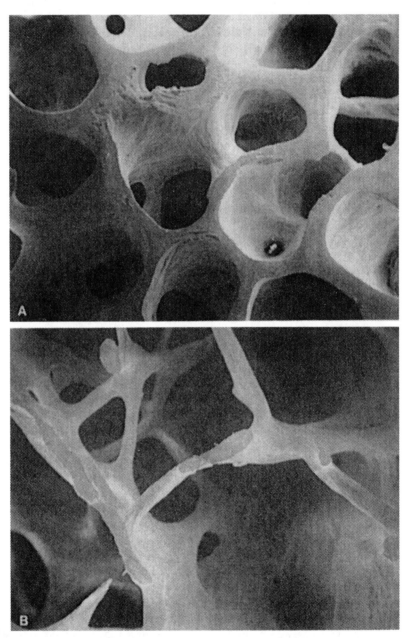

Figure 11–2. Scanning electron micrograph of an iliac crest biopsy from (A) a normal subject and (B) a woman with osteoporosis. Contrast the normal contiguous vertical and horizontal trabeculae with the thinning decreased number and loss of continuity of the trabecular plates in osteoporosis. (From Dempster DW, et al: A simple method for correlative light and scanning electron microscopy of human iliac crest bone biopsies: Qualitative observations in normal and osteoporotic subjects. J Bone Min Res 1(1):15, 1986, with permission.)

fracture, even in the presence of a relatively normal amount of bone mineral.[13] This is an important consideration when prescribing exercise for older women.

Types and Rates of Bone Loss

As mentioned above, there are two types of bone: cortical and trabecular. Cortical (compact) bone is found primarily in the appendicular skeleton (for example, in the femur, tibia, and fibula of the lower limbs, and in the humerus, ulna, and radius of the arms). Cortical bone constitutes 80% of the total skeleton but is metabolically less active than trabecular bone. About 10% of the cortical bone is remodeled each year.

Trabecular (cancellous) bone is found in the axial skeleton, primarily in the vertebral bodies (70% to 95%), with lesser concentrations in areas such as the neck of the femur (25% to 35%) and the distal radius (5% to 20%). The remodeling process is far more active in trabecular bone, in part because the architectural arrangement of the bone plates provides a larger exposed surface area for exchange with the extracellular compartment. Approximately 40% of trabecular bone is remodeled each year. Because of this greater activity, vertebral osteoporosis occurs more frequently than hip (cortical-related) fractures. It may also account for the increased susceptibility of the vertebrae to the bone mineral loss noted in female long-distance runners.[14]

After longitudinal bone growth has been completed, the bone mineral content and mass of bone further increase until about the age of 35 years, at which point the individual is said to have achieved her maximal cortical bone mass. From this age until the onset of menopause, it is considered normal for women to lose at least 0.12% of cortical bone per year (as measured by single- and dual-photon absorptiometry); after menopause and until age 65, the rate of bone loss increases to at least 1% per year, slowing down after age 65 to 0.18% per year. This "physiologic" bone loss averages out to a 25% decrease in cortical bone mass over the

30 years from age 50 to age 80.[13] Trabecular bone accrual reaches its maximum during the mid to late 20s and is followed thereafter by a linear loss of bone.[15] Others maintain that the trabecular bone loss pattern equals that of cortical bone, with a loss of at least 0.19% per year before menopause and at least 1.1% thereafter. Thus an estimated 31.7% of trabecular bone is lost during the 50-year span between 30 and 80 years of age.[13] The greater the bone mineral content at bone mass maturity (maximum), of course, the more an individual can afford to lose, so there is a need to focus on the accrual of bone during youth rather than on the treatment of a reduced bone mass in the postmenopausal period.

How to Acquire More Bone

Mechanical force plays an important role in bone formation and function, but it is not known how much exercise is needed and whether there is an optimal form of exercise for bone accrual. It has been postulated[16] that there is a physiologic "band" of activity that is site-specific: immobilization can lead to severe bone loss at some sites, whereas repeated loading at appropriate strain magnitudes can result in bone hypertrophy. The frequency and degree of activity is important: repeated and prolonged exercise causes bone fatigue and microscopic fractures.[16] Given appropriate intervals between periods of exercise, however, normal bone turnover will repair these microfractures and even strengthen the bone.[16] Excessive activity is known to have an adverse effect, with stress fractures a common reality in long-distance runners.[16]

Gravity. Bone mineral is lost with the inactivity of simple bed rest. The average rate appears to be 4% per month during the early phase of bed rest; although subjects with higher initial bone mass lose bone more rapidly than those with lower values, all immobilized patients seem to end up with a similar bone mass.[17] Lack of force on bones plays a major role in bone loss, with trabecular bone being more sensitive than cortical bone. Three hours a day of quiet standing is partially effective in restoring bone mineral, while 4 hours of walking prevents the bone loss associated with 20 hours of bed rest.

Osteogenesis in long bones requires mechanical stress; when electrodes are placed on opposite sides of bone, bending results in a negative electrical potential on the concave side relative to the convex side.[18] The resulting piezoelectricity stimulates new bone cell growth. It is therefore not surprising that isometric or horizontal exercise—which does not "bend" bone and thereby stimulate this piezoelectricity—is not able to restore bone loss associated with immobilization.

Systemic versus Local Effect. It is important to differentiate the amount of exercise needed to maintain bone mass from that needed to increase it. This difference is well illustrated by a study that compared male professional tennis players with age-matched casual tennis players. The former group was found to have an overall greater bone mass, but in addition, the cortical thickness in the playing arm of the professional tennis players was 34.9% greater than in the nondominant arm. The same was found in female professional tennis players; cortical thickness in the dominant arm was 28.4% greater than in the nondominant arm.[19] Exercise thus seems to have both a systemic and a local effect and appears to be related to the type of exercise performed. When combined with the effect of gravity, weight-bearing activity is more osteogenic than weight-supported exercises such as swimming. However, both male and female swimmers have been shown to have greater vertebral bone mineral content than do their sedentary counterparts of the same sex.[20] Although the differences between male swimmers and sedentary men were statistically significant, the differences between female swimmers and sedentary women did not achieve significance, probably because of the smaller numbers of women studied (58 male swimmers, 78 sedentary men; 35 female swimmers, 20 sedentary women).

Age. Age is yet another significant factor: bone mass accrual occurs more readily in "growing" than in "mature" bone.[21] Both animal experimentation and clinical experience have shown that the accumulation of appropriate mechanical damage can stimulate bone hypertrophy. This requires the exposure of adult bone to cyclic strain levels of 2000 microstrain or more.[22] However, there is an optimal level beyond which increasing strain levels will no longer enhance bone mass and may even have a negative effect.[22] Thus, the type and intensity of exercise prescribed must be tailored to the age of the individual.

Exercise Prescription. In presenting an osteogenic exercise program, two additional criteria should be met: (1) the activity should be diverse and vigorous, but nonrepetitive,[23] and (2) the exercise program should be enjoyable, in order to ensure long-term compliance. In addition, a program that will simultaneously improve cardiovascular fitness would provide an added incentive and advantage. By extrapolating from animal data,[24] it has been suggested that aerobic exercise at an intensity associated with 65% to 80% of maximal heart rate is osteogenic.

Exercise and Osteogenesis: Clinical Research

Several investigators have studied the effects of exercise programs upon bone mineral density in postmenopausal women, using various protocols for exercise. Some of these studies have included hormone replacement therapy in the protocol, and some have also quantified calcium intake. Disparate results reflect differences in protocols and populations.

When interpreting the efficacy of a given program, the method of bone strength measurement needs to be considered. Most assessments are based on radiologic techniques, single- and dual-photon absorptiometry, and/or CT scanning. A qualitative improvement in bone strength resulting from aerobic exercise may also derive from an engineering rather than a biologic principle—an increase in bone width. Radial expansion of long bones is an important determinant of bone strength. The so-called cross-sectional moment of inertia (CSMI) is what determines bone's resistance to bending. An increase in the external diameter of the bone, brought about by increased periosteal (outer layer) new bone formation, can compensate for the inevitable loss in the quality of bone tissue that occurs with aging. Cavanaugh and Cann[25] have demonstrated that a moderate brisk walking program of 1 year's duration does not prevent loss of vertebral bone density in early postmenopausal women. Kirk and colleagues[26] reported similar vertebral bone densities for postmenopausal runners and age-matched sedentary women. Although the calcium intake of the runners was higher (1145 mg/d versus 707 mg/d), neither group consumed adequate amounts by current standards. These data suggest that exercise cannot compensate for an estrogen deficiency in preventing bone loss.

Relatively brief exercise programs have been shown to have a positive effect on vertebral bone mineral. Sixteen healthy women (mean age 61 ± 6 years) participated in an exercise program that involved walking, running, and calisthenics for 1 hour twice weekly. At the end of 8 months, the vertebral bone mineral content (measured by dual-photon absorptiometry) increased by 3% to 5%, whereas in an age-matched control group it decreased by 2.7%. The bone mineral content of the distal radius, however, showed an average decrease of 3.5%.[27] The authors concluded that physical exercise inhibits or reverses bone loss from the lumbar vertebrae in normal women, but that the changes in the forearm were independent of these exercises.

These results are divergent from another study that examined bone mineralization by x-ray densitometry (middle phalanx of the fifth finger and os calcis) and photon absorptiometry (distal and midshaft) in 42 normally menstruating marathon runners (mean age 37.7 ± 0.82 years) and 38 sedentary controls (mean age 39.6 ± 1.0 years). Mean values of the mineral content and the bone density of the marathon runners' radial midshaft and middle phalanx (representative of cortical bone) were significantly greater, but the mean density of the os calcis (trabecular bone) was higher in the physically inactive women.[28] Women with moderate exercise had greater cortical but less trabecular bone mineral contents, indicating that the increase in cortical bone through exercise came at the "expense" of trabecular bone.

Although anatomically distinct, the metabolic functions of the cortical and trabecular bone compartments are shared—a gain in one compartment may be matched by a loss in another. These two studies raise the question: can one exercise too much, and if so, will this result in a compromise of the trabecular skeleton? Hypoestrogenic, amenorrheic runners have been shown to have a reduced amount of trabecular bone in their lumbar vertebrae (as measured by dual-photon absorptiometry) but normal or minimally reduced cortical bone (as measured by single-photon absorptiometry and radiogrammetry).[14,29–31] Lower bone density in these women correlates with estrogen deficiency, inadequate dietary calcium, and reduced body weight. Calcium intake obviously plays a very important role. When reported, calcium intake was inadequate in most osteopenic groups, regardless of estrogen and exercise status. The menstruating marathon runners referred to previously lost trabecular bone despite an intact hypothalamic pituitary ovarian axis; another study has shown that physically active women with anorexia nervosa (all of whom were amenorrheic and obviously hypoestrogenic) had significantly greater bone mass than a similar group of inactive anorectics.[32]

Unpublished results from a study at the Center for Climacteric Studies comparing different forms of exercise in natural and surgically menopausal women reflect on some of the aforementioned issues—age, type and intensity of exercise, and an "intact" estrogen milieu. Bone mineral content in this study was measured by dual-photon absorptiometry of the total skeleton. Naturally menopausal women participating in aerobic (walking on a treadmill, riding a stationary bicycle) and muscle-strengthening (Nautilus) exercises, none of whom were receiving hormonal therapy, had less bone loss over a 1-year period than did a control group that did not exercise. The controls lost 9.9% of their bone mineral content, compared with 3.8% in the Nautilus exercise group and 0.5% in the bicycle-riding group. The treadmill subjects gained 0.4%.[33]

Heikkinen and associates[34] showed that weight training for 40 minutes in one session per week was insufficient to enhance the beneficial effect of estrogen and progestogen on bone mineral density in postmenopausal women, nor was there any improvement in bone density in a control group not treated with hormonal therapy. However, a study performed at the Center for Climacteric Studies demonstrated increased bone mineral density of the spine when a group of surgically menopausal women were treated with both estrogen and intense Nautilus weight training for 45 to 60 min/wk, divided into three sessions.[35] In this study, the increase in vertebral bone mineral density (measured by dual-photon absorptiometry) was statistically significant for the estrogen-plus-Nautilus group, compared to baseline, but the increase did not reach statistical significance for the estrogen-only group, or for the between-group comparison (Fig. 11–3). It is likely that this lack of significance resulted from the small numbers studied (n = 9 for estrogen plus Nautilus; n = 11 for estrogen only). All subjects ingested a minimum of 1400 mg of calcium daily during the 12-month study. These studies suggest that an estrogen-replete state might be needed for an osteogenic effect in women involved in intense exercise programs, and that more moderate levels of activity can conserve and maintain bone independent of the estrogen milieu (Table 11–1). However, more studies are needed to delineate the frequency, intensity, and duration of exercise necessary.

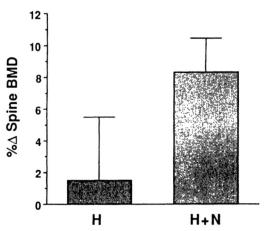

Figure 11–3. Percentage change (mean ± SEM) in the bone mineral density (BMD) of surgical menopausal women after 1 year of hormone therapy alone (H) or hormone therapy plus Nautilus exercise (H + N). The probability (one-tailed t-test) associated with the change in spine BMD measures within the exercising group was p = 0.002. The probability (one-tailed t-test) associated with the change in spine BMD measures within the hormone-only group was p = 0.44. Changes between groups were not significant. (From Notelovitz et al,[35] p 587, with permission.)

Exercise and Calcium Intake

The precise mechanism whereby exercise stimulates new bone formation is not clearly established. Mechanical load, muscular activity, and gravity serve as extracellular stimuli that are transmitted to bone cells to initiate their genetic program for growth and differentiation. Intermediaries include events such as the generation of piezoelectricity, which stimulates cyclic nucleotide

Table 11–1. EFFECT OF EXERCISE AND HORMONE REPLACEMENT THERAPY ON BONE MASS IN POSTMENOPAUSAL WOMEN

HRT*	Moderate Exercise (Aerobic)	Intense Exercise (Nautilus)	Effect on Bone Mass
No	Yes		0
No		Yes	0
Yes		Yes	+

*Hormone replacement therapy.
Source: From Notelovitz et al,[33] with permission.

activity, prostaglandin synthesis, and other matrix-derived bone growth factors.

It has been established that exercise is directly associated with the laying down of matrix on the remodeling surface of bone's trabeculae and cortices. The matrix is composed primarily of collagen. Chvapil and colleagues[36] showed that the amount and concentration of collagen in the femurs of adult rats increased with exercise, but there was no effect on the calcium content. This experiment illustrates a most important point: to benefit from exercise and its osteogenic stimulus, it is necessary to ensure an adequate supply of the substrate (mainly calcium) needed to mineralize and mature the newly formed bone. It is well known that fluoride therapy without simultaneous calcium supplementation will increase mineralization of the axial skeleton, but at the expense of the cortical bone and with an increase in hip fractures.[37] A similar situation may be true for exercise-induced osteogenesis, except that in this instance it is the cortical bone that benefits at the expense of the trabecular compartment. This may prove to be one of the reasons why the amenorrheic women reported by Drinkwater and associates[14] had lower spinal, but not cortical, bone mineral content when compared with the eumenorrheic controls. Although both groups met the current recommended dietary allowance of 800 mg of elemental calcium per day, the amenorrheic subjects fell short of the recommended amount needed to maintain calcium balance in low estrogen states (1500 mg), whereas the eumenorrheic women exceeded their daily requirement of 800 mg.

Established Osteoporosis

Exercise in women with established osteoporosis has to be modulated because pre-existing microfractures and discontinuity between the trabecular plates, especially in the axial skeleton, may be aggravated by weight-bearing exercise. Furthermore, even though individual fragments of the horizontal trabecular plates may be hypertrophied

by exercise, the bone may not improve in strength in response to stress because their continuity (and hence structural integrity) has been lost. Nevertheless, light to moderate exercise in older women has resulted in an improvement of the cortical bone mass. Smith and co-workers[38] designed an exercise program for older women (mean age 81 years) that oriented activity (1.5 to 3.0 METs in intensity) around a chair. (One MET equals an oxygen uptake of $3.5 \ mL \cdot min^{-1} \cdot kg^{-1}$, the average value of effort during chair rest.) Over 3 years, the exercise group demonstrated a 2.9% increase in midshaft radius bone mineral content, whereas a matched, nonexercising control group showed a 3.29% decrease.

Inadequate attention is given to the prescription of exercise for women with established osteoporosis, most of whom will present to the physician during the late climacteric. Key is discouraging activities that involve flexion of the back. Long-term follow-up of patients with radiologically confirmed osteoporosis revealed concurrent fractures in 16% of women practicing back extension exercises, 89% in a flexion program, 53% in a combined extension and flexion regimen, and 67% in a nonexercising control group.[39] Posture is also important. Avoidance of flexion during sedentary activities, such as sewing, can prevent further stress on already weakened vertebrae.[40] Instruction should also be given to avoid back straining by twisting, lifting, and making sudden, forceful movements. To remove the strain from the lower back when lifting or reaching lower objects, the large muscles of the legs (i.e., the hamstrings and quadriceps) should be used, by bending the knees and keeping the back vertical during these activities.

Walking is the safest form of exercise for women with osteoporosis. Also safe and effective are group activities such as square dancing, ballroom dancing, and folk dancing, as well as other activities such as riding a three-wheel bike or an exercycle. Swimming is an excellent exercise that allows patients to regain their confidence in being physically active, and at the same time allows them to increase the flexibility and mobility of their joints. Osteoporotic or markedly osteopenic women should be advised to avoid activities such as aerobic (jazz) dance classes that jar the spine and emphasize flexibility. In evaluating these women, care should be taken to test for balance and for orthostatic hypotension, and to advise them about practical measures such as the type of shoes they wear.

Additional information about bone concerns may be found in Chapter 5.

ATHEROGENIC DISEASE AND CARDIORESPIRATORY FITNESS

Premature cessation of ovarian function has been shown to increase the risk of myocardial infarction. Women who had a bilateral oophorectomy before age 35 were estimated to have a 7.2 times greater risk of being hospitalized for a myocardial infarction than age-matched normal premenopausal women.[41] Other studies have also observed high rates of coronary disease in women who experience an early menopause.[7,42,43] There is a general consensus that the postmenopausal period is associated with well-defined high-risk factors for atherogenesis: increased total plasma cholesterol and increased low-density lipoprotein (LDL) levels.[7] This is a biologic, not a chronologic, event. A Swedish study compared women aged 50 and older, of whom some were still menstruating and others had reached menopause; serum cholesterol and triglycerides were significantly higher in the postmenopausal group, and these levels increased with postmenopausal age.[44]

The pathogenesis of atherosclerosis is characterized by two factors: (1) endothelial desquamation with later smooth muscle cell proliferation, and (2) cholesterol deposition within these cells. Inhibition of LDL internalization and deposition in the smooth muscle cell by high-density lipoproteins (HDL) cholesterol is said to be a key factor in the prevention or slowing down of the atherogenic process.[45] Exercise has a beneficial effect on the lipoprotein moiety, especially regarding the HDL cholesterol.[46]

Physical inactivity has also been linked to atherogenic disease. Men who are physically active have fewer stigmata of coronary heart disease, and when they do occur, they are less severe and appear at an older age.[47] The same is true for women.[48] Despite some previous claims that physical inactivity contributed only indirectly to cardiovascular disease risk, there is now considerable evidence that low physical fitness stands as an independent risk factor, in both men and women, for all-cause mortality, cardiovascular disease mortality, and cancer mortality.[49,50] In addition to the direct role demonstrated after controlling for other known risk factors,[50] regular physical exercise probably also plays an indirect role by reducing other known risk factors for coronary heart disease, such as serum lipid concentrations and ratios,[51] hypertension,[51] hyperinsulinemia,[52] diabetes mellitus,[51,53,54] and abdominal fat.[55,56] The type, intensity, and duration of exercise linked to a potential decrease in coronary heart disease varies. There appears to be a threshold of activity needed to achieve a benefit. This has been estimated to be 300 kcal/d above normal activity and requires 30 to 60 minutes of moderately intensive exercise per day.[57] Earlier speculation that women,[58] especially older women, would not be able to achieve this goal has been disproved.

Based on the previous observations, two practical aspects of physical activity and cardiovascular health can be objectively measured: (1) the response of biochemical parameters such as cholesterol and HDL cholesterol, and (2) measures of physical fitness and exercise quantity—maximal oxygen uptake ($\dot{V}O_2$max) and total exercise time.

Lipids, Lipoproteins, and Exercise

The plasma lipoproteins are the means whereby endogenous synthesized lipids are transported in the circulation. They are classified according to their gravitational density into four basic classes: chylomicrons, very low density lipoproteins (VLDL), LDL, and HDL. The latter are frequently subfractionated into HDL_2 and the more dense HDL_3. The HDL_2 cholesterol component is higher in women[59] and is inversely related to the development of coronary heart disease.[60] Exercise stimulates HDL_2, which is higher in both male and female runners than in sedentary controls. In one study, for example, male runners had HDL_2 cholesterol values of 119 versus 53 mg/dL for sedentary men; in women the values for active and sedentary subjects were 218 versus 122 mg/dL.[59] The HDL-elevating effect of exercise is thought to be due to an increase in lipoprotein lipase, an enzyme responsible for the catabolism of triglyceride-rich lipoproteins. Lipoprotein lipase is found in greater concentrations in the skeletal muscle fibers (slow-twitch) of endurance athletes.[61]

The adverse effects of estrogen deficiency on low-density lipoprotein cholesterol levels tend to be offset by aerobic training. However, the beneficial effects of strenuous exercise on plasma apolipoprotein levels can be reversed, in premenopausal women, by exercise-induced amenorrhea and decreased serum estradiol levels.[62]

Table 11–2 lists the serum cholesterol values found in a cross-sectional study of women conducted at the Center for Climacteric Studies, showing an age- and menopause-related increase.[63] To determine whether this change would be improved by exercise, a group of 50 healthy women between the ages of 40 and 65 were invited to participate in a 12-week program of exercise, discussion sessions, or both. The dis-

cussion group served as the controls. Levels of serum cholesterol, triglycerides, total HDL, and HDL_{2a} and HDL_{2b} were monitored at baseline, at 6 weeks, and at 12 weeks. The exercise groups were instructed to walk-jog for 30 minutes (after a 15-minute warm-up session) and to pace their activity in order to maintain their heart rate at 70% to 80% of their predicted maximum heart rate. One exercise session each week was supervised by a group therapy leader, and the women exercised on their own during two other sessions per week. Cardiorespiratory function was determined at baseline and at 12 weeks by having subjects walk on a motorized treadmill until they declared fatigue or reached their predicted maximal heart rate. The exercising group had a significantly greater increase in $\dot{V}O_2$max, time spent on the treadmill, and time required to attain 90% of maximal oxygen consumption ($p < 0.01$), but did not show a statistically significant difference in the lipid or lipoprotein fractions at either 6 or 12 weeks.[64] This disappointing result was confirmed by Franklin and associates,[65] who exercised their subjects four times a week as part of a 12-week conditioning program. These discrepant results may be explained by the duration of the exercise program and intensity of the exercise. For example, when the weekly running mileage of 22 women was increased from 3.5 miles to 44.9 miles (over a 7-month period), their mean HDL cholesterol increased from 53.5 to 58.5 mg/dL ($p < 0.01$).[66]

In another study, hysterectomized postmenopausal women who exercised thrice weekly in 30-minute sessions of aerobic exercise at a minimum of 70% of maximal heart rate had a significant reduction in total serum cholesterol and LDL cholesterol.

Table 11–2. SERUM CHOLESTEROL (mg/dL) OF WOMEN, RELATED TO AGE AND MENOPAUSE

	Premenopausal		Postmenopausal		
Age range	35–45	46–55	46–55	56–65	66–75
N	30	24	23	24	10
Cholesterol (mean ± SEM)	170.5 ± 4.3	203.2 ± 7.6	233.8 ± 5.9	230.1 ± 6.9	238.8 ± 6.7

Source: From Notelovitz et al.[63]

However, this effect was not greater than that induced by oral estrogen alone.[67]

Like their younger counterparts, postmenopausal women who engage in regular endurance exercise have higher HDL cholesterol levels than inactive women.[68-70] Postmenopausal long-distance runners and joggers had significantly greater levels of HDL cholesterol compared with a control group of relatively inactive women—79.8, 73.5, and 61.8 mg/dL, respectively. The lipid-lipoprotein profiles were minimally affected by exercise in a simultaneously studied group of exercising premenopausal women,[70] raising the issue of whether it is possible to make "normal" *more* normal.

It appears that the cardioprotective HDL cholesterol level improves after only 3 months of moderate activity (e.g., running 10 to 15 miles/wk) or low-level activity (e.g., walking 30 miles/wk).[59] As with men, exercise training in women lowers total cholesterol slightly or not at all.[65,66]

Aerobic Power

With the advent of the "fitness craze," women have come into their own and have exploded the myth that women are "frail"; physical fitness in young women has now become socially acceptable and, in many circles, even desirable. Until fairly recently, however, it was felt that exercise would not benefit middle-aged people, and that the decline in cardiorespiratory function with aging would reduce the expected benefit from exercise.[58] Furthermore, it was postulated that menopause per se could be responsible for the decrease in aerobic power in women over the age of 50.[71,72]

As with men, cardiorespiratory fitness does decrease with age, but this decline is not related to the hormonal changes of the climacteric. Figure 11–4 shows that a decrement of 5.5% of $\dot{V}O_2max$ occurred with each succeeding decade between ages 35 and 75 in a study of 163 healthy sedentary women.[73] This observation approximates with the generalization that sedentary individuals have a 1% loss of $\dot{V}O_2max$ per year

with age, especially after age 50. Women usually achieve maximal $\dot{V}O_2max$ values in their 20s; by age 50 to 65 years, the values are decreased by almost 30%.[74] This loss of aerobic power is not related to menopause per se, however. In a recent study, women aged 45 to 55 had their $\dot{V}O_2max$ predicted by means of a submaximal bicycle ergometer test.[73] They were divided into premenopausal and postmenopausal groups, as confirmed by hormonal analysis and by their menstrual pattern: postmenopausal women were required to have been amenorrheic for at least 1 year. As reflected in Table 11–3, serum LH and FSH were significantly higher in the postmenopausal women ($p < 0.0001$), and the estradiol and estrone levels were significantly lower ($p < 0.0001$). The premenopausal women were slightly younger (48.7 ± 0.4 years versus 52.2 ± 0.4), but the difference was not statistically significant. No significant difference was found in the estimated $\dot{V}O_2max$ for the two groups ($p > 0.05$).[73]

The observed decline in $\dot{V}O_2max$ with age probably reflects a loss of functional capacity due both to a natural age-related deterioration and to a decrease in physical activity. The age-associated reduction in cardiorespiratory efficiency at submaximal exercise, however, is due primarily to weight gain rather than to actual systems degeneration.[75] The rate of decline is slower in

Table 11–3. MEAN ESTIMATED MAXIMAL O_2 UPTAKE VALUES AND HORMONAL STATUS ($\pm$ SD) OF PREMENOPAUSAL AND POSTMENOPAUSAL WOMEN AGE 46–55 YR

Parameter	Premeno-pausal (n = 28)	Postmeno-pausal (n = 30)
Estimated $\dot{V}O_2max$ ($mL \cdot kg^{-1} \cdot min^{-1}$)	27.4 ± 6.3	26.3 ± 4.7
LH (mIU/mL)	23.5 ± 3.6	62.8 ± 3.5
FSH (mIU/mL)	12.6 ± 2.6	55.7 ± 3.5
Estrone (pg/mL)	107.5 ± 11.5	62.9 ± 3.9
Estradiol (pg/mL)	146.2 ± 18.7	19.5 ± 3.5

Source: From Notelovitz et al,[73] with permission.

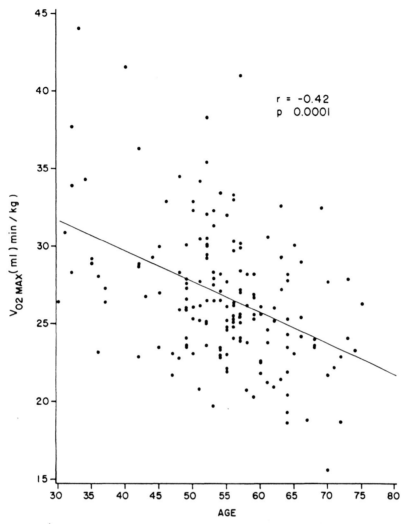

Figure 11–4. Measured $\dot{V}_{O_2}$max (mL·kg·min) in 163 healthy climacteric women, who first were screened for cardio-vascular normalcy by a 12-lead ECG stress test and physical examination. The $\dot{V}_{O_2}$max was elicited using a modified Balke treadmill procedure, and was directly measured using a Beckman Metabolic Measurement Cart. (From Notelovitz et al.,[73] with permission.)

physically active men[76] and women.[76,77] This raises the issue of whether menopausal women can be efficiently trained. Premeno-pausal women (mean age 41 years) who trained for 9 weeks improved their $\dot{V}_{O_2}$max by 12.1%, while similarly trained postmeno-pausal women (mean age 57 years) im-proved their $\dot{V}_{O_2}$max by 19%.[78] This result has been confirmed by others,[79] including two studies conducted at the Center for Cli-macteric Studies in Gainesville, Florida. Moderate exercise (walk-jogging three

times a week for 12 weeks) resulted in a sig-nificant increase in maximal oxygen con-sumption, time on the treadmill, and the time to reach 90% of maximal oxygen con-sumption, when compared with age-matched female controls who did not exer-cise.[80] More recently, 63 postmenopausal women were evaluated over a 1-year period, during a structured program that involved three weekly 20-minute treadmill, ergome-ter, or Nautilus (muscle-strengthening) ses-sions. Two nonexercising groups were

Table 11–4. RESPONSE OF CLIMACTERIC WOMEN—MEAN AGE 56 YR—TO INTENSIVE STRUCTURED EXERCISE,[81] MEAN ($\pm$ SD) MAXIMAL O_2 UPTAKE ($mL \cdot kg^{-1} \cdot min^{-1}$)

Group	Age	n	Baseline	3 Mo	6 Mo	12 Mo	% Difference Baseline vs 12 Mo
Nautilus	59.3 $\pm$ 6.7	13	26.0 $\pm$ 5.2	26.1 $\pm$ 4.7	26.5 $\pm$ 4.0	26.2 $\pm$ 3.9	0.8
Treadmill	54.9 $\pm$ 6.9	10	27.1 $\pm$ 2.7	29.5 $\pm$ 2.8	30.5 $\pm$ 2.8	29.5 $\pm$ 2.4	8.9
Ergometer	55.9 $\pm$ 6.9	10	26.7 $\pm$ 4.7	28.9 $\pm$ 4.1	30.2 $\pm$ 4.1	30.0 $\pm$ 4.8	12.4
Control	62.0 $\pm$ 7.1	14	26.5 $\pm$ 4.7	26.1 $\pm$ 6.0	25.9 $\pm$ 5.9	26.2 $\pm$ 5.8	−1.1
Hormone	48.4 $\pm$ 7.2	16	26.6 $\pm$ 3.9	26.3 $\pm$ 3.7	26.4 $\pm$ 4.2	25.1 $\pm$ 3.9	−5.6

Source: From Notelovitz et al,[81] with permission.

included: an age-matched nontreatment group and a slightly younger group on hormone replacement therapy. Aerobically trained subjects were exercised at 70% to 85% of the maximal heart rate. Significant improvements in both $\dot{V}O_2max$ and time on the treadmill were recorded and maintained only by the bicycle and treadmill groups (Tables 11–4 and 11–5).[81]

The anticipated degree of improvement in aerobic power is inversely related to the subject's initial level of fitness, but at all initial levels, the greater the intensity and frequency of the training program, the greater the improvement. For example, the postmenopausal women in Cowan and Gregory's study[78] had a 19% improvement in $\dot{V}O_2max$ (from 12.6 $mL \cdot kg^{-1} \cdot min^{-1}$ to 15.0 $mL \cdot kg^{-1} \cdot min^{-1}$), compared with a 10.7% improvement in the Gainesville study[81] (from 26.9 $mL \cdot kg^{-1} \cdot min^{-1}$ to 29.8 $mL \cdot kg^{-1} \cdot min^{-1}$).

An intriguing observation in both of these studies is the considerably greater improvement in total exercise time versus $\dot{V}O_2max$.

Cowan and Gregory[78] noted a 29.6% increase in total walking time; in the Gainesville study,[81] the time for treadmill walkers increased 21.5%, and for bicyclists, 17.4%. Premenopausal women exposed to the same exercise regimen had an improvement rate of 10.9% in total exercise time.[78] Since the heart rate and stroke volume response to exercise was appropriate in postmenopausal women, there is a possibility that the lesser percentage response in $\dot{V}O_2max$ compared with percentage improvement in exercise time might be accounted for by partially compromised lung ventilation, lung diffusion capacity for oxygen, and/or oxygen utilization by the tissues in the postmenopausal period.

Less attention has been directed to older women. When 10 healthy women of mean age 72.0 years exercised three times per week for 20 minutes per session, at 70% of maximum heart rate, for 26 weeks, maximum oxygen uptake increased 8.4% and total exercise time increased 25.4%, compared to a 6.1% decrease in maximum oxy-

Table 11–5. RESPONSE OF CLIMACTERIC WOMEN—MEAN AGE 56 YR—TO INTENSIVE STRUCTURED EXERCISE,[81] MEAN ($\pm$SD) TOTAL EXERCISE TIME (MIN)

Group	Age	n	Baseline	3 Mo	6 Mo	12 Mo	% Difference Baseline vs. 12 Mo
Nautilus	59.3 $\pm$ 6.7	13	12.1 $\pm$ 3.2	12.2 $\pm$ 2.5	12.9 $\pm$ 2.4	12.5 $\pm$ 2.4	5.3
Treadmill	54.9 $\pm$ 6.9	10	12.5 $\pm$ 1.6	14.2 $\pm$ 2.1	15.2 $\pm$ 2.0	15.3 $\pm$ 2.1	21.5
Ergometer	55.9 $\pm$ 7.9	10	13.0 $\pm$ 3.1	14.1 $\pm$ 3.0	14.5 $\pm$ 3.0	15.2 $\pm$ 3.3	17.4
Control	62.0 $\pm$ 7.1	14	12.2 $\pm$ 3.3	11.6 $\pm$ 3.6	12.2 $\pm$ 4.0	12.1 $\pm$ 3.4	−0.95
Hormones	48.4 $\pm$ 7.2	16	13.4 $\pm$ 2.4	12.6 $\pm$ 2.3	13.0 $\pm$ 2.3	12.3 $\pm$ 2.2	−7.7

Source: From Notelovitz et al,[81] with permission.

Table 11–6. IMPROVEMENT OF MAXIMAL O_2 UPTAKE FOLLOWING AEROBIC TRAINING PROGRAMS IN WOMEN OVER AGE 50

Author	n	Duration of Exercise per Session (min)	Frequency of Exercise per Week	Intensity of Exercise	Duration of Training Program (wk)	%Gain in Maximal O_2 Uptake
Kilbom[58]	13	30	2–3	70%*	7	8
Adams and DeVries[133]	17	50	3	85%†	12	20.8
Sidney et al.[134]	25	60	4	120–150‡	7	>30
Sidney and Shephard[135]	28	55	3	60–80%†	14	17
Cowan and Gregory[78]	14	50	4	80%†	9	18.9
Notelovitz et al[81]	10 (T)	20	3	70–85%†	52	8.9
	10 (E)	20	3	70–85%	52	12.4
Probart et al[82]	10	20	3	70%†	24	8.4

*$\dot{V}o_2$max.
†Maximum heart rate.
‡Heart rate.
T = treadmill; E = ergometer.
Source: Adapted from Cowan and Gregory.[78]

gen uptake and a 5.4% decrease in total exercise time in six age-matched controls who did not exercise.[82] These data and others (Table 11–6) indicate that older women can certainly expect to improve fitness and exercise capacity with aerobic training.

In the studies summarized in Table 11–6, the percentage gain in aerobic power ranges from 8% to 30%. With only one exception, the duration of these training programs was less than 14 weeks. The best improvement was obtained in programs whose duration of exercise exceeded 30 minutes in each session. The study that continued for 12 months demonstrated that most of the improvement attained by 12 months had been achieved by 3 months of training. These results, however, do not reflect the true potential of older women engaged in long-term, intensive exercise programs, nor do they consider a most important practical, real-life issue of exercise: compliance.

Measurements of aerobic fitness may help to motivate some sedentary women. Kirk and co-workers[26] reported higher levels of fitness (maximal oxygen consumption) among postmenopausal runners compared to age-matched sedentary women. In an-

other cross-sectional study,[83] active women had a fitness gain of one decade when compared to sedentary women. The mean $\dot{V}o_2$max of active 40- to 49-year-old women was higher than sedentary 30- to 39-year-old women; active 50- to 59-year-old women had values similar to sedentary women in their 40s. One way of encouraging women to exercise is to use cardiorespiratory fitness assessments as a means of demonstrating improvement in aerobic function before the physical benefits of exercise are appreciated. Bruce and colleagues[84] reported that 63% of their patients attributed a change in one or more adverse health habits to a graded exercise test. Persons with an abnormal result were motivated the most.

Maximal oxygen uptake tests need to be performed in a specially equipped laboratory and are not suited to everyday clinical practice. Submaximal testing, on the other hand, is more suited to the practicing physician. Several studies have shown that predicted maximum $\dot{V}o_2$ values (using a bicycle ergometer) correlate well with observed maximal testing when corrected for age,[85,86] but none of these studies have involved climacteric women. To test this relationship in postmenopausal women, 29 women (mean age 55.6 ± 9.1 years) participating in an ongoing exercise program had both a maximal treadmill test and a submaximal ergometry test.[73] The interval between the two tests was less than 1 month, and the order of testing was randomly selected. The measured $\dot{V}O_2max$ was 28.6 ± 4.9 mL·kg^{-1}·min^{-1}, and the predicted $\dot{V}O_2max$ 32.5 ± 5.3 mL·kg^{-1}·min^{-1}. When the latter result was calculated using the recommended Åstrand age correction factor, the mean predicted $\dot{V}O_2max$ was 23.4 ± 4.9 mL·kg^{-1}·min^{-1}. This correlated closely with the directly measured result (r = 0.789; Fig. 11–5).

Submaximal testing can thus be used both as a screen to determine the cardiorespiratory fitness of climacteric women and as a way of monitoring the response to prescribed exercise. Patients at high risk for cardiovascular disease and those classified as having fair to poor fitness (as measured by ergometry) require more detailed evaluation before embarking on a prescribed exercise program. A nomogram is also very useful (Figs. 11–6 and 11–7); when used together with age-adjusted tables listing cardiorespiratory fitness for women (Table 11–7), potential exercise candidates can obtain a good index of both their current fitness status and the goals they should reach. Because postmenopausal women appear to show a greater response to a given exercise program in total exercise time than in maximum oxygen uptake, the total exercise nomogram (Fig. 11–7) may be used as the primary indicator of exercise response and improvement.

In view of the laziness inherent in most people, any program that can produce improved results for little effort is more likely to be successful and lead to a greater degree of compliance than a program that requires great effort and discipline. Schoenfeld and co-workers[87] examined the efficiency of walking with a backpack load as a method for improving physical fitness of sedentary men. They showed that it was possible to increase $\dot{V}O_2max$ by 15% to 30% by walking for 3 to 4 miles with a 3- or 6-kg backpack. When we compared the effects of treadmill walking with and without extra weight in a small group of postmenopausal women, we found greater improvement in the aerobic capacity of the load-bearing group.[88] However, confirmatory studies with larger numbers are needed to determine whether load-bearing enhances the efficacy of aerobic training or modifies the perceived effort.

MUSCLE TISSUE AND STRENGTH

Age-Related Loss of Muscle Tissue and Strength

Muscle mass and muscle strength decline with aging, and muscle weakness can greatly reduce the quality of life and self-sufficiency of many older women. The age-related decline in lean body mass correlates with several changes: a decline in endogenous growth hormone (GH),[89] a decline in pituitary responsiveness to growth hormone releasing hormone (GHRH),[90] loss of muscle fibers,[91] neuromuscular alterations, inactiv-

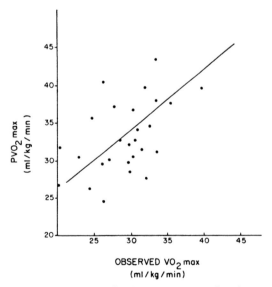

Figure 11–5. Correlation between measured and predicted $\dot{V}O_{2max}$ in climacteric women. (From Notelovitz et al.,[73] with permission.)

AGE VS. $\dot{V}O_{2max}$

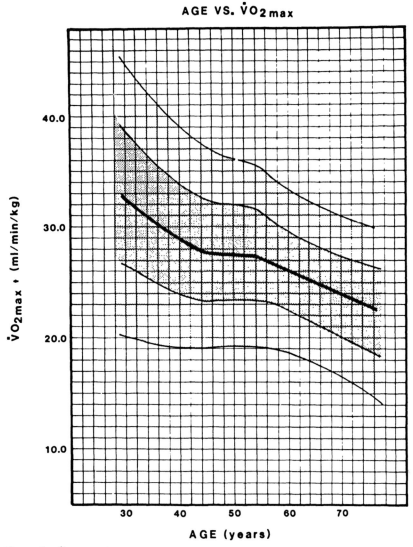

Figure 11–6. Normative $\dot{V}O_2$max values for climacteric women. Mean ± 1 and 2 SD for each age group. (From Notelovitz M, Fields C, et al: Unpublished data. Center for Climacteric Studies, Gainesville, FL, with permission.)

ity, and other age-related changes. Premenopausal women have significantly greater pituitary response to GHRH than do men of the same age, but postmenopausal women do not;[90] this finding suggests that postmenopausal estrogen deficiency accelerates the age-related decline in GH secretion and may also accelerate the loss of muscle tissue that occurs as women age. Although Rudman and his co-workers[92] reported that older men increased both lean body mass and skin thickness and de-

Table 11–7. GUIDELINES FOR FITNESS ASSESSMENT BY $\dot{V}O_2$max $(mL \cdot kg^{-1} \cdot min^{-1})$ OF HEALTHY WOMEN AGE 30–70

Age	Poor	Fair	Average	Good	Excellent
30–39	<20	20–27	28–33	33–44	45+
40–49	<17	17–23	24–30	31–41	42+
50–59	<15	15–20	21–27	28–37	38+
60–69	<13	13–17	18–23	24–34	35+

Source: Adapted from Exercise Testing and Training in Apparently Healthy Individuals: A Handbook for Physicians, published by the Committee on Exercise, The American Heart Association, Dallas, TX, 1972.

AGE vs TET

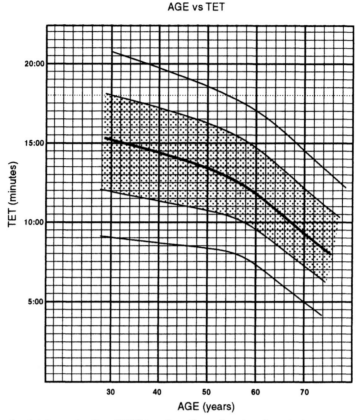

Figure 11–7. Normative total exercise time (TET) to exhaustion values for climacteric women, using modified Balke method. Mean ± 1 and 2 SD for each age group. (From Notelovitz M, Fields C, et al: Unpublished data. Center for Climacteric Studies, Gainesville, FL, with permission.)

creased adipose tissue mass during GH treatment, this has not been studied in older women. Furthermore, the safety of such therapy has not been demonstrated.

Several cross-sectional studies also have shown a loss of muscle strength with age, beginning after the third decade of life and amounting to a decline of 16.5% or more.[93] The loss is greater in women.[94] Loss of muscle tissue is related to a number of important metabolic activities. For example, Tzanoff and Norris[95] maintain that the decrease in muscle mass may be wholly responsible for the age-related decrease in basal metabolic rate (BMR). The average $\dot{V}O_2$max of older men was 22% lower when compared with younger men, but this difference decreased to only 8% when the values were expressed

in terms of milliliters per kilogram per minute of muscle, as determined by 24-hour urine creatinine measurements. Increasing muscle mass can thus play an important role in determining energy expenditure: a 2-kg increase in a woman's lean body mass results in an additional expenditure of about 50 kcal/d, the equivalent of about 5 lb of body fat per year.

Muscle is also an important determinant of carbohydrate utilization. The rate of glucose removal from muscle is more rapid in physically active persons, and the amount of insulin needed is significantly reduced.[96] This effect is reputed to be due to the enhanced sensitivity of insulin receptors in skeletal (and adipose) tissue. Obesity and diabetes are two age-related conditions that are prevalent in the late climacteric. Van Dam and colleagues[96a] have shown improvement in glucose tolerance among postmenopausal women following aerobic exercise training.

Strength Training

Weight training in women has been shown to improve strength with a loss of adipose tissue and with relatively little muscle hypertrophy. These studies have involved young women, trained athletes, or both, however.[97–99] It is not known whether muscle strengthening exercises will enhance the metabolic function of postmenopausal skeletal muscle, and if so, to what degree. Extrapolation from data collected in male subjects suggests that the accumulation of greater mass will lead to greater energy expenditure. Strength training does not improve cardiorespiratory function (see Table 11–4), a finding confirmed by studies done in middle-aged men.[100] Weight training stresses muscles far more than do most aerobic exercises. It is safe to start an aerobic exercise program and then, many months later, to start lifting weights.

OTHER MENOPAUSAL PROBLEMS: VASOMOTOR SYMPTOMS

Very few studies have addressed the relationship between menopausal vasomotor symptoms ("hot flushes") and exercise. In one study, Hammar and co-workers[101] found vasomotor symptoms to be less common among exercising menopausal women than among inactive women. Since exercise has not been shown to relieve symptoms, however, this finding may reflect a self-selection bias, representing differences between the two groups questioned.

Although the etiology of the menopausal vasomotor flush remains enigmatic, estrogen remains the most effective form of therapy available.[102] When estrogen is contraindicated, medroxyprogesterone acetate[103] or megestrol acetate[104] (synthetic progesto-

gens) will provide relief for most women. It should be noted that medroxyprogesterone acetate has not been approved, in the United States, for use in women with breast cancer.

OTHER AGE-RELATED CHANGES

Exercise and Adipose Tissue

Most people add adipose tissue with aging. There is no evidence that accumulation of adipose tissue is related to menopause, estrogen deficiency, or any other alterations in reproductive hormones, but many women first notice this accumulation around the time of menopause. Menopause also has not been shown to affect the distribution of body fat,[105] but there is a progressive age-related increase in upper and central body fat deposition, which tends to accelerate in postmenopausal women.[106] However, it remains to be shown whether this change is related to menopause, aging, or both.

Levels of adipose tissue lipoprotein lipase (LPL) correlate directly with body mass index (in kilograms per square meter of body surface) and affect the maintenance of adipocyte size, body weight, and obesity.[107] Adipocyte size is similar at mammary, abdominal, and femoral sites and is similar for premenopausal and postmenopausal women.[108] It has been shown[108] that femoral LPL activity is much higher among premenopausal women than among postmenopausal women and that, among premenopausal women, it is much higher than it is at mammary or abdominal locations. Treatment of postmenopausal women with estradiol and a progestogen leads to an increase in femoral LPL activity.[109] When percutaneous progesterone is applied to the femoral region of premenopausal women during the follicular phase of a natural menstrual cycle, LPL activity rises locally.[110] These data suggest that progesterone is an important determinant of femoral LPL activity.[111]

Regional fat distribution has achieved importance since it was demonstrated that abdominal fat is a risk factor for cardiovascular disease and diabetes, while femoral fat is not.[55,56] Aerobic exercise facilitates the loss of abdominal fat more readily than fat at other sites, and promotes fat loss more readily in men than in women.[112-115] It is fortunate that abdominal fat is so sensitive to exercise, since this facilitates reduction in disease risk. However, the relative resistance of femoral fat depots to exercise may discourage many women with a preponderance of femoral fat.

Inactivity is the most common cause of obesity, and it accelerates the accumulation of body fat that occurs naturally with aging. Cowan and Gregory[78] have reported a loss of body fat during a 9-week training program in women, confirming that exercise can certainly help older women to lose fat. Control of weight and body fat is discussed more thoroughly in Chapter 2.

Exercise and Osteoarthrosis

The articular cartilage that covers the bone ends in joints is rich in collagen and the mucopolysaccharide proteoglycan. This collagen layer acts as a barrier preventing the leakage of proteoglycan from the deeper layers into the joint space, and at the same time it inhibits potential harmful enzymes in the synovial fluid from perfusing into the deeper cartilage.[116] Loss or damage to the cartilage layer leads to joint degeneration and the development of osteoarthritis.

Osteoarthritis is a highly prevalent disease: 86% of women over the age of 65 show radiologic evidence of the condition,[117] although only 25% to 30% of individuals with diagnosed osteoarthritis are symptomatic. There are conflicting opinions regarding the role of microtrauma to the joint surface in the pathogenesis of osteoarthritis. Impulse loading causes trabecular microfracture with subsequent healing by sclerosis, resulting in stiffened bone that increases the stress on the articular cartilage, with eventual damage to the cartilage and joint degeneration. These changes appear on roentgenogram as osteophytes, sclerosis of the subchondral bone, cyst formation, and narrowing of the joint space.

Postmenopausal women have decreased amounts of collagen in skin and bone,[118] and it is most likely that the same is true for the collagen content of their articular surfaces. The collagen in the skin (and possibly also in the bone) of postmenopausal women is responsive to estrogen replacement. Although arthralgia is a common symptom in the late climacteric, a direct linkage between menopause and joint disease has not been established. However, a study has demonstrated that noncontraceptive hormonal therapy does help some women with rheumatoid arthritis.[119]

With the increased interest in jogging, a question arises of whether damage to the musculoskeletal-articular system exceeds the benefit of exercise. Lane and associates[120] recently studied female long-distance runners over age 50 and compared them with age-matched nonactive community controls. The female runners did have more sclerosis and spur formation in the weight-bearing areas of the spine and knees, but not in the hands. These changes were not found in men studied in the same and other investigations.[121]

Given the asymptomatic nature of these changes and the difficulty of extrapolating cross-sectional data into "real-life" terms, it cannot be concluded that jogging has an adverse effect on the joints of middle-aged women. The absence of joint changes in age-matched and hormone-replete men, however, suggests the possibility that an estrogen-primed articular surface (with an improved collagen content) might be similarly resilient to mechanical stress.

EXERCISE AND WELL-BEING

The administration of exogenous estrogens, especially parenteral estrogen therapy, to postmenopausal women is frequently associated with a mood-elevating effect. Exercise is also known to induce a state of well-being and, according to some studies, a reduction in symptoms such as depression and anxiety. The early work of Weber and Lee[122] demonstrated that vigorous activity in animals had a positive influence on psychologic measures and that this was probably due to alterations in brain neurotransmitter levels or activity, or both.[123] Studies in humans have been less clear, and there is some question whether the "runner's high" really exists.[124]

Part of the controversy lies in the fact that much of the research has been conducted in nondepressed subjects. Greist and colleagues[125] demonstrated that aerobic exercise performed for 12 weeks reduced depression (in patients complaining of mild to moderate depression) to a greater degree than traditional psychotherapy. Additional advantages noted by the authors included less expense, no need to use antidepressant medication, and the persistence of a depression-free state when evaluated 12 months later, whereas half the patients receiving psychotherapy returned earlier for additional treatment. The reader is referred to an excellent review by Dunn and Dishman[126] of the relationship between exercise and depression.

One of the most distressing symptoms expressed by menopausal women is anxiety. Vigorous physical activity reduces muscle tension and is also associated with a significant decrease in anxiety.[127] This effect was noted only when the exercise was intense enough to provoke significant elevations in plasma epinephrine and norepinephrine, however,[128] and did not occur if light to moderate exercise was performed.

Another common problem associated with the menopausal syndrome—insomnia—may be positively influenced by exercise. Healthy subjects who engaged in static exercise (e.g., contraction of a hand dynamometer at 40% of maximal level for 40 minutes, separated by a 10-minute rest at mid-session) 2 hours before bedtime were shown to have a significantly reduced time to onset of sleep relative to nonexercise nights. The improvement in sleep was associated with increased slow-wave sleep and decreased movement time during sleep,

factors that contribute to a "refreshing" sleep period.[129]

To evaluate the effect of exercise on psychologic well-being, preprogram and postprogram psychosocial measures were obtained by questionnaire and standardized tests in a group of healthy women (age 40 to 64 years) participating in a 12-week exercise program. Methods of evaluation included a self-report of physical activity, a somatization scale, the multidimensional health locus of control inventory, the Profile of Mood States Scale, and a social support questionnaire. Members of the exercised group were required to walk-jog for 30 minutes three times a week for 12 weeks, and they were compared with matched women participating in discussion groups and a nonintervention control group. The only noted apparent benefit of exercise was a decrease in intake of stimulants (e.g., coffee) among exercisers, whereas there was an increase in intake among the nonexercisers.[80] These results are similar to the report of Penny and Rust,[130] whose subjects participated in a walk-jog program involving 1½ miles of exercise twice a week for 15 weeks. A comparison of personality scales measured by the MMPI showed no difference from a control nonexercising group. Despite these negative results, discussions with individuals who exercised elicited commonly observed responses: "feeling better, enjoying social functions more, participating in more extracurricular activities, and not being tired at day's end."[130] The operative factors appear to be the frequency, intensity, and duration of exercise, and patience. The last is most important, as the benefits of exercise rarely occur before 10 weeks of training, the time when most individuals drop out of exercise programs.

In summary, although the chemical basis of the mood improvement induced by physical activity is not known, fairly strong evidence suggests that acute and chronic vigorous exercise is associated with an improvement in affective states, especially anxiety and moderate depression.

Psychomotor speed is one well-recognized behavior that is slowed by aging. This is especially true for response speed that occurs in reaction time, performance of tasks that require the coordination of two simultaneous movements, writing speed, and simple tasks such as tapping in place.[131] The quicker the response, the higher the perceptual speed score. Perceptual speed was evaluated in healthy aging women as part of a large study examining age-related changes, and a progressive decrease was noted with both chronologic and biologic aging.[63] As shown in Table 11-8, the perceptual speed score decreased from a mean score of 64.4 ± 2.1 in 40-year-old premenopausal women to 48.0 ± 2.6 in 68-year-old women (p < 0.0001; r = −0.41). An interesting observation is the difference in the perceptual speed score between premenopausal and postmenopausal women aged 46 to 55. Although the premenopausal women were only a few years younger, their mean perceptual speed score was significantly higher than that of the postmenopausal group, whose score was similar to the score of women 5 or more years past their menopause.

Further analysis of these data revealed that, within the groups, physical fitness was positively correlated with the perceptual speed score. The greater the degree of fitness, the more functionally competent the individual.[63] This raises the issue of whether exercise may prevent premature aging of the central nervous system and compensate for possible alterations in the neurohormonal milieu of postmenopausal women. A number of investigators have shown that people who exercise consistently have a faster reaction time, and that this difference is related to

generalized rather than specific exercise. For example, the reactive speed of the fingers is improved in runners, who primarily exercise their legs.[132] It is not clear whether this exercise-induced improvement affects central nervous system processing time, or motor speed. As with the psychologic response to exercise, CNS function (e.g., short-term memory) that is not impaired in a particular individual cannot be expected to be improved by exercise. With this caveat in mind, it is fair to conclude that "exercise seems to be one way for people to achieve maximal plasticity in aging, approximating full vigor and consistency of performance until life's end."[132]

SUMMARY

"Menopause," an often-misused term, is actually the duration of a woman's final menstrual period. The 15 years leading up to and following this event are known more properly as the "climacteric."

Women lose a small percentage of bone as a natural phenomenon in the aging process. However, the greater the bone mineral content at bone mass maturity, the more one can afford to lose. Thus, women should be encouraged during, and even before, the early climacteric to accrue as much bone as possible, through an appropriate calcium intake and an osteogenic exercise program. Likewise, such practices can be used to avoid excessive bone loss during the climacteric. For women who have osteoporosis, a regimen of walking may be the safest type of

Table 11–8. CHANGES IN PERCEPTUAL SPEED SCORE ASSOCIATED WITH CHRONOLOGIC AND BIOLOGIC AGING IN WOMEN

	Premenopausal		Postmenopausal		
Age range	35–45	46–55	46–55	56–65	66–75
Mean age (± SEM)	40.9 ± 0.5	48.7 ± 0.4	52.2 ± 0.4	59.3 ± 0.5	68.5 ± 0.5
N	30	29	30	29	27
Perceptual speed score (mean ± SEM)	64.4 ± 2.1	61.1 ± 1.9	56.6 ± 1.8	55.3 ± 1.3	48.0 ± 2.6

Source: From Notelovitz et al,[63] with permission.

exercise program. These women should avoid exercises that emphasize flexion of the back.

The postmenopausal period has been associated with an increased plasma total cholesterol level and an increased LDL level—both risk factors for atherosclerotic disease. A regular, long-term exercise program promotes beneficial changes in lipoprotein cholesterol levels, aerobic fitness, exercise time, and coronary heart disease risk.

Exercise also adds to a feeling of well-being and may counteract clinical depression and anxiety experienced by some women in this stage of life.

REFERENCES

1. Jaszman LJB: Epidemiology of the climacteric syndrome. In Campbell S (ed): The Management of the Menopause and Postmenopausal Years. University Book Press, Baltimore, 1976, p 11.
2. Notelovitz M: Climacteric medicine and science: A societal need. In Notelovitz M, and van Keep P (eds): The Climacteric in Perspective. MTP Press Ltd, Lancaster, England, 1986, p 19.
3. Cummings SR, Rubin SM, and Black D: The future of hip fractures in the United States: Numbers, costs, and potential effects of postmenopausal estrogen. Clin Orthop 252:163, 1990.
4. Lewinnek G, Kelsey J, White A, et al: Significance and comparative analysis of the epidemiology of hip fractures. Clin Orthop 152:35, 1980.
5. Keene JS, and Anderson CA: Hip fractures in the elderly, discharge predictions with a functional rating scale. JAMA 248:564, 1982.
6. NCHS. Advance report of final mortality statistics, 1989. Hyattsville, Maryland: US Department of Health and Human Services, Public Health Service, CDC (Monthly vital statistics report, vol. 40, no. 8, suppl. 2), 1992.
7. Public Health Service. Healthy people 2000: National health promotion and disease prevention objectives—full report, with commentary. Washington DC: US Department of Health and Human Services, Public Health Service, DHHS publication no. (PHS)91-50212, 1991.
8. Council on Scientific Affairs: Exercise programs for the elderly. JAMA 252:544, 1984.
9. Health United States, US Dept of Health and Human Services, DHHS Pub No (PHS) 85-1232, 1984.
10. Cohn SH, Abesamis C, Yasumura S, et al: Comparative skeletal mass and radial bone mineral content in black and white women. Metabolism 26:171, 1977.
11. Parfitt AM: The cellular basis of bone remodeling: The quantum concept re-examined in light of recent advances in cell biology of bone. Calcif Tissue Int 36:S37, 1984.
12. Katz JL, Yoon HS, Lipson S, et al: The effects of remodeling on the elastic properties of bone. Calcif Tissue Int 36:531, 1984.
13. De Deuxchaisnes C, Nagant: The pathogenesis and treatment of involutional osteoporosis. In Dixon AHJ, Russel RGG, and Stamp TCB (eds): Osteoporosis: A Multidisciplinary Problem. The Royal Society of Medicine. Academic Press, London, 1983, p 291.
14. Drinkwater BL, Nilson K, Chestnut III C, et al: Bone mineral content of amenorrheic and eumenorrheic athletes. N Engl J Med 311:277, 1984.
15. Riggs BL, Wahner HW, Dunn WL, et al: Differential changes in bone mineral density of appendicular and axial skeleton with aging: Relationship to spinal osteoporosis. J Clin Invest 67:328, 1981.
16. Editorial: Osteoporosis and activity. Lancet 2:1365, 1983.
17. Whedon GC: Interrelation of physical activity and nutrition on bone mass. In White PL, and Mondeika T (eds): Diet and Exercise: Synergism in Health Maintenance. American Medical Association, Chicago, 1982, p 99.
18. Basset CA, and Becker RO: Generation of electric potentials by bone in response to mechanical stress. Science 137:1063, 1962.
19. Jones HH, Priest JD, Hayes WC, et al: Humeral hypertrophy in response to exercise. J Bone Joint Surg 59A:204, 1977.
20. Orwoll ES, Ferar J, Oviatt SK, et al: The relationship of swimming exercise to bone mass in men and women. Arch Intern Med 149:2197, 1989.
21. Carter DR: Mechanical loading histories of bone remodelling. Calcif Tissue Int 36:S19, 1984.
22. Lanyon LE: Functional strain as a determinant for bone remodelling. Calcif Tissue Int 36:S56, 1984.
23. Lanyon LE, and Rubin CT: Regulation of bone mass in response to physical activity. In Dixon AHJ, Russel RGG, and Stamp TCB (eds): Osteoporosis: A Multidisciplinary Problem. The Royal Society of Medicine. Academic Press, London, 1983, p 51.

24. Woo SLY, Kuei SC, Amiel D, et al: The effect of prolonged physical training on the properties of long bone. J Bone Joint Surg 63A:780, 1980.

25. Cavanaugh DJ, and Cann CE: Brisk walking does not stop bone loss in postmenopausal women. Bone 9:201, 1988.

26. Kirk S, Sharp CF, Elbaum N, et al: Effect of long-distance running on bone mass in women. J Bone Min Res 4:515, 1989.

27. Krølner B, Toft B, Nielsen SP, et al: Physical exercise as prophylaxis against involutional vertebral bone loss: A controlled trial. Clin Sci 64:541, 1983.

28. Brewer V, Meyer BM, Keele MJ, et al: Role of exercise in prevention of involutional bone loss. Med Sci Sports Exerc 15:445, 1983.

29. Linnell J, Stager JM, Blue PW, et al: Bone mineral content and menstrual regularity in female runners. Med Sci Sports Exerc 16:343, 1984.

30. Marcus R, Cann C, Madvig P, et al: Menstrual function and bone mass in elite women distance runners. Ann Intern Med 102:158, 1985.

31. Myerson M, Gutin B, Warren MP, et al: Total body bone density in amenorrheic runners. Obstet Gynecol 79:973, 1992.

32. Rigotti NA, Nussbaum SR, Herzog DR, et al: Osteoporosis in women with anorexia nervosa. N Engl J Med 311:1601, 1984.

33. Notelovitz M, et al: Unpublished data.

34. Heikkinen J, Kurttila-Matero E, Kyllonen E, et al: Moderate exercise does not enhance the positive effect of estrogen on bone mineral density in post-menopausal women. Calif Tissue Int (Suppl)49:S83, 1991.

35. Notelovitz M, Martin D, Tesar R, et al: Estrogen therapy and variable-resistance weight training increase bone mineral in surgically menopausal women. J Bone Min Res 6:583, 1991.

36. Chvapil M, Bartos D, and Bartos F: Effect of long-term physical stress on collagen growth in the lung, heart and femur of young and adult rats. Gerontologia 19:263, 1973.

37. Inkovaara J, Heikinheimo R, Jarvinen K, et al: Prophylactic fluoride treatment and aged bones. Br Med J 3:73, 1975.

38. Smith EL, Reddan W, and Smith PE: Physical activity and calcium modalities for bone mineral increase in aged women. Med Sci Sports Exerc 13:60, 1981.

39. Sinaki M, and Mikkelsen BA: Postmenopausal spinal osteoporosis: Flexion versus extension exercises. Arch Phys Med Rehabil 65:593, 1984.

40. Goodman CE: Osteoporosis: Protective measures of nutrition and exercise. Geriatrics 40:59, 1985.

41. Rosenberg L, Hennekens CH, Rosner B, et al: Early menopause and the risk of myocardial infarction. Am J Obstet Gynecol 139:47, 1981.

42. Szajderman B, and Oliver MF: Spontaneous premature menopause, ischemic heart disease and serum lipids. Lancet 1:962, 1963.

43. Robinson RW, Higano N, and Cohen WD: Increased incidence of coronary heart disease in women castrated prior to menopause. Arch Intern Med 104:908, 1959.

44. Bengtsson C, and Lindquist O: Menopausal effects on risk factors for ischemic heart disease. Maturitas 1:165, 1979.

45. Miller G, and Miller N: Plasma high density lipoprotein concentration and development of ischaemic heart disease. Lancet 1:16, 1975.

46. Haskell WL: The influence of exercise on the concentrations of triglyceride and cholesterol in human plasma. In Terjung RL (ed): Exercise and Sports Sciences Reviews. Collamore Press, Lexington, MA, 1984, p 205.

47. Paffenbarger RS, Hyde RT, Wing AL, et al: A natural history of athleticism on cardiovascular health. JAMA 252:491, 1984.

48. Salonen JT, Puska R, and Tuomilehto J: Physical activity and risk of myocardial infarction, cerebral stroke and death: A longitudinal study in eastern Finland. Am J Epidemiol 115:526, 1982.

49. Leon AS, Connett J, Jacobs DR, and Rauramaa R: Leisure-time activity levels and risk of coronary heart disease and death. The Multiple Risk Factor Intervention Trial. JAMA 258:2388, 1987.

50. Blair SH, Kohl HW III, Paffenbarger RS, et al: Physical fitness and all-cause mortality: A prospective study of health men and women. JAMA 262:2395, 1989.

51. Castelli WP: Epidemiology of coronary heart disease. The Framingham Study. Am J Med 76:4, 1984.

52. Ducimetière P, Eschwege E, Papoz L, et al: Relationship of plasma insulin levels to the incidence of myocardial infarction and coronary heart disease in a middle-aged population. Diabetologia 19:215, 1980.

53. Manson JE, Rimm EB, Stampfer MJ, et al: Physical activity and incidence of non-insulin-dependent diabetes mellitus in women. Lancet 338:774, 1991.

54. Manson JE, Nathan DM, Krolewski AS, et al: A prospective study of exercise and incidence of diabetes among US male physicians. JAMA 268:63, 1992.

55. Lapidus L, Bengtsson C, Larsson B, et al: Distribution of adipose tissue and risk of cardiovascular disease and death: A 12 year follow-up of participants in the population

study of women in Gothenburg, Sweden. Br Med J 289:1257, 1984.

56. Larsson B, Svärdsudd K, Welin L, et al: Abdominal adipose tissue distribution, obesity, and risk of cardiovascular disease and death: 13 year follow-up of participants in the study of men born in 1913. Br Med J 288:1401, 1984.

57. Haskell WL, and Superko R: Designing an exercise plan for optimal health. Family and Community Health, p 72, May 1984.

58. Kilbom A: Physical training in women. Scand J Clin Lab Invest 28(Suppl 119):1, 1971.

59. Wood P, and Haskell W: The effect of exercise on plasma high-density lipoproteins. Lipids 14:417, 1979.

60. Goffman J, Young W, and Tandy R: Ischemic heart disease, atherosclerosis and longevity. Circulation 34:679, 1966.

61. Jacobs I, Lithell H, and Karlson J: Dietary effects on glycogen and lipoprotein lipase activity in skeletal muscle of men. Acta Physiol Scand 115:85, 1982.

62. Lamon-Fava S, Fisher EC, Nelson ME, et al: Effect of exercise and menstrual cycle status on plasma lipids, low density lipoprotein particle size, and apolipoproteins. J Clin Endocrinol Metab 68:17, 1989.

63. Notelovitz M, Dougherty M, Resnick J, et al: The psychosocial and biologic adaptation to aging in women. Final Report NIA #R01 AG00796-03, 1982.

64. Busby J, Notelovitz M, Putney K, et al: Exercise, high density lipoprotein cholesterol and cardiorespiratory function in climacteric women. South Med J 78:769, 1985.

65. Franklin B, Buskirk E, Hodgson J, et al: Effects of physical conditioning on cardiorespiratory function, body composition and serum lipids in relatively normal weight and obese middle-aged women. Int J Obes 3:97, 1979.

66. Rotkis T, Boyden TW, Pamenter RW, et al: High density lipoprotein cholesterol and body composition of female runners. Metabolism 30:994, 1981.

67. Notelovitz M, Feldman E, Larsen S, and Khan F: Lipids and lipoproteins in postmenopausal women: Effect of route of estrogen administration and aerobic exercise. In Christiansen C, and Overgard K (eds): Osteoporosis. Third International Symposium on Osteoporosis, Copenhagen, Denmark, October 1990, p 1822.

68. Moore CE, Hartung GH, Mitchell RE, et al: The effect of exercise and diet on high-density lipoprotein cholesterol levels in women. Metabolism 32:189, 1983.

69. Vodak PA, Wood PD, Haskell WL, et al: HDL-cholesterol and other plasma lipid and lipoprotein concentrations in middle-aged male and female tennis players. Metabolism 29:745, 1980.

70. Harting GH, Moore CE, Mitchell R, et al: Relationship of menopausal status and exercise level to HDL cholesterol in women. Exp Aging Res 10:13, 1984.

71. Drinkwater B, Horvath S, and Wells C: Aerobic power of females ages 10 to 68. J Gerontol 30:385, 1975.

72. Plowman S, Drinkwater B, and Horvath S: Age and aerobic power in women: A longitudinal study. J Gerontol 34:512, 1979.

73. Notelovitz M, Fields C, Caramelli K, et al: Cardiorespiratory fitness evaluation in climacteric women: Comparison of two methods. Am J Obstet Gynecol 154:1009, 1986.

74. DeVries HA: Exercise and the physiology of aging. In DeVries HA: Exercise and Health. American Academy of Physical Education Papers, No. 17. Human Kinetics Publishers, Champaign, IL, p 76, 1984.

75. Zauner C, Notelovitz M, Fields CD, et al: Cardiorespiratory efficiency at submaximal work in young and middle-aged women. Am J Obstet Gynecol 150:712, 1984.

76. Dehn MM, and Bruce RA: Longitudinal variations in maximum oxygen intake with age and activity. J Appl Physiol 33:805, 1972.

77. ¡Astrand I: Aerobic work capacity in men and women with special reference to age. Acta Physiol (Scand) 49:45, 1960.

78. Cowan MM, and Gregory LW: Responses of pre- and postmenopausal females to aerobic conditioning. Med Sci Sports Exerc 17:138, 1985.

79. White MK, Yenter RA, Martin RB, et al: Effects of aerobic dancing and walking on cardiovascular function and muscular strength in postmenopausal women. J Sports Med 24:159, 1984.

80. Gill AA, Veigl VL, Shuster J, et al: A well-woman's health maintenance study comparing physical fitness and group support programs. Occup Ther J Res 4:286, 1984.

81. Notelovitz M, Fields C, Caramelli K, et al: Alternatives to hormone therapy. Presented at XIth World Congress of Obstetrics and Gynecology, October 1985.

82. Probart CK, Notelovitz M, Martin D, et al: The effect of moderate aerobic exercise on physical fitness among women 70 years and older. Maturitas 14:49, 1991.

83. Profant GR, Early RG, Nilson KL, et al: Response to maximal exercise in healthy middle-aged women. J Appl Physiol 33:595, 1972.

84. Bruce RA, DeRouen TA, and Hossack KF: Pilot study examining the motivational ef-

fects of maximal exercise testing to modify risk factors and health habits. Cardiology 66:111, 1980.

85. Glassford RG, Baycroft GHY, Sedgwick AW, et al: Comparison of maximal oxygen uptake values determined by predicted and actual methods. J Appl Physiol 20:509, 1965.

86. Cink RE, and Thomas TR: Validity of the Åstrand-Rhyming monogram for predicting maximal oxygen uptake. Br J Sports Med 15:182, 1981.

87. Shoenfeld Y, Keven G, Shimoni I, et al: Walking. A method for rapid improvement of physical fitness. JAMA 243:2062, 1980.

88. Caramelli KE, and Notelovitz M: Effect of load-bearing during treadmill walking in women aged 57 to 67 years (abstr). Maturitas 6:95, 1984.

89. Zadik Z, Chalew SA, McCarter RJ, et al: The influence of age on the 24-hour integrated concentration of growth in normal individuals. J Clin Endocrinol Metab 60:513, 1985.

90. Lang I, Schernthaner G, Pietschmann P, et al: Effects of sex and age on growth hormone response to growth hormone-releasing hormone in healthy individuals. J Clin Endocrinol Metab 65:535, 1987.

91. Grimby G, and Saltin B: The aging muscle. Clin Physiol 3:209, 1983.

92. Rudman D, Feller AG, Nagraj HS, et al: Effects of growth hormone in men over 60 years old. N Engl J Med 323:1, 1990.

93. Fisher MB, and Birren JE: Age and strength. J Appl Psychol 31:490, 1947.

94. Montoye HJ, and Lamphiear DE: Grip and arm strength in males and females age 10–69. Res Q 48:109, 1977.

95. Tzanoff SP, and Norris AH: Effect of muscle mass decrease on age-related BMR changes. J Appl Physiol 43:1001, 1973.

96. Joman VR, Veikko AK, Deibert D, et al: Increased insulin sensitivity and insulin binding to monocytes after physical training. N Engl J Med 301:200, 1979.

96a. Van Dam S, Gillespy M, Notelovitz M, and Martin AD: Effect of exercise on glucose metabolism in postmenopausal women. Am J Obstet Gynecol 159:82, 1988.

97. Wells JB, Jokl E, and Bohanen J: The effect of intensive physical training upon body composition of adolescent girls. J Assoc Phys Mental Rehab 17:68, 1963.

98. Brown CH, and Wilmore JH: The effects of maximal resistance training on strength and body composition of women athletes. Med Sci Sports Exerc 6:174, 1974.

99. Wilmore JH: Alterations in strength, body composition and anthropometric measurements consequent to a 10-week weight training program. Med Sci Sports 6:133, 1974.

100. Hurley BF, Seals AA, Ehsani AA, et al: Effects of high-intensity strength training on cardiovascular function. Med Sci Sports Exerc 16:483, 1984.

101. Hammar M, Berg G, and Lindgren R: Does physical exercise influence the frequency of postmenopausal flushes? Acta Obstet Gynecol Scand 69:409, 1990.

102. Tataryn IV, Lomax P, Meldrum DR, et al: Objective techniques for the assessment of postmenopausal hot flashes. Obstet Gynecol 57:340, 1981.

103. Schiff I, Tulchinsky D, Cramer D, et al: Oral medroxyprogesterone in the treatment of postmenopausal symptoms. JAMA 244:1443, 1980.

104. Erlik Y, Meldrum DR, Lagasse LD, et al: Effect of megestrol acetate on flushing and bone metabolism in post-menopausal women. Maturitas 3:167, 1981.

105. Lanska DJ, Lanska MJ, Hartz AJ, and Rimm AA: Factors influencing anatomic location of fat tissue in women. Int J Obes 9:29, 1985.

106. Shimokata H, Tobin JD, Muller DC, et al: Studies in the distribution of body fat: I. Effects of age, sex and obesity. J Gerontol 44:M66, 1989.

107. Eckel RH: Lipoprotein lipase. A multifunctional enzyme relevant to common metabolic diseases. N Engl J Med 320:1060, 1989.

108. Rebuffé-Scrive M, Eldh J, Hafström L-O, and Björntorp P: Metabolism of mammary, abdominal, and femoral adipocytes in women before and after menopause. Metabolism 35:792, 1986.

109. Rebuffé-Scrive M, Lönnroth P, Mårin P, et al: Regional adipose tissue metabolism in men and postmenopausal women. Int J Obes 11:347, 1987.

110. Rebuffé-Scrive M, Basdevant A, and Guy-Grand B: Effect of local application of progesterone on human adipose tissue lipoprotein lipase. Horm Metab Res 15:566, 1983.

111. Rebuffé-Scrive M: Steroid hormones and distribution of adipose tissue. Acta Med Scand (Suppl)723:143, 1988.

112. Després JP, Bouchard C, Savard R, et al: The effect of a 20-week endurance training program on adipose tissue morphology and lipolysis in men and women. Metabolism 33:235, 1984.

113. Tremblay A, Després JP, Leblanc C, and Bouchard C: Sex dimorphism in fat loss in response to exercise-training. J Obes Weight Regul 3:193, 1984.

114. Tremblay A, Després JP, and Bouchard C: Alteration in body fat and fat distribution during growth and later health consequences. In Bouchard C, and Johnston FE:

Current Topics in Nutrition and Disease, Vol 17. Alan R Liss, New York, 1988.

115. Després JP, Tremblay A, Nadeau A, and Bouchard C: Physical training and changes in regional adipose tissue distribution. Acta Med Scand (Suppl)723:205, 1988.

116. Bullough PG: Pathologic changes associated with the common arthritides and their treatment. Pathol Annu 14:69, 1979.

117. Gordon T: Osteoarthritis in U.S. adults. In Bennett BH, and Wood PHN (eds): Population Studies in the Rheumatic Diseases. Excerpta Medica, New York, 1968, p 391.

118. Brincat M, Moniz CT, Studd JWW, et al: Skin thickness and skin collagen mimic an index of osteoporosis in the postmenopausal woman. In Christiansen C, Arnaud CD, Nordin BEC, et al (eds): Osteoporosis. Copenhagen International Symposium on Osteoporosis, June 3–8, 1984, p 353.

119. Vandenbroucke JP, Witteman JC, Valkenburg HA, et al: Noncontraceptive hormones and rheumatoid arthritis in perimenopausal and postmenopausal women. JAMA 255:1299, 1986.

120. Lane NE, Bloch DA, Jones HH, et al: Long-distance running, bone density and osteoarthritis. JAMA 255:1147, 1986.

121. Panush RS, Schmidt C, Caldwell JR, et al: Is running associated with degenerative joint disease? JAMA 255:1152, 1986.

122. Weber JC, and Lee RA: Effects of differing pre-puberty exercise programs on the emotionality of male albino rats. Res Q 39:748, 1968.

123. Olson EB Jr, and Morgan WP: Rat brain monoamine levels related to behavioral assessment. Life Sci 30:2095, 1982.

124. Levin DC: The runner's high: Fact or fiction? JAMA 248:24, 1982.

125. Greist JH, Klein MH, Eicchens RR, et al: Running as treatment for depression. Comp Psychiatry 20:41, 1979.

126. Dunn AL, and Dishman RK: Exercise and the neurobiology of depression. Exerc Sport Sci Rev 19:41, 1991.

127. Morgan WP: Anxiety reduction following acute physical activity. Psychiatr Annu 9:36, 1979.

128. Morgan WP, Horstman DH, Cymerman A, et al: Facilitation of physical performance by means of cognitive strategy. Cog Ther Res 7:251, 1983.

129. Browman CP: Sleep following sustained exercise. Psychophysiology 17:577, 1980.

130. Penny GD, and Rust JO: Effect of a walking-jogging program on personality characteristics of middle-aged females. J Sports Med 20:221, 1980.

131. Spirduso WW: Exercise as a factor in aging motor behavior plasticity in exercise and health. American Academy of Physical Education Papers, No. 17. Human Kinetics Publishers, Champaign, IL, 1984, p 89.

132. Spirduso WW, and Clifford P: Replication of age and physical activity effects in reaction and movement time. J Gerontol 33:26, 1978.

133. Adams G, and DeVries H: Physiological effects of an exercise training regimen upon women aged 52 to 79. J Gerontol 28:50, 1973.

134. Sidney K, Shephard R, and Harrison J: Endurance training and body composition of the elderly. Am J Clin Nutr 30:326, 1977.

135. Sidney K, and Shephard R: Frequency and intensity of exercise training for elderly subjects. Med Sci Sports Exerc 10:125, 1978.

III

Special Issues and Concerns

CHAPTER 12

The Breast

CHRISTINE E. HAYCOCK, M.D.

Wearing a bra can provide two useful functions during exercise—providing support and limiting breast motion.[1,2] This can help reduce discomfort and impact of the breast against the anterior chest wall. Padding can be added to help prevent traumatic injuries, such as that from a hockey stick or an elbow.

There is no evidence that free-swinging breasts are more likely to be damaged during exercise. However, women in primitive cultures who never wear bras do develop long pendulous breasts, whereas those in modern society who frequently wear bras are less likely to develop these changes.

BREAST SUPPORT

In an effort to ascertain the injury potential for the female athlete in the early 1970s, two surveys were conducted in more than 300 physical education departments throughout the country. The first questionnaire, performed by Joan Gillette, A.T.C., and published in 1975 in *The Physician and Sportsmedicine*,[3] asked for the numbers and types of injuries seen by coaches and trainers. I sent out a more detailed questionnaire to cover the 1974 to 1975 season, with more emphasis on the types of injuries rather than on just the numbers and associated sports. The combined results of the two surveys were published in 1976.[4] The surveys indicated that, in general, the types and numbers of injuries to these female athletes were essentially the same as to their male counterparts. Of particular interest to me was the fact that, of all injuries reported, those to the breast were least common. Other studies have confirmed these findings.[5-7]

The results of the earlier surveys prompted me to undertake a third survey,[8] specifically asking if female athletes reported tenderness or soreness in their breasts or injuries such as scratches from metallic parts or allergies to the materials in their bras. Thirty-one percent of the respondents indicated sore or tender breasts after exercise. Of these, 52% reported specific minor injuries to the breasts.

A study was undertaken by Haycock, Shierman, and Gillette[9] to ascertain what factors cause breast injury and discomfort. To determine if a bra is necessary to control breast motion, a test was instituted to measure breast movement during exercise.

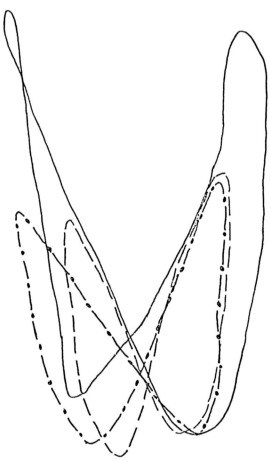

Figure 12-1. The subject wore a size D cup. The *solid* line represents the range of motion with no bra; the *dash-dot-dash* line, the subject's own bra, which had fairly good support; and the *dash* line, the specially fitted bra, showing the best support.

Twelve female athletes with different breast sizes were fitted with special supportive bras. They were encouraged to use these garments during athletic competition and to note how they compared in comfort and support with the bras they had been using previously. Most of the women felt that the bulky test bras provided better support than their own. The women who benefited the most had size B cups or larger. Five volunteers were filmed with a high-speed (100 frames per minute), 16-mm camera while walking and running on a treadmill and while jumping to simulate the motion of shooting a basketball into the hoop. A marker was placed on each nipple so that line studies made by tracing each frame could be drawn. Each marker was placed either on the bra or on the breast itself, since the athletes were filmed wearing their own bras, wearing the special bras or wearing no bras.

The films showed that during running, the breast moves considerably up and down, and during jumping, the breasts roll in a spiral motion (Fig. 12-1). Although the force of breast impact upon the chest wall was not measured, it was estimated to be between 60 and 80 foot pounds per square inch, with the largest breasts exerting the greatest force. Although both sets of bras limited motion, the specially fitted ones did the best job, corroborating the increased support and comfort reported by the athletes themselves.

These findings are consistent with the original expectations of the authors. The natural support of the breasts is minimal. The breast is composed mostly of adipose tissue. It is held in place by the skin and some deep fascial structures, which loosely attach the glands to the underlying muscles, blood vessels, and nerves. Cooper's ligaments do not support the breasts. They are merely connective tissue strands extending between the skin and the pectoralis fascia and separating the glandular structures.[8] As a result of this study, the following recommendations regarding sports bras can be made:[9]

1 A bra should be made of firm, mostly nonelastic material with good absorptive qualities (about 60% cotton plus about 40% synthetic materials for fast drying and easy laundering). More elasticity provides less support.

2 It should be constructed to limit motion in all directions and provide firm support. There should be either no seams over the nipples or smooth seams that will not irritate.

3 Some provision should exist for insertion of padding, if indicated to reduce the risk of traumatic injury. Obviously, a bra intended only for use during running does not need these features.

4 All metal or plastic hooks or catches should be well covered to protect the wearer from skin irritation or abrasion.[8,10,11] Various types of bras have been studied.[12-16] In the most recent study, Dr. Deana Lorentzen of Utah State University at Logan[17] compared eight of the most popular bras currently on the market. Her findings were in agreement with the previous recommendations. Dr. Lorentzen also suggested adding an underwire. Many athletes prefer this type of bra, as do many larger-breasted women, regardless of their exercise habits.

NIPPLE INJURY

"Runners' nipples" is a condition in which the nipples are irritated, abraded, and/or lacerated[18-20] by the rubbing of clothing on the nipple during activity over a prolonged period of time. Any type of rough-surfaced cloth or seam can cause this problem. Male runners can wear Band-Aids over their nipples to prevent this from happening to them. Female runners can wear well-designed bras to protect their nipples. An abrasion of the nipple can lead to infection.

Exposure to cold can damage the nipples, too. A combination of moisture from perspiration with evaporation and wind chill can lower nipple temperature to injure the nipples and cause soreness and sensitivity to touch and temperature change. The use of windbreaking material over the chest area helps prevent this type of injury. There is no treatment for cold injury to nipples, except for supportive measures. Athletes should be cautioned to prevent such injury by avoiding cold exposure.[21,22]

TRAUMA

Blows to the breasts by field hockey sticks, pucks, elbows, kicks, and other objects certainly occur but seldom result in more than mild contusions. This superficial capillary damage may look significant but usually responds well to the simple application of cold for 10 to 20 minutes. Edema and ecchymosis gradually resolve within weeks.

A severe blow to the breast may cause a hematoma owing to subcutaneous bleeding from deeper vessels. Hemostasis usually is attained spontaneously, and most breast hematomas resolve spontaneously too. A breast hematoma should be evacuated only if accompanied by increasing pain, increasing size, or possible infection. If a fibrous nodule remains after resolution or evacuation of a hematoma, its removal may be necessary.

There is no evidence that trauma to the breast causes cancer.[23-25] However, breast injury usually leads to careful examination, and previously undetected masses are more likely to be appreciated as a result of more careful scrutiny.

BREAST AUGMENTATION AND REDUCTION

Cosmetic surgery involving either augmentation or reduction of the breast can cause special problems. Following breast augmentation, a swimmer was unable to swim at her previous freestyle speed despite regaining all her previous skills and strength and regaining her previous backstroke speed. Her larger breasts increased her resistance against the water. She was able to accept this loss of speed because she felt an increase in her breast size from 32A to 34B more than compensated psychologically. However, a more competitive swimmer probably would not have been content to sacrifice speed for the emotional benefit of a more personally satisfying appearance.[26] Dr. K. Barthels of California showed that simulated augmentation of the breasts slowed swimmers with specific heights and weights but did not slow others.[27]

Athletes in contact sports probably should not undergo breast augmentation. Blunt chest trauma can cause rupture of the prosthesis, with resultant hemorrhage and deformity of the breasts.[28]

There are no studies to show whether a reduction in breast size improves swim speed in large-breasted swimmers, but this possibility has been suggested.[27] Theoretically, breast reduction might improve the performance of large-breasted athletes, particularly those in nonaquatic endurance sports. Several top track coaches feel that large-breasted women do not perform as well as small-breasted women in running events. This impression remains anecdotal and unconfirmed and, if real, may relate to carrying less fat weight as well as having altered contours and resistance factors.

PREGNANCY AND LACTATION

Physiologic breast enlargement during pregnancy has not been shown to hinder athletic performance, which usually declines during pregnancy, particularly for sports requiring speed. It is impossible to isolate the effects of breast enlargement, abdominal enlargement, weight gain, altered center of gravity, and hormonal changes in determining causal relationships. A good supporting bra is certainly useful to the pregnant exerciser.[29]

Several studies of the effects of exercise upon lactation have shown no adverse effects. Wallace and Rabin[30] have reported transient increases in the concentration of lactic acid in breast milk following maximal exercise, but it is not known whether this alteration is of any significance. Lovelady, Lonnerdal, and Dewey[31] demonstrated no differences in milk composition between exercising and sedentary lactating women. The exercising women in this study tended to have greater milk energy and volume, but the differences were not statistically significant, possibly because of the small numbers of subjects studied (n = 8 in each group).

PREMENSTRUAL CHANGES AND FIBROCYSTIC BREASTS

Many female athletes experience breast discomfort premenstrually. This may be reduced by wearing a supportive bra and by taking bromocriptine or danazol orally, if indicated. Premenstrual mastalgia may also occur in women who have fibrocystic changes. About 50% of women have some clinical evidence of this process. No specific therapy has proved effective, although some investigators have advocated a reduction of methylxanthine consumption or administration of vitamin E or of danazol.[32-34] (See Chapter 13 for additional discussion.) A supportive bra is helpful for these women, too. In addition to wearing it during exercise, athletes with nocturnal discomfort may find it helpful to wear it while sleeping as well.

Any breast masses should be evaluated with mammography and probably also sonography. Diagnostic needle aspiration of breast cysts may be therapeutic. If a cyst resolves completely following aspiration, biopsy is not necessary. Persistence of a cyst following attempted needle aspiration requires excisional biopsy for diagnosis.

All athletes should practice monthly breast self-examination. This is best performed at the end of menses, when palpable physiologic changes from hormonal influence are minimal. The American Cancer Society, the American College of Radiology, the American Medical Association, the College of American Pathologists, and the National Cancer Institute have endorsed the following guidelines for screening mammography:

1 Onset or baseline mammography by age 40

2 Mammography every 1 to 2 years between ages 40 and 49

3 Annual mammography thereafter.[35]

EXERCISE FOLLOWING TRAUMA OR SURGERY

Appendix A discusses the appropriate return to exercise following various types of breast surgery, as well as trauma.

SUMMARY

Breast problems in the female athlete can at times be of serious import to the participant, but usually they fall more into the category of a nuisance to performance, when size and resultant discomfort are a factor. Trauma and tumors are responsible for the more disturbing conditions.

The use of good supporting bras for the large-breasted athlete is certainly indicated and can make athletic events more enjoyable for these individuals. Cosmetic surgery is best relegated to the postathletic phase of life.

REFERENCES

1. Haycock C: Supportive bras for jogging. Med Aspects Hum Sexuality. 14:6, 1980.
2. Haycock C: The female athlete and sportsmedicine in the 70's. J Florida M A 67:411, 1980.
3. Gillette J: When and where women are injured in sports. Phys Sportsmed 3(5):61, 1975.
4. Haycock C, and Gillette J: Susceptibility of women athletes to injury: Myths vs reality. JAMA 236:163, 1976.
5. Whiteside PA: Men's and women's injuries in comparable sports. Phys Sportsmed 8(3):130, 1980.
6. Eisenberg I, and Allen WC: Injuries in a women's varsity athletic program. Phys Sportsmed 6(3):112, 1978.
7. Zelisko JA, Noble B, and Porter M: A comparison of men's and women's professional basketball injuries. Am J Sports Med 10:297, 1982.
8. Haycock C: A need to know: Joggers' breast pain. Response. Phys Sportsmed 7(8):27, 1979.
9. Haycock C, Shierman G, and Gillette J: The female athlete—does her anatomy pose problems? Proceedings of the 19th Conference on the Medical Aspects of Sports, AMA, 1978.
10. Haycock CE: Breast support and protection in the female athlete. AAHPER Research Consortium Symposium Papers 1:50, 1978.
11. Report: Female athletes need good bras, MD reports. Phys Sportsmed 5(8):15, 1977.
12. Baynes JD: Pro+ Tec Protective Bra. J Sports Med Phys Fitness 8:34, 1968.
13. Hunter L: The bra controversy: Are sports bras a necessity? Phys Sportsmed 10(11):75, 1982.
14. Gehlsen G, and Albohm M: Evaluation of sports bras. Phys Sportsmed 8(10):89, 1980.
15. Schuster K: Equipment update: Jogging bras hit the streets. Phys Sportsmed 7(4):125, 1979.
16. Survey: Women marathoners describe bra needs. Phys Sportsmed 5(12):12, 1977.
17. Lorentzen D, and Lawson L: Selected sports bras: A biomechanical analysis of breast motion while jogging. Phys Sportsmed 15(5):128, 1987.
18. Levit F: Jogger's nipples. N Engl J Med 297:1127, 1977.
19. Cohen HJ: Jogger's petechiae. N Engl J Med 279:109, 1968.
20. Corrigan AB, and Fitch KD: Complications of jogging. Med J Aust 2:363, 1972.
21. Powell B: Bicyclist's nipples. JAMA 249:2457, 1983.
22. Adrian MJ: Proper clothing and equipment. In Haycock CE (ed): Sports Medicine for the Athletic Female. Medical Economics Book Div, Oradell, NJ, 1980, p 61.
23. Karon SE: Medical testimony in a trauma and breast cancer case, showing the direct and cross-examinations of the plaintiff's internist and the defendant pathologist. Med Trial Tech Q 13:361, 1967.
24. Stevens M: Traumatic breast cancer. Med Trial Tech Q 25:1, 1978.
25. Dziob JS: Trauma and breast cancer, or the anatomy of an insurance claim. RI Med J 63:37, 1980.
26. Levine NS, and Buchanan RT: Decreased swimming speed following augmentation mammoplasty. Plast Reconstr Surg 71:255, 1983.

27. Barthels KM: Discussion—decreased swimming speed following augmentation mammoplasty. Plast Reconstr Surg 71:257, 1983.

28. Dellon AL: Blunt chest trauma: Evaluation of the augmented breast. J Trauma 20:982, 1980.

29. Shangold M: Gynecological and endocrinological factors. In Haycock C (ed): Sports Medicine and the Athletic Female. Medical Economics Book, Oradell, NJ, 1980.

30. Wallace JP, and Rabin J: The concentration of lactic acid in breast milk following maximal exercise. Int J Sports Med 12:328, 1991.

31. Lovelady CA, Lonnerdal B, and Dewey KG: Lactation performance of exercising women. Am J Clin Nutr 52:103, 1990.

32. Minton JP, Abou-Isaa H, Reiches N, et al: Clinical and biochemical studies on methyl-xanthine related fibrocystic breast disease. Surgery 90:301, 1981.

33. Ernster VL, Mason L, Goodson WH, et al: Effects of caffeine-free diet on benign breast disease: A randomized trial. Surgery 91:263, 1982.

34. London RS, Sundaram GS, Schultz M, et al: Endocrine parameters and alpha-tocopherol therapy of patients with mammary dysplasia. Cancer Res 41:3811, 1981.

35. Mammography screening urged: Major medical groups agree on guidelines. ACR Bull 45:1, 1989.

CHAPTER 13

Gynecologic Concerns in Exercise and Training

MONA M. SHANGOLD, M.D.

CONTRACEPTION
Oral Contraceptives
Intrauterine Devices (IUDs)
Mechanical (Barrier) Methods
Norplant
Choosing a Contraceptive

DYSMENORRHEA

ENDOMETRIOSIS

PREMENSTRUAL SYNDROME

FERTILITY

STRESS URINARY INCONTINENCE

POSTOPERATIVE TRAINING AND
RECOVERY

EFFECT OF MENSTRUAL CYCLE
ON PERFORMANCE

Athletic women have many concerns about the effects of regular training upon various gynecologic conditions, the effects of various gynecologic conditions and their treatments upon exercise performance, and the effects of endogenous and exogenous hormones upon exercise and health parameters. Menstrual and hormonal changes associated with exercise and training are discussed comprehensively in Chapter 9. This chapter will address what is known about other gynecologic concerns of the athlete, including contraception, dysmenorrhea, premenstrual syndrome, fertility, stress urinary incontinence, and cyclic changes in exercise performance.

CONTRACEPTION

Although oral contraceptives have been reported to be the most popular form of contraception among American women,[1] two surveys have found that runners prefer diaphragm use.[2,3] In a survey of the 1841 women who entered the 1979 New York City Marathon, Shangold and Levine[2] reported that 37% of the 394 respondents were diaphragm users, while only 6% were oral contraceptive users. Jarrett and Spellacy[3] surveyed runners through a newspaper advertisement and found that 44% of the 70 respondents used diaphragms, while only 13% used oral contraceptives. Thus, based on these survey data, it seems that at the time of these studies runners preferred the diaphragm over any other form of contraception.

Oral Contraceptives

Many women are concerned about side effects and complications associated with oral contraceptive use, and such fears have undoubtedly limited the use of these agents. However, most of the reported and publicized side effects and complications were associated with higher-dose pills than are generally prescribed now. Studies have shown that the low-dose pills, each containing 30 to 35 μg of ethinyl estradiol, are much safer than the pills containing 50 or more μg of ethinyl estradiol, offering reductions in cardiovascular and thromboembolic risks. Many of the adverse effects of oral contraceptives on thrombosis, arterial disease, and lipid and carbohydrate metabolism are related to the progestin content of the pill.[4-8] As described in an excellent review article by Mishell,[9] despite the detrimental effects associated with steroid contraceptives, women who take these agents actually have a reduced incidence of heavy bleeding, irregular bleeding, endometrial cancer, several types of benign breast disease, ovarian carcinoma, rheumatoid arthritis, and salpingitis, compared with women who do not take oral contraceptives.

Low-dose oral contraceptive agents were first introduced in 1973 and have grown in availability since then. They are probably used more widely now than at the time of the surveys cited. Progestin-only pills were first marketed in 1973 and were intended for those women for whom estrogen is contraindicated; these pills have a high incidence of breakthrough bleeding, and their use is rarely indicated. Oral contraceptive agents containing less than 30 μg of estrogen also have a high incidence of breakthrough bleeding and are poorly tolerated by most women as a result. Biphasic preparations were first introduced in 1982 and were followed by the introduction of triphasic preparations in 1984. In these pills, the doses of progestin, and occasionally of estrogen, are different on different days. These newest agents have not been proved to offer consistent advantages over the standard (monophasic) pills containing 30 to 35 μg of estrogen and seem to lead to more breakthrough bleeding and confusion.

Because of the beneficial effects of endurance training upon some parameters affected adversely by oral contraceptives (e.g., coagulation, lipid metabolism, and carbohydrate metabolism), several investigators have studied the combined effects of exercise and oral contraceptives on these variables.

Oral contraceptives are associated with a number of changes in coagulation and fibrinolytic factors in both sedentary and trained women. Plasma plasminogen activator, which converts plasminogen to plasmin, is increased by oral contraceptive use and is further increased by exercise.[10] Huisveld and co-workers[11] reported that oral contraceptive users have increased total plasminogen and free plasminogen levels, increased factor XII and decreased C1-inactivator and increased factor XII–dependent fibrinolytic activity, higher activity levels of normal euglobulin fraction-fibrinolytic activity and extrinsic (tissue-type) plasminogen activator, and decreased urokinase-like fibrinolytic activator activity. Hedlin, Milojevic, and Korey[12] confirmed the increased fibrinolytic activity induced by exercise or oral contraceptive use or both, and they have also shown that exercise raises antithrombin III activity, whereas oral contraceptive use lowers it. In this study, the hemostatic change induced by oral contraceptives was offset by exercise. It is probable that exercise and training offset any net tendency toward increased coagulability induced by oral contraceptive use.

Powell and colleagues[13] demonstrated that several different oral contraceptive agents alter lipoprotein lipid levels adversely, raising total triglyceride, total cholesterol, and low-density lipoprotein (LDL) cholesterol significantly. However, the report by Gray, Harding, and Dale[14] showed that runners taking oral contraceptives have lipid profiles similar to those of runners taking no hormonal medication, suggesting that exercise may offset the adverse effects of oral contraceptive agents upon lipid levels.

In view of the many beneficial effects known about oral contraceptive use, it remains unclear why these agents are not chosen by more female athletes. It is likely that many avoid using them because of unfounded fears based on reported side effects of the higher-dose oral contraceptive agents (containing 50 μg or more of estrogen). However, the weight gain, bloating, depression, and mood changes associated with higher dosages are uncommon with pills containing less than 50 μg of estrogen. The two major side effects associated with use of the lower-dose agents are breakthrough bleeding (i.e., bleeding on the days of hormone ingestion) and amenorrhea (i.e., lack of withdrawal bleeding at the end of each hormone cycle). Each of these is a nuisance but not of serious consequence. Breakthrough bleeding may resolve spontaneously within three cycles; if it does not, it may resolve with additional hormone therapy, either transiently or permanently. Amenorrhea rarely resolves spontaneously but usually resolves with short-term or long-term ingestion of additional estrogen or less progestin.

Intrauterine Devices

Intrauterine contraceptive devices (IUDs) were associated with an increased prevalence of menorrhagia (heavy menstrual bleeding) and dysmenorrhea (painful menstruation), each of which could impair athletic performance. Only two IUDs currently are available in the United States: ParaGard, which contains copper, and Progestasert, which contains progesterone. Manufacture of all other IUDs that previously were available has been discontinued for economic reasons, primarily expensive litigation (mostly unwarranted). An IUD is an acceptable contraceptive choice for the athlete who is in a monogamous relationship and has never had a pelvic infection, provided that menorrhagia and/or dysmenorrhea do not ensue and impair the athletic performance.

Mechanical (Barrier) Methods

Mechanical methods of contraception are acceptable for all women who are motivated and reliable enough to use them. Diaphragms and condoms are more effective when used in combination with contraceptive foam or jelly. The sponge is no more effective than the diaphragm and has been reported to be associated with more local irritation and other side effects. The main disadvantages of mechanical (barrier) methods of contraception are their messiness, inconvenience, and disruption of sexual activity. Since athletes tend to be motivated and disciplined, these deterrents are usually considered minor. However, leakage of vaginal contraceptive jellies or foams during exercise may be uncomfortable. When added to vaginal secretions and semen, the volume of such discharge may be substantial and annoying during exercise. This problem may be remedied by placing a second, smaller diaphragm distal to the first, by inserting a vaginal tampon, or, preferably, by wearing a minipad.

Diaphragm use requires vaginal retention of the diaphragm for 6 to 8 hours following the last vaginal ejaculation. Some athletes may find it uncomfortable to exercise with a diaphragm in the vagina; such women may benefit from refitting with a slightly smaller diaphragm, which will provide equal contraceptive efficacy and greater comfort.

Norplant

Norplant is a subdermal implant system that recently has been approved for long-term contraception.[15] It is made up of six slender capsules containing levonorgestrel, which are implanted in the upper arm. The levonorgestrel in each capsule is released slowly, providing contraception for about 5 years. The primary mechanism of action is suppression of ovulation, and the major side effects are irregular bleeding and headaches. The major advantages of this subdermal implant are its long effectiveness, comfort, lack of requirement for attention, and safety for use in women for whom estrogen is contraindicated. Its major disadvantages are its expense, invasive insertion and removal, and frequency of associated irregular bleeding. Although no changes in carbohydrate metabolism, blood coagulation, or liver function have been reported, it is unknown whether Norplant contraception affects exercise performance or endurance.

Choosing a Contraceptive

The choice of an optimal contraceptive agent for any athlete rarely should be affected by exercise habits but should include consideration of medical history and life-

Table 13–1. FIRST-YEAR FAILURE RATES OF BIRTH CONTROL METHODS

	Lowest Reported*	Typical†
Female sterilization	0.0	0.4
Male sterilization	0.0	0.15
Implant (Norplant)	0.0	0.04
Injectable progestogen (Depo-Provera)	0.0	0.3
Birth control pill	0.0–1.1	3
IUD	0.5–1.9	3
Condom	4.2	12
Diaphragm	2.1	18
Sponge	14–28	18–28
Cap	8	18
Withdrawal	6.7	18
Periodic abstinence	2–14	20
Spermicides	0.0	21
Chance	43	85

*In the literature on contraceptive failure, the *lowest reported* percentage who experienced an accidental pregnancy during the first year following initiation of use (not necessarily for the first time) if they did not stop use for any other reason.

†Among *typical* couples who initiated use of a method (not necessarily for the first time), the percentage who experienced an accidental pregnancy during the first year if they do not stop use for any other reason.

Source: Modified from Hatcher et al,[16] with permission.

style. Women who have coitus once weekly or less frequently probably should use barrier methods of contraception, unless there is an additional reason to use oral contraceptives (e.g., hormone deficiency or treatment of acne or hirsutism). It is reasonable for women who have coitus twice weekly or more frequently to use oral contraceptives, unless there is some contraindication to their use (see Tables 9–5 and 9–6). Oral contraceptives have not been shown to alter athletic performance.

Failure rates for various contraceptive methods are listed in Table 13–1.[16]

DYSMENORRHEA

Dysmenorrhea is caused by myometrial ischemia during myometrial contractions induced by prostaglandin $F_{2\alpha}$, which is produced by the endometrium. Synthesis of this chemical can be prevented by any of several prostaglandin synthetase inhibitors (Table 13–2).

Although many women have noticed less dysmenorrhea during exercise or training or both, most of these observations remain anecdotal and unsupported by well-controlled scientific studies. The nature of studies involving exercise as the independent

Table 13–2. PROSTAGLANDIN INHIBITORS

Generic Name	Brand Name	Recommended Dose
Aspirin		650 mg every 4 h
Naproxen	Naprosyn	500 mg, then 250 mg every 6–8 h
Naproxen sodium	Anaprox, Anaprox-DS	550 mg, then 275 mg every 6–8 h or 550 mg every 12 h
Ibuprofen	Motrin, Advil, Nuprin	400 mg every 4–6 h
Mefenamic acid	Ponstel	500 mg, then 250 mg every 6 h
Ketaprofen	Orudis	25–50 mg every 6–8 h

variable and perception of pain as the dependent variable makes double-blinding impossible. Theories proposed to explain the apparent reduction of pain by exercise and training include an exercise-induced increase in pain-preventing endorphins, an exercise-induced increase in vasodilating prostaglandins, and exercise-induced vasodilatation. The truth remains to be elucidated.

Athletes who experience dysmenorrhea should be treated with prostaglandin inhibitors. Exercise-induced relief from dysmenorrhea should not be expected, since responses are variable and unpredictable. Prostaglandin inhibitors often cause reduced menstrual blood loss as an additional benefit, due to the vasoconstriction caused by the inhibition of vasodilating prostaglandins.

ENDOMETRIOSIS

Endometriosis is a condition in which functioning endometrial tissue exists outside the endometrial cavity. Its most common symptoms are pain and infertility, although it may produce no symptoms. In a multicenter study, Cramer and associates[17] reported that women who had exercised regularly since age 25 or younger and for more than 2 hours weekly had a decreased risk of developing endometriosis. Conditioning exercises such as jogging seemed most associated with this decreased risk.

Women who have endometriosis may be treated medically or surgically. Surgical treatment depends on the severity of disease and may include fulguration of endometriotic implants, resection of endometriotic tissue or cysts, or hysterectomy with bilateral salpingo-oophorectomy.

Medical treatment is most effective with a gonadotropin-releasing hormone (GnRH) analog or danazol. Several synthetic GnRH analogs are available today, including leuprolide acetate (Lupron), which is administered by daily or monthly injections, and nafarelin acetate (Synarel), which is admin-

istered by nasal spray. These agents usually lead to significant pain relief. Major side effects include hot flushes, decreased libido, vaginal dryness, headaches, emotional lability, acne, myalgia, and reduced breast size. Synarel side effects also include nasal irritation. Because these drugs produce a pseudomenopausal state with low estrogen levels, their most serious side effect is bone loss. Treatment with GnRH analogs may be continued for a maximum of 6 months, during which time significant bone loss is unlikely.

Danazol is a derivative of testosterone, and it has expected androgenic and anabolic properties. Within 6 months of danazol therapy, women have a significant loss of adipose tissue and a significant increase in lean body mass.[18] These changes persist longer than 6 months after discontinuing therapy.[18] Other major side effects include hot flushes, headaches, emotional lability, acne, reduced breast size, edema, seborrhea, and weight gain. Danazol does not lead to bone loss. Although the changes in body composition during danazol use are desirable for an athlete, muscle cramps may potentially impair athletic training. Anecdotally, athletes treated with danazol for endometriosis have noticed improved performance, but this has not been investigated scientifically. Drug testing would detect danazol use.

Although reduced distal radial bone mass has been reported in untreated women with endometriosis,[19] the bone mineral density of the lumbar spine has been found to be normal in a population-based cross-sectional study of untreated women with endometriosis.[20]

PREMENSTRUAL SYNDROME

Premenstrual syndrome (PMS) is a condition in which women experience emotional and/or physical symptoms during the 3 to 5 days prior to the onset of menstruation. In some cases, it may last even longer. Symptoms may include anxiety, depression, mood swings, increased appetite, headaches, mastalgia, and edema and may vary in severity as well as in duration. The multitude and variability of symptoms in this syndrome have made it difficult to define this entity precisely, and this problem has led Magos and Studd[21] to propose the following working definition for investigators and clinicians: "distressing physical, psychological, and behavioral symptoms, not caused by organic disease, which regularly recur during the same phase of the menstrual/ovarian cycle, and which disappear or significantly regress during the remainder of the cycle."

Although the cause of PMS remains to be elucidated, it is probably related to hormone levels and/or changes at that time of the menstrual cycle. No laboratory tests can diagnose this condition, since no laboratory measurements have been shown to correlate with symptomatology during any given cycle or to vary between affected and unaffected individuals. The diagnosis of PMS is a historic one, made solely by reviewing a calendar record of when symptoms and menstruation occur. Those women whose symptoms occur solely premenstrually have PMS, and those whose symptoms occur randomly throughout the cycle do not. This seemingly clear picture is confused somewhat by the fact that some women who have symptoms throughout the cycle note a premenstrual exacerbation of symptomatology.

It has been reported that women who exercise are less likely to experience PMS and that women are less likely to experience PMS when exercising regularly. Prior, Vigna, and Alojado[22] have shown that conditioning exercise decreases premenstrual symptoms. However, it is difficult to design controlled studies in which women are blinded to the fact that they are exercising. Thus, it remains difficult to isolate exercise as a variable and difficult to confirm that exercise prevents or relieves PMS symptoms. It is probable that the mood elevation and general feeling of well-being associated with exercise may play a role.

Optimal treatment of PMS remains to be determined. Although several drugs relieve symptoms, only a few of these have been shown to be more effective than placebo. The high placebo response in this entity makes it difficult to evaluate the effectiveness of all treatments. Spironolactone has been shown to be more effective than placebo[23] and is associated with very few side effects. Although pharmacologic doses of progesterone are prescribed by many clinicians to treat PMS, there is no evidence that PMS is caused by a progesterone deficiency or that progesterone therapy in physiologic doses is more effective than placebo in treating it. Luteal phase deficiency is not associated with a more severe PMS than a normal luteal phase.[24] Progesterone in pharmacologic doses has been shown in only one study to be more effective than placebo;[25] other studies have found this agent to be no more effective than placebo.[26,27]

A few studies showed bromocriptine to be more effective than placebo in relieving some PMS symptoms, particularly mastodynia[28]; but other studies have failed to confirm this.[28] Danazol has been reported to relieve PMS symptoms,[29,30] but this has been tested in only one double-blind, controlled study to date.[30] (The side effects associated with danazol are listed in the preceding section.) A GnRH agonist (Lupron) has been shown to relieve PMS symptoms while inducing amenorrhea.[31] Since this drug and other analogs and antagonists of GnRH promote bone loss as a result of the hypoestrogenic state they induce,[32] these agents alone may not be promising for long-term use in this condition. Alprazolam has also been shown to be more effective than placebo in relieving the severity of several symptoms of PMS; its reported low incidence of side effects may make it a good choice for many women unresponsive to other therapies.[33] It remains to be shown whether any of these medications will affect athletic performance.

Despite claims to the contrary, there is no evidence that PMS is caused by any dietary deficiency or excess, or that dietary manipulation will consistently relieve symptoms. However, salt restriction may alleviate symptoms in some PMS sufferers and certainly will harm no one. Furthermore, Wurtman and co-workers[34] have shown improvement in mood when PMS sufferers consumed a high carbohydrate diet.

At the present time, athletes who are inconvenienced by significant PMS symptoms probably should be treated with spironolactone (25 to 100 mg daily). It may be reassuring for some of them to know that 75% of all women experience at least some premenstrual symptoms, probably due to hormonal changes that reflect normal reproductive function (i.e., regular ovulation). Studies now in progress may help us to understand the etiology of PMS and lead us to optimal therapy.

FERTILITY

No studies to date have shown that infertility is more prevalent among athletes than among the general population. It is true that luteal phase deficiency, oligomenorrhea, and amenorrhea are more prevalent among athletes, and infertility is more prevalent among women who have these conditions. However, the definition of infertility includes a desire for pregnancy. Since many athletes are not actively seeking pregnancies at the time of intensive training, when they are most likely to experience menstrual dysfunction, these women technically are not infertile, even though their fertility, if tested, might be impaired. Many of these women resume having regular ovulatory menses when they decrease intensive training. It is probable that transient infertility is associated with intensive training, but this has not been documented to date.[2]

Even if temporary infertility is associated with training, athletes who do not desire pregnancy should not presume that conception is impossible. As discussed in Chapter 9, reliable contraception should be used by even amenorrheic athletes who do not want a pregnancy. Many anecdotal reports of amenorrheic athletes with unsuspected and unwanted pregnancies support this recommendation. Hypothalamic-pituitary-ovarian dysfunction can resolve spontaneously, and ovulation can occur prior to the first subsequent menstrual period. The cause of the amenorrhea in such cases changes from hypothalamic-pituitary-ovarian dysfunction to pregnancy, but the symptom of amenorrhea continues. Thus, the amenorrheic athlete may not detect an unplanned, unwanted pregnancy until it is advanced enough to produce a significant increase in abdominal girth.

Infertile athletes and their partners should undergo the same comprehensive evaluation that would be recommended for any infertile couple. Rarely should treatment be modified because of exercise or training.

STRESS URINARY INCONTINENCE

Many women experience stress urinary incontinence during exercise.[35] Involuntary urine leakage results when intravesical pressure is higher than intraurethral pressure.

Although stress incontinence is most likely to occur in women who have an anatomic defect in the posterior urethrovesical angle, even women with normal anatomy can experience stress urinary incontinence when intravesical pressure increases enough. Physical activity involving a Valsalva maneuver increases intra-abdominal pressure. Because changes in intra-abdominal pressure are not always transmitted equally to both bladder and urethra, physical activities like running and jumping may raise intravesical pressure above intraurethral pressure, leading to urine leakage during exercise.[36] Although stress urinary incontinence is more common during exercise than during rest, exercise-induced increases in intra-abdominal pressure are transient and do not produce chronic pressure alterations or anatomic abnormalities.

Genital prolapse includes several anatomic abnormalities marked by loss of support, including cystocele, urethrocele, rectocele, and uterine descent. These anatomic defects have been reported to be associated with prior trauma during vaginal delivery and with endogenous joint hypermobility.[37] Such joint laxity may also predispose women to joint injury.

Many women who have stress urinary incontinence may be able to control leakage by avoiding fluid ingestion for 3 hours prior to exercising and emptying their bladders immediately prior to exercising. However, they must be careful to avoid dehydration during prolonged exercise sessions lasting more than 1 hour. Such women should replace fluid loss immediately after cessation of exercise.

Many women who experience involuntary urine leakage may benefit from practicing Kegel exercises. These are done by contracting the pubococcygeus muscle at any time, or specifically during urination, thereby stopping the urinary stream. Women who lose urine during exercise may decrease their discomfort and embarrassment by wearing a minipad. No medication will alleviate this condition. Those who have anatomic defects and who cannot relieve their symptoms to a satisfactory degree by practicing Kegel exercises or wearing a minipad should consider surgical correction of the anatomic defect. Postoperatively, such women may be at increased risk of recurrence due to the pressure changes during exercise and to persistence of the endogenous tissue factors that caused the original problem. No studies are available to confirm or disprove this suspicion, but these women probably should be cautious when exercising postoperatively.

POSTOPERATIVE TRAINING AND RECOVERY

The traditional recovery period following abdominal or other major surgery has been 6 to 10 weeks. Recommendations for recovery should be site- and sport-specific. However, athletes should aim to recover cardiovascular fitness as soon as possible, while avoiding excessive stress on the surgical site. As a general rule, postoperative avoidance of pain will lead to avoidance of injury or damage. Those who have greater strength in muscles far from the operative site can gain mobility early by using those muscles rather than the muscles near the operative site.

A surgical wound begins to heal immediately following closure. By the 21st postoperative day, the wound has gained nearly as much strength as it will ultimately have (although it will never be as strong as it was preoperatively). Based on the fact that it takes 21 days for a surgical wound to regain nearly all of its ultimate strength, it is probably reasonable for athletes to postpone submaximal resistance training that involves the operative site for 21 days following a surgical procedure. Lighter work can probably be done safely prior to this time, particularly if the wound is not stressed. Avoidance of pain remains a reasonable goal for the exercising patient postoperatively, and exercises that do not cause pain are probably safe. Overzealous athletes should be cautioned to use moderation in training postoperatively and to notice subtle body perceptions of discomfort and fatigue.

Although there are no studies to indicate when exercise can be safely resumed following surgery, I propose the following guidelines for earliest safe resumption of exercise:

- Following a dilatation and curettage or a first-trimester abortion, weighttraining and aerobic exercise, except water sports, may be resumed the same or the next day; water sports should be avoided until bleeding has ceased. Tampon use also should be avoided until bleeding has ceased.
- Following a vaginal delivery or a second-trimester abortion, weighttraining may be resumed the same day; aerobic exercise, except water sports, may be resumed in 2

days; water sports may be resumed when bleeding has ceased. Tampon use should be avoided until bleeding has ceased.

- Following a diagnostic laparoscopy, aerobic exercise in and out of water and weighttraining may be resumed after 1 to 2 days. Following operative laparoscopy, aerobic exercise in and out of water and weighttraining should be postponed at least 21 days, depending upon the complexity of the procedure. Avoidance of pain may not provide sufficient limitation of activity for safety.
- Following a cesarean delivery or other abdominal surgery (requiring an incision), light aerobic exercise outside of water and light weighttraining may be resumed in 7 days; intense aerobic exercise (speed work), submaximal weighttraining, and water sports should be postponed at least 21 days.

It must be emphasized that these are the *earliest* times I recommend resuming exercise postoperatively. Delays may enhance healing despite potential hindrance of training. Exercise should never be resumed if it causes pain. All situations should be individualized, and each patient should follow the advice of her surgeon.

EFFECT OF MENSTRUAL CYCLE ON PERFORMANCE

Many investigators have studied the effect of the menstrual cycle on performance, including specific measurements of strength, speed, endurance, fatigability, and perceived exertion and cognitive, perceptual, and motor skills at different phases of the menstrual cycle, reflecting different levels and ratios of estrogen and progesterone. For a thorough review of these reports, the reader is referred elsewhere.[38] The findings of these studies have been inconsistent but suggest that menstrual cycle phase does not have a significant effect on any of these parameters. Very few such studies have been published in peer-reviewed journals, but a recent well-designed study by DeSouza and colleagues[39] concluded that neither menstrual phase (follicular versus luteal) nor menstrual status (eumenorrheic versus amenorrheic) alters or limits exercise performance in female athletes.

It is rarely advisable or necessary to manipulate an athlete's menstrual cycle to enhance her performance. However, some women *do* perform better during the follicular phase than at other times, and others perceive or believe that they do. If such women are elite athletes, it may be appropriate to manipulate the menstrual cycle for special events of great importance; I believe that such manipulation should be reserved for world-class athletes (e.g., Olympic competition).

The simplest and least invasive method of manipulating an athlete's menstrual cycle involves administering low-dose oral contraceptives for several months prior to the competitive event, continuing the hormone-containing pills until 10 days before the competitive event. The athlete can expect to have withdrawal bleeding within 3 days after cessation of the pills. She should postpone restarting the pills (if she plans to do so) until the competitive event has passed. This plan will give her a predictable bleeding pattern during training and will leave her with low levels of both estrogen and progesterone at the time of the important event. For world-class athletes in their prime, this regimen can be repeated every few months for the events of great importance. It also provides hormonal protection to those athletes who are deficient in one or both hormones (estrogen and progesterone) during training, and it provides contraception to all athletes, regardless of menstrual status.

The only undesirable side effects associated with this plan are the potential risks of breakthrough bleeding during training and of impaired training during oral contraceptive use, in certain individuals. However, I believe these risks are small and are outweighed by the benefits of this plan.

An alternative method of management involves administering only a progestogen (e.g., medroxyprogesterone acetate 5 mg) for 5 to 10 days, ending 10 days prior to the important event. This is most likely to be effective in women with chronic anovulation, and it may produce undesirable bloating and a sensation of "heaviness," which may impair training. This method provides no contraception. As I have indicated, I prefer to prescribe low-dose oral contraceptives to athletes in need of menstrual manipulation.

SUMMARY

The choice of an optimal contraceptive agent should be made on the basis of a patient's lifestyle and medical history but is rarely affected by the fact that a patient is an athlete. Oral contraceptives have not been shown to alter athletic performance.

Athletes who experience dysmenorrhea should be treated with prostaglandin inhibitors, which often reduce menstrual blood loss as an additional benefit.

Women who have endometriosis may be treated medically or surgically. Some of these treatment modalities may affect athletic performance.

Premenstrual syndrome, if severe, may disrupt athletic training. Exercisers are less likely than sedentary women to experience PMS, optimal treatment for which remains to be determined.

Infertile athletes and their partners should undergo a thorough evaluation. Treatment rarely should be modified because of exercise or training.

Although stress urinary incontinence is more common during exercise than during rest, exercise-induced increases in intra-abdominal pressure are transient and do not produce chronic alterations in pressure or anatomy.

Recommendations for postoperative recovery following abdominal or pelvic surgery should be site-specific and sport-specific. Exercise should never be resumed if it causes pain. All situations should be individualized and should follow the advice of the patient's surgeon.

It is rarely advisable or necessary to manipulate an athlete's menstrual cycle to enhance her performance. If manipulation is considered, it should be reserved for special events of great importance to elite athletes.

REFERENCES

1. Forrest JD, Fordyce RR: U.S. women's contraceptive attitudes and practice: How have they changed in the 1980s? Fam Plan Perspect 20(3):112, 1988.
2. Shangold MM, and Levine HS: The effect of marathon training upon menstrual function. Am J Obstet Gynecol 143:862, 1982.
3. Jarrett JC, and Spellacy WN: Contraceptive practices of female runners. Fertil Steril 39:374, 1983.
4. Plunkett ER: Contraceptive steroids, age, and the cardiovascular system. Am J Obstet Gynecol 142:747, 1982.
5. Mann JI: Progestogens in cardiovascular disease: An introduction to the epidemiologic data. Am J Obstet Gynecol 142:752, 1982.
6. Kay CR: Progestogens and arterial disease—Evidence from the Royal College of General Practitioners' study. Am J Obstet Gynecol 142:762, 1982.
7. Wynn V, and Niththyananthan R: The effect of progestins in combined oral contraceptives on serum lipids with special reference to high-density lipoproteins. Am J Obstet Gynecol 142:766, 1982.
8. Spellacy WN: Carbohydrate metabolism during treatment with estrogen, progestogen, and low-dose oral contraceptives. Am J Obstet Gynecol 142:732, 1982.
9. Mishell DR: Noncontraceptive health benefits of oral steroidal contraceptives. Am J Obstet Gynecol 142:809, 1982.
10. Hedlin AM, Milojevic S, and Korey A: Plasminogen activator levels in plasma and urine during exercise and oral contraceptive use. Thromb Haemost 39:743, 1978.
11. Huisveld IA, Kluft C, Hospers AJH, et al: Effect of exercise and oral contraceptive agents on fibrinolytic potential in trained females. J Appl Physiol 56:906, 1984.
12. Hedlin AM, Milojevic S, and Korey A: Hemostatic changes induced by exercise during oral contraceptive use. Can J Physiol Pharmacol 56:316, 1978.

13. Powell MG, Hedlin AM, Cerskus I, et al: Effects of oral contraceptives on lipoprotein lipids: A prospective study. Obstet Gynecol 63:764, 1984.

14. Gray DP, Harding E, and Dale E: Effects of oral contraceptives on serum lipid profiles of women runners. Fertil Steril 39:510, 1983.

15. Shoupe D, and Mishell DR: Norplant: Subdermal implant system for long-term contraception. Am J Obstet Gynecol 160:1286, 1989.

16. Hatcher RA, Stewart F, Trussell J, et al: Contraceptive Technology 1990–1992, 15th rev ed. Irvington, New York, 1990, p 134.

17. Cramer DW, Wilson E, Stillman RJ, et al: The relation of endometriosis to menstrual characteristics, smoking, and exercise. JAMA 255:1904, 1986.

18. Bruce R, Lees B, Whitcroft SIJ, et al: Changes in body composition with danazol therapy. Fertil Steril 56:574, 1991.

19. Comite F, Delman M, Hutchinson-Williams K, et al: Reduced bone mass in reproductive-aged women with endometriosis. J Clin Endocrinol Metab 69:837, 1989.

20. Lane N, Baptista J, and Orwoll E: Bone mineral density of the lumbar spine in women with endometriosis. Fertil Steril 55:537, 1991.

21. Magos AL, and Studd JWW: The premenstrual syndrome. In Studd JWW (ed): Progress in Obstetrics and Gynaecology, Vol 4. Churchill Livingstone, Edinburgh, 1984, p 334.

22. Prior JC, Vigna Y, and Alojado N: Conditioning exercise decreases premenstrual symptoms—A prospective controlled three month trial. Eur J Appl Physiol 55:349, 1986.

23. O'Brien PMS, Craven D, Selby C, et al: Treatment of premenstrual syndrome with spironolactone. Br J Obstet Gynecol 86:142, 1979.

24. Ying Y-K, Soto-Albors CE, Randolph JF, et al: Luteal phase defect and premenstrual syndrome in an infertile population. Obstet Gynecol 69:96, 1987.

25. Dennerstein L, Spencer-Gardner C, Gotts G, et al: Progesterone and the premenstrual syndrome: A double-blind crossover trial. Br Med J 290:1617, 1985.

26. Sampson GA: Premenstrual syndrome: A double-blind controlled trial of progesterone and placebo. Br J Psychiatr 135:209, 1979.

27. Freeman E, Rickels K, Sondheimer SJ, and Polansky M: Ineffectiveness of progesterone suppository treatment for premenstrual syndrome. JAMA 264:349, 1990.

28. Andersch B: Bromocriptine and premenstrual symptoms: A survey of double blind trials. Obstet Gynecol Surv 38:643, 1983.

29. Day J: Danazol and the premenstrual syndrome. Postgrad Med J 55(Suppl 5):87, 1979.

30. Sarno AP, Miller EJ, and Lundblad EG: Premenstrual syndrome: Beneficial effects of periodic, low-dose danazol. Obstet Gynecol 70:33, 1987.

31. Muse KN, Cetel NS, Futterman LA, et al: The premenstrual syndrome: Effects of "medical ovariectomy." N Engl J Med 311:1345, 1984.

32. Abbasi R, and Hodgen GD: Predicting the predisposition to osteoporosis: Gonadotropin-releasing hormone antagonist for acute estrogen deficiency test. JAMA 255:1600, 1986.

33. Smith S, Rinehart JS, Ruddock VE, et al: Treatment of premenstrual syndrome with alprazolam: Results of a double-blind crossover clinical trial. Obstet Gynecol 70:37, 1987.

34. Wurtman JJ, Brzezinski A, Wurtman RJ, and Laferrere B: Effect of nutrient intake on premenstrual depression. Am J Obstet Gynecol 161:1228, 1989.

35. Nygaard I, DeLancey JOL, Arnsdorf L, and Murphy E: Exercise and incontinence. Obstet Gynecol 75:848, 1990.

36. James ED: The behavior of the bladder during physical activity. Br J Urol 50:387, 1978.

37. Al-Rawi ZS, and Al-Rawi ZT: Joint hypermobility in women with genital prolapse. Lancet 1:1439, 1982.

38. Brooks-Gunn J, Gargiulo J, and Warren MP: The menstrual cycle and athletic performance. In Puhl JL, and Brown CH (eds): The Menstrual Cycle and Physical Activity. Human Kinetics, Champaign, IL, 1986, p 13.

39. DeSouza MJ, Maguire MS, Rubin KR, and Maresh CM: Effects of menstrual phase and amenorrhea on exercise performance in runners. Med Sci Sports Exerc 22:575, 1990.

CHAPTER 14

Orthopedic Concerns

LETHA Y. GRIFFIN, M.D., Ph.D.

With the growth of women's athletics, many observers predicted an increase in the number and types of injuries occurring as women became more aggressive and competitive in sports.[1] Early injury studies of female athletes actually reported that a greater number of injuries were sustained by female than by male athletes.[2,3] However, this reflected a lack of adequate conditioning in women rather than any true physiologic weakness and predisposition to injury. As women became more serious in their sport participation, training and conditioning techniques improved, and injury rates decreased.[4] Recent studies surveying injury rates in conditioned female athletes demonstrate that their injury rates are no higher than those of their male counterparts.[5-7]

A review of injuries in professional and recreational athletes demonstrated sprains and strains to be the most common injuries and the knee and ankle to be the most frequently traumatized areas in both men and women.[8] Injuries are more sport-specific than sex-specific; that is, injury types and rates are similar for men and women in the same sport, but they differ for female athletes participating in different sports.[9]

Certain conditions, however, occur more commonly in women—in some cases owing to anatomic differences, in others owing to greater participation in specific sports. We have elected to focus in this chapter on those conditions more commonly seen in women (patella pain, impingement syndromes, Achilles tendinitis, shin splints, stress fractures, low back pain, bunions, and Morton's neuroma), and refer the reader to other more general texts on athletic injuries for a discussion of such injuries as sprains, dislocations, fractures, and inflammation of muscle origins. Table 14-1 briefly lists some common musculoskeletal injuries and the women's sports in which they are commonly seen.

PATELLA PAIN

Anatomy of the Patella

The patella or kneecap is a sesamoid bone, which means it is completely surrounded by fascial extensions (retinaculum) of the four components of the quadriceps muscle—the vastus medialis, the vastus lateralis, the rectus femoris, and the vastus intermedius (Fig. 14-1). Fascial terminations of these muscles arise just superior to the patella, extend over it, and continue inferiorly from the patella to the tibial tubercle as the patella tendon. The patella lies in the distal femoral groove formed where the medial and lateral femoral condyles join at the knee. The patella is guided in the femoral groove during knee flexion and extension by the powerful group of quadriceps muscles. Since the quadriceps muscle courses along the long axis of the femur while the patella tendon inserts into the tibial tubercle, patella tracking in the femoral groove is also very much influenced by the tibial-femoral angle. This angle (the Q angle) is measured by drawing a line through the center of the quadriceps muscle and noting its intersection with a line drawn through the center of the tibial tuberosity (Fig. 14-2). Because the gynecoid pelvis of the woman is wider than the narrow android pelvis of the man, this angle is generally greater in women than in men and may explain the increase in patella tracking problems and patella pain in women (Fig. 14-3). In fact, patella pain is one of the most common complaints of female athletes.

Although the anterior surface of the patella is flat, the posterior surface is composed of two facets which intersect longitudinally (Fig. 14-4). The medial facet is generally smaller than the lateral. The facets are lined with hyaline cartilage and articulate with the hyaline cartilage–covered su-

Table 14-1. SPECIFIC SPORTS COMMONLY ASSOCIATED WITH ORTHOPEDIC INJURIES

Injury	Sport
Shoulder subluxation	Swimming
	Throwing sports
Sprains	
Thumb	Skiing
Ankle	Running sports
	Uneven ground (field hockey, soccer, softball, cross-country)
	Basketball, volleyball (one-foot landings)
	Ice skating
Knee	Basketball, volleyball
Tendinitis	
First dorsal compartment	Gymnastics (squeezing poles or bars)
Achilles tendon	Track, basketball, skiing, ice skating, rollerskating
Biceps	Tennis, other racquet sports, throwing sports
Lateral epicondylitis (tennis elbow)	Tennis, other racquet sports, throwing sports
Shin splints	Running
Impingements	
Shoulder	Swimming,* throwing sports, racquet sports
Ankle	Gymnastics, ballet, diving, ice skating
Wrist	Gymnastics, crew, racquet sports
Low back pain	Gymnastics, diving, skating
Stress fractures (pars intra-articularis)	Running, gymnastics, ice skating, diving

*In greater numbers than male counterparts.

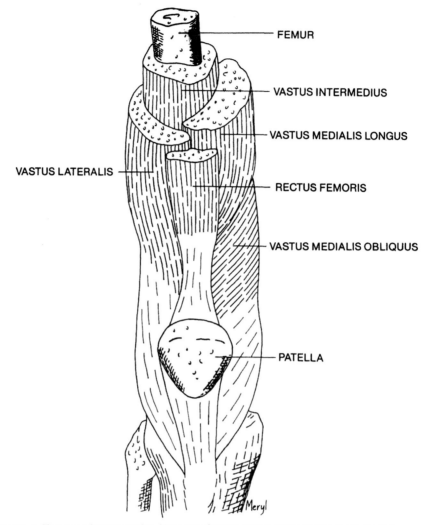

Figure 14–1. The quadriceps muscles. Note the oblique course of the vastus medialis obliquus muscle. (From Scott WN, Nisonson B, Nicholas JA, et al: Principles of Sports Medicine. Williams & Wilkins, Baltimore, 1984, p 274, with permission.)

perior extensions of the femoral condyle, forming the patellofemoral joint (Fig. 14–5).

Sources of Pain

Forces across the joint have been the subject of much investigation, since patellofemoral pain is a common source of discomfort in many activities, especially in sports that require multiple flexion-extension maneuvers (running, kicking, climbing). Forces across the joint change with increasing flexion of the knee (Fig. 14–6), and as previously discussed, are greatly influenced by the quadriceps pull and the tibial-femoral angle.

Patella tracking in the patellofemoral groove may also be influenced by foot strike. Pronation of the foot increases the knee valgus angle and may lead to an increase or at least an alteration in lateral patellofemoral forces (Fig. 14–7). If the patella does not track anatomically in the femoral groove,

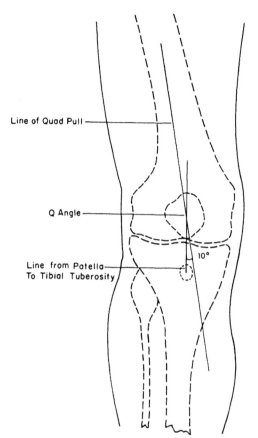

Figure 14–2. The Q angle is an angle formed by the intersection of a line drawn longitudinally through the middle of the quadriceps and a line drawn from the middle of the patella to the center of the tibial tuberosity. (From O'Donoghue DH: Treatment of Injuries to Athletes, ed 4. WB Saunders, Philadelphia, 1984, p 510, with permission.)

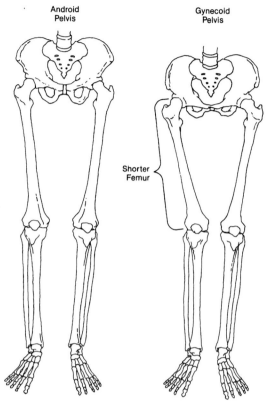

Figure 14–3. Android pelvis and gynecoid pelvis. Note that the female (gynecoid) pelvis is wider, with a greater varus angle of the femoral neck, resulting in a greater valgus angle at the knee when compared with the typical male (android) pelvis.

forces created during quadriceps contraction may not be adequately dissipated between the two facets, causing abnormally high forces on a small area of the articular surfaces and resulting in patella pain (patellofemoral stress syndrome).

Athletes who have sustained multiple subluxations or dislocations of their patellae may have pain secondary to traumatic loss of the hyaline cartilage during such episodes, that is, chondromalacia. If the cartilage is thinned or absent or chemically unable to absorb the forces applied to it, these forces are transferred to the bone beneath, resulting in pain.

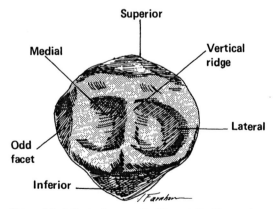

Figure 14–4. Posterior aspect of the patella, illustrating the two patellar facets. (From Norkin CC and Levangie PK: Joint Structure and Function, ed 2. FA Davis, Philadelphia, 1992, p 367, with permission.)

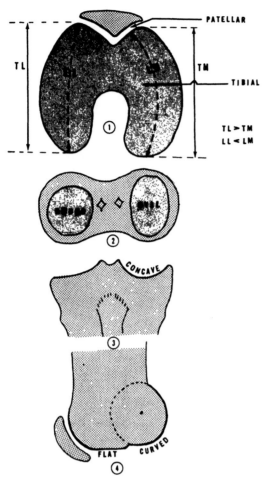

Figure 14–5. Patellofemoral joint. (*1*) Femoral condyle surfaces of the right knee. TL = anteroposterior length of the lateral condyle; TM = length of the medial condyle. The length of the medial condyle (LM) is greater than the length of the lateral condyle (LL), because of its curved surface. (*2*) Superior surface of the right tibia. The lateral articular surface is round and the medial articular surface is oval. (*3*) The medial tibial articular surface is deeper and more concave than is the lateral. (*4*) Side view of the femur showing the flat anterior surface and the curved posterior surface. The two articulations are illustrated in part 1: the patellar surface, in which the patella articulates with the anterior femur and the tibial surface, which then glides upon the tibia. (From Cailliet R: Knee Pain and Disability, ed 3. FA Davis, Philadelphia, 1992, p 2, with permission.)

Evaluating Patella Pain

In evaluating the athlete who complains of a painful knee, one must always consider the patella as a potential source of the pain. The athlete who sustains a traumatic patella dis-

location with spontaneous relocation may not report that her "kneecap jumped out of joint" but may perceive only severe knee pain following her twisting injury. Similarly, an athlete who complains of give-way or locking of her joint may not have a mechanical locking of her knee from a torn meniscus or loose body but may have pseudolocking or give-way on the basis of patella pain.

Observation

The first step in evaluating the patella is to observe the knee: does the patella sit higher in the femoral groove than usual (patella alta), or is it lower (patella baja)? Athletes whose patellas sit higher in the femoral groove have a greater tendency to patella subluxation,[10] whereas those with low-lying patellas may have increased forces across the patellofemoral joint, especially with repetitive flexion-extension activities.

Does the patella lie centrally in the femoral groove, or is it tipped laterally (Fig. 14–8)? Since an increased Q angle and poorly developed vastus medialis are associated with an increased incidence of patella pain, the Q angle should be measured, and the quadriceps mechanism assessed, especially its more medial oblique fibers, known as the vastus medialis obliquus.

Palpation and Manipulation

The retinaculum around the patella's medial, lateral, and superior borders should be palpated to check for tenderness. The athlete who has just sustained an acute patella subluxation or dislocation with spontaneous relocation will have a great deal of tenderness at the insertion of the vastus medialis on the medial border of the patella. In addition, she may have ecchymoses along the fibers of the muscles, from having stretched or disrupted part of the fibers at the time of the subluxation or dislocation.

Next, the patella should be tipped medially, and the examiner should feel under the medial facet (Fig. 14–9). Athletes with patellofemoral stress syndrome or chondroma-

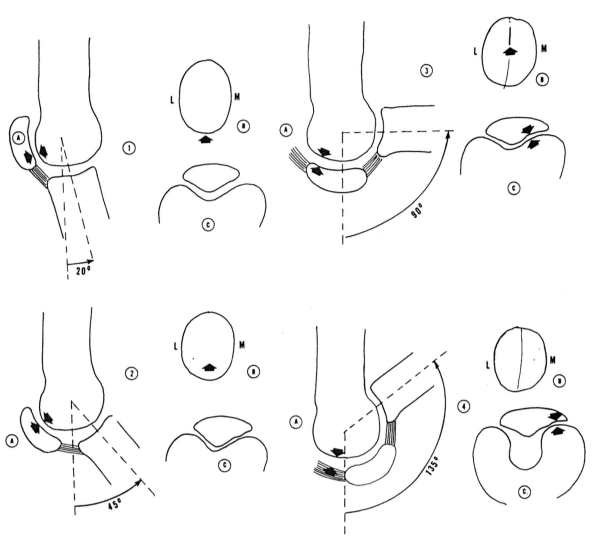

Figure 14–6. Patellar contact areas with femoral condyles during knee flexion. (*1*) Knee flexed 20°: (*A*) Lateral view of the patellofemoral joint. Arrows depict site of contact. (*B*) Area of contact of the patella (*shaded area*) (L = lateral; M = medial). (*C*) Superior view showing patella within femoral condyles. At 20° flexion, there is contact symmetrically of the lateral condyle. (*2*) Knee flexed 45°: Pressure upon the patella is in the broader central zone (*C*). As above, pressure on the medial and lateral patellar facets is symmetrical. (*3*) Knee flexed 90°: There is broad contact with the superior area of the medial and lateral patellar facets (*B*). As shown by (*C*), there is beginning to be more contact of medial facets. (*4*) Knee flexed 135° (full flexion): The patellar facets contact both femoral condyles, and the patella shifts (*C*) so that the odd facet contacts the medial condyle more firmly. (From Cailliet R: Knee Pain and Disability, ed 2. FA Davis, Philadelphia, 1983, pp 88–89, with permission.)

lacia will experience pain with this maneuver. Then the examiner should place a hand firmly above the patella and ask the patient to contract her quadriceps (Fig. 14–10). In this maneuver, called an inhibition test, athletes with patellofemoral stress syndrome or chondromalacia will have give-way symptoms after beginning the contraction.

This action mimics the give-way sensations reported by women with these entities.

Next, one should palpate the patella tendon to check for its intactness and to examine for tenderness at its origin off the inferior surface of the patella or at its attachment to the tibia. In the very young patient (age 6 to 9 years), inflammation of

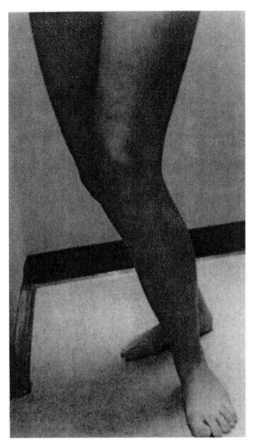

Figure 14-7. As the foot goes into pronation, the valgus angle of the knee and lateral tracking of the patella are accentuated.

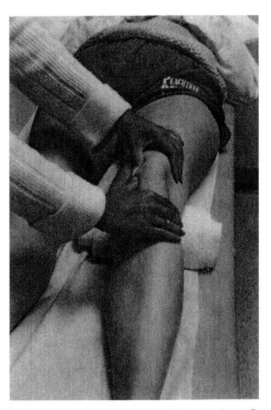

Figure 14-9. Palpation of the medial patella facet. Patients with patellofemoral stress frequently have tenderness along the medial border of the patella at the retinaculum or under the medial facet of the patella.

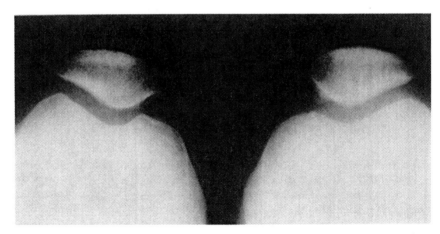

Figure 14-8. Radiograph of laterally tipped patellas. Note the very short medial condylar flare and the elongated lateral flare, corresponding to the increased width of the lateral patella facet when compared with the medial one.

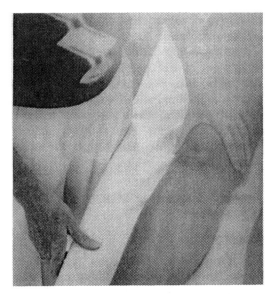

Figure 14-10. In the inhibition test, the examiner applies pressure above the patella as the patient contracts the quadriceps muscle. This maneuver frequently reproduces the pain of the athlete with patellofemoral stress syndrome.

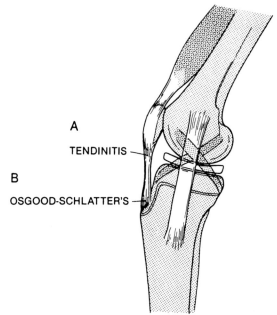

Figure 14-11. (*A*) The patient with patella tendinitis will have pain at the origin of the patella tendon. (*B*) The patient with Osgood-Schlatter's disease (seen in the teenager with open growth centers) will have irritation at the insertion of the patella tendon into the tibial apophysis. (From Andrish JT: Knee injuries in gymnastics. In Weiker GG (ed): Gymnastics. Clin Sports Med 4:120, 1985, with permission.)

the patella tendon at its origin off the inferior surface of the patella may be associated with irregularities of the lower patella apophyseal pole (Fig. 14-11). Similarly, irritation of the attachment of the patella tendon to the tibial apophysis when it is developing (approximately age 11 to 13 years) can result in its inflammation or apophysitis, a condition termed Osgood-Schlatter's disease (Fig. 14-11).

Aspiration of Fluid

If there is fluid within the knee joint, it may be aspirated. A hemarthrosis, or blood in the knee, may result from a traumatic patella dislocation with spontaneous relocation. (Remember that the athlete who has had a spontaneous relocation of her patella may not have perceived her injury as a patella dislocation.) Other diagnoses associated with a hemarthrosis include anterior cruciate ligament tear, peripheral meniscal tear, and intra-articular fracture.

Yellow synovial fluid aspirated from the joint may indicate that the knee joint has been or is irritated. Patella abnormalities that can result in an increase in synovial fluid include patella subluxations or abnormalities of the hyaline cartilage of the retropatellar surface (chondromalacia).

Radiographic Evaluation

Many different radiographic techniques have been designed to evaluate the patella and its relationship to the femur in the patellofemoral groove. The ratio of a line drawn longitudinally through the patella to a line drawn from the tip of the patella to the tibial tubercle measured on a lateral radiograph, with the knee in 50 degrees of flexion, can be used to estimate patella alta or baja. A ratio greater than 1.2 is indicative of patella alta (Fig. 14-12), whereas a ratio of less than 1.0 is associated with patella baja.

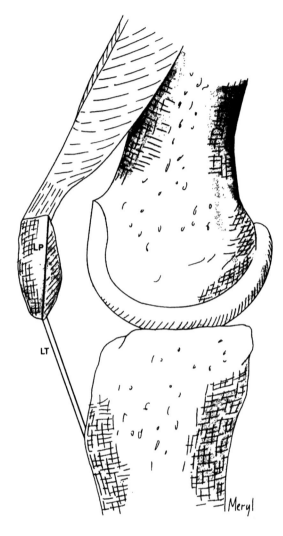

PATELLA ALTA

Figure 14–12. Objective confirmation of patella alta is obtained by using a lateral radiograph and determining the length of the patella (LP) and the length of the patella tendon (LT). If the tendon length exceeds the patella length by 20%, then patella alta is present (i.e., LP/LT ≤ 0.8). (From Scott WN, Nisonson B, Nicholas JA, et al: Principles of Sports Medicine. Williams & Wilkins, Baltimore, 1984, p 312, with permission.)

A view of the patella taken with the knee flexed to 30 degrees and the cassette held perpendicular to the radiograph tube is called a skyline view of the patella (Fig. 14–13). It is used to assess the patella's position in the femoral groove, as well as to detect the presence of patella spurs and to note the

thickness of the articular cartilage of the patellofemoral joint.

Another helpful study used to assess the intactness of the patellofemoral cartilage and the position of the patella in the femoral groove is computerized axial tomography done following injection of contrast material into the knee joint. The contrast material nicely coats the articular surface for visualization (Fig. 14–14).

Acute Traumatic Patella Dislocation

Diagnosis

If spontaneous relocation has not occurred, the diagnosis of a dislocation of the patella is obvious from observation. The patella typically lies lateral to the knee joint, and the injured athlete usually will hold her knee partially flexed because of pain. To confirm the diagnosis and make certain there are no fractures, radiographs should be taken.

Initial Treatment

First, the intactness of the neurovascular structures should be assessed. After medication has been given to decrease pain (giving intravenous morphine as an analgesic is often extremely helpful), the examiner should gently extend the patient's leg while exerting a medial force on the patella. The patella will relocate with an audible sound, resulting in rapid relief of pain. A dislocated patella can sometimes be reduced on the field or court without medication, but it is usually wiser to first radiographically document the diagnosis and make certain there are no associated fractures.

Following relocation, one should apply a compressive wrap with lateral pads to hold the patella medially. The knee is then supported in a soft knee immobilizer which keeps the knee extended. The intent of the lateral pad and the immobilization in extension is to bring the patella in close approximation to the vastus medialis fibers so that they can heal securely back to the patella.

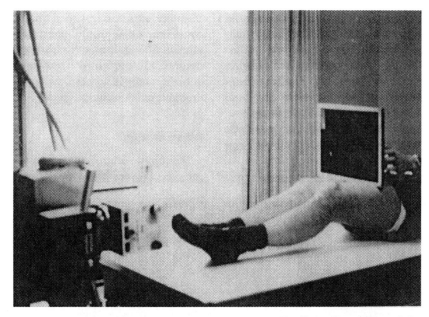

Figure 14-13. Technique for obtaining skyline view of the patella. (From Hunter LY, et al: Common orthopedic problems of female athletes. In Frankel VH (ed): Instructional Course Lectures. American Academy of Orthopedic Surgeons, CV Mosby, St. Louis, 1982, p 131, with permission.)

The physician should instruct the athlete to ice and elevate the extremity and should place her on crutches, so that she bears only partial weight on the affected leg. If she develops a marked hemarthrosis over the next several days, it can be aspirated to increase comfort and to decrease stretching of the already injured medial retinaculum.

Some physicians recommend immediate arthroscopic examination of the joint to evacuate the hemarthrosis and to check for the presence of a chondral fracture off the

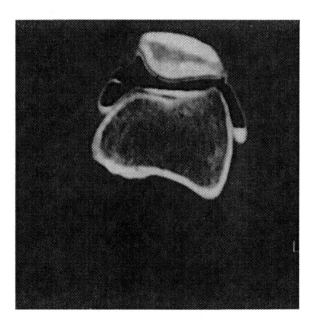

Figure 14-14. The patellofemoral joint as viewed by computed axial tomography after injection of contrast material into the knee joint.

posterior surface of the patella or the opposing lateral femoral condyle. Cartilage fractures are not recognized on routine radiographs unless the fracture extends into bone (an osteochondral fracture). Fracture fragments, whether cartilage alone or cartilage and bone, need to be removed, because they will become loose bodies that can intermittently catch in the joint, causing severe pain and locking.

Physicians who do not recommend immediate arthroscopy feel that if an athlete develops loose body symptoms following patella dislocation, arthroscopy can be performed at that time. However, performed acutely, such a procedure may merely increase quadriceps atrophy.

Rehabilitation

The knee is kept wrapped with a lateral pad and immobilized in the extended posi-

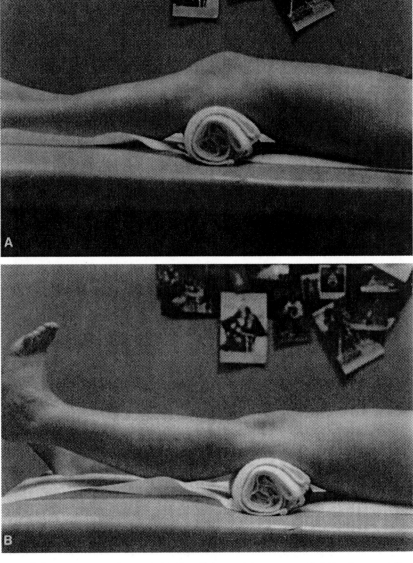

Figure 14–15. Short arc extension exercises increase quadriceps strength following a patella dislocation.

tion for approximately 3 to 6 weeks, to allow the torn medial retinaculum to heal. Isometric exercises can be done by the athlete while she is in the immobilizer. Some physicians will use muscle-stimulating units during this period to help strengthen the vastus medialis.

At the end of this time, short arc extension exercises, as well as functional strengthening activities such as walking, bike riding, or using a stair climber can be started. If an exercise bike is used, the seat should be set as high as possible and tension kept on medium to low. If biking outdoors, a bike that has at least 3 gears, but preferably 5 or 10, should be used. The athlete should be instructed to use low gears (rapid pedaling at low tension) and to avoid hills. Again, seat height should be set so the athlete's knee is completely extended on the downstroke. Similarly, if a stair climber is used, the athlete should set the tension of the machine on low and perform rapid small steps.

Short arc extension exercises are performed by placing a rolled towel beneath the knee, so that the exercise is begun at approximately 30 degrees of knee flexion. In a rhythmic fashion, the athlete performs multiple extensions from this flexed starting position (Fig. 14–15). Initially, no ankle weights should be used; as the athlete progresses in her exercise program, up to 5 lb of weight may be added. Usually sets of 10 to 15 repetitions are done at one time and incorporated into a total strengthening program for the lower extremities. The partially flexed starting position and use of minimal weights minimize the forces over the patellofemoral joint, while the exercises increase quadriceps strength.

As rehabilitation proceeds, a lateral patella pad or one of the many braces designed for patella stabilization can be used. The braces typically incorporate a lateral or horseshoe pad to stabilize the patella medially (Fig. 14–16). These same braces may be used by the athlete when she returns to her sport. Following acute patella dislocation, however, it may be as much as 6 months before an athlete can fully participate in pivotal sports.

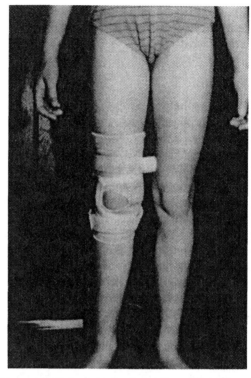

Figure 14–16. An example of a patella-stabilizing brace. Note pad encircling the patella. (From Walsh WM, et al: Overuse injuries in girls' gymnastics. In Walsh WM (ed): The Athletic Woman. Clin Sports Med 3:841, 1984, with permission.)

The athlete who sustains a patella dislocation is at greater risk for redislocation. A quadriceps-strengthening program as well as brace support may be helpful in minimizing that risk. Athletes with recurrent patella dislocation may require operative procedures to help stabilize the patella. (See Surgery, under Patella Subluxation.)

Patella Subluxation

Athletes whose patellas sit laterally or who have small, high-riding patellas (patella alta) are more predisposed to patella subluxation. During an episode of subluxation, the patella slides laterally with twisting movements of the knee (especially lateral twists or valgus stresses) but does not frankly dislocate or come completely out of its femoral groove. In principle, the greater the Q angle, the more easily the patella can slip laterally. Medial patella subluxation theoretically can occur, but practically is rarely found.

Symptoms

Athletes with patella subluxation may complain merely of knee pain with kicking, twisting, or running maneuvers. The whip kick or frog kick in swimming may be painful. Even though both patellas are high-riding, small, and easily subluxable, frequently only the dominant knee is symptomatic and so the athlete may not complain of pain in both knees. Like the athlete with patellofemoral stress syndrome, she may state that she has give-way episodes when going downstairs (an activity that increases patellofemoral forces) or may complain of locking or catching of her knee. She may not localize her pain to the patella and may never have experienced an episode of frank patella dislocation.

The pain experienced by the athlete with chronic patella subluxation may result from inflammation of the parapatellar retinaculum as it is stretched when the patella rides laterally, or it may be secondary to abnormal forces on the hyaline cartilage surface of the patella. In fact, some women with chronic subluxable patellas may develop fibrillation or even fissuring of the hyaline cartilage, eventually have erosion and loss of the hyaline cartilage surface, and hence develop patellofemoral arthritis.

Family History

The history from the athlete with subluxable patellas may reveal a sister, mother, grandmother, or even a male relative who has had knee problems. The predisposition for patella symptoms is based on anatomic factors.

Physical Examination

As indicated previously, the patella is frequently small and high-riding. The vastus medialis obliquus may be poorly developed.

In fact, the whole vastus medialis may be poorly developed.

Women with patella subluxation frequently have an ectomorphic body type, with slender, poorly muscled lower extremities. The examiner observing active and passive knee flexion can see the patella riding laterally and/or sitting high in the femoral groove.

Palpating the medial retinaculum or the medial facet of the patella will frequently cause discomfort. The athlete generally will be apprehensive if one moves her patella laterally. In fact, this sign is so characteristic of the patient whose patella subluxes or dislocates that it is believed to be diagnostic of this condition. Frequently, the examiner may be able to completely dislocate the patella by putting a direct lateral force on it with the knee in extension.

Treatment: Conservative

Treatment of the athlete with symptomatic chronic patella subluxation is difficult. Exercise to strengthen the quadriceps, especially the vastus medialis and particularly its oblique fibers, so that the patella will ride more medially in the patellofemoral groove, may be helpful. When the athlete is acutely symptomatic with pain, the anti-inflammatory agents, such as aspirin (two taken four times a day) or one of the other nonsteroidal anti-inflammatory drugs, may be helpful.

Intra-articular injection of steroids is not recommended in the young athlete, as this may cause softening of the hyaline cartilage.

Treatment: Surgical

If all conservative measures fail—including activity modification to avoid rapid pivotal sports—operative procedures to better centralize the patella can be performed. Incising (releasing) the lateral retinaculum arthroscopically or with a small parapatellar lateral incision may help the patella to track more medially. Theoretically this weakens the pull of the vastus lateralis muscles on the patella. However, this procedure must be linked with a rehabilitation program designed to strengthen the vastus medialis muscles.

Other operative procedures transfer the bony attachment of the patella tendon more medially on the tibia. This decreases the Q angle and should better centralize the patella, preventing subluxation. Such a procedure may be combined with lateral retinacular release.

Care must be taken not to move the patella tendon attachment distally on the tibia, as this will increase patellofemoral forces and lead to patella cartilage softening or chondromalacia.[11]

Patellofemoral Stress Syndrome

Patellofemoral stress syndrome is very common, particularly in the teenaged female athlete. This diagnosis is used to describe a syndrome in which there is patella pain with activities that load the patellofemoral joint such as kneeling, kicking, running (especially downhill running), climbing, or sitting for a prolonged period of time with the knee acutely flexed. The syndrome does not include athletes with subluxable or dislocatable patellas.

Symptoms

The athlete with patellofemoral stress syndrome may have symptoms similar to those of the athlete with patella subluxation. She may present with increasing aching discomfort in the knee, with or without associated effusion, or she may present with an acute episode of knee pain with locking or giving way. Effusions are more typically associated with patella subluxations or dislocations.

Physical Examination

On physical examination, although she may have a patella that rides laterally in the patellofemoral groove, with an increased Q angle, a woman with patellofemoral stress syndrome is not apprehensive when the examiner tries to force her patella laterally. Moreover, although her patella may sit laterally in the patellofemoral groove, it is stable in its position, and the examiner will not have the feeling that it could be dislocated by being pushed too firmly laterally.

The athlete with patellofemoral stress syndrome will have a positive patella inhibition test; that is, she will experience pain if the examiner puts a hand firmly above the patella and asks the athlete to contract her quadriceps. This test increases patellofemoral forces, and hence, reproduces the athlete's pain and give-way episodes.

The examiner should note the degree of vastus medialis development, as frequently athletes with patellofemoral stress syndrome, like those with patella subluxation or dislocation, have a poorly developed vastus medialis. Hamstring tightness has also been reported to increase patellofemoral forces—when the athlete fully extends the knee, the tight hamstrings create a "bowstring" effect.

Note should be made of the footstrike in the athlete with patella pain. Check to see if the feet appear to have no arches, due to excessive inward rolling of the feet at the ankles. Many people who have "flat feet" may have normal arches. Their feet may appear flat because they pronate excessively. Such athletes (overpronators) may be at an increased risk of developing patella pain during running. During running, the foot strikes the ground on the lateral part of the sole and rolls medially prior to toeing off. If there is excessive pronation associated with this medial roll, the patella may be forced laterally in the patellofemoral groove, resulting in abnormal distribution of patellofemoral forces.

Treatment

Alteration of patella tracking is the fundamental principle in all treatment programs for patellofemoral stress syndrome. Quadriceps-strengthening exercises, designed to minimize patellofemoral force while increasing quadriceps strength, are recommended. Short arc extensions and biking, as described above, are two ways of achieving this objective. Another is straight leg lifts, with minimal weights and maximal repetitions. A stair-stepper machine can also be used, but only with small, rapid steps at low tension settings.

Devices that limit pronation are often useful in treating patella pain. Many track shoes have varus wedges (thicker heels medially than laterally). Arch supports incorporated into insoles or custom-ordered orthotics to alter foot strike may be helpful. For an orthotic to limit pronation effectively, it must be used in a shoe that has a tight counter to grip the heel and a saddle to keep the foot from slipping over the orthotic.

Icing the parapatellar area following exercise may help decrease inflammation, and hence, pain. Oral anti-inflammatory agents, either aspirin, ibuprofen, or other prescription nonsteroidal drugs, may be useful in the patient who is acutely symptomatic.

Braces like those previously described for use in athletes with patella subluxation or dislocation can also help to alter patella tracking.[12] In addition, there are patella straps or bands of material that fasten about the proximal tibia at the level of the patella tendon. Theoretically, these bands are designed to alter the resting length of the quadriceps-patella tendon unit, and hence, decrease the force this unit can generate at the patellofemoral joint, much like tennis elbow bands are thought to alter the force generated by the wrist extensor mechanism, and hence, decrease the stress placed on the lateral epicondyle.

The symptomatic athlete should be instructed to avoid prolonged knee flexion; that is, she should not sit "Indian-style" for long periods of time, and she should stretch her legs frequently while riding in a car or sitting in the theater or at her desk. Her training routines should be reviewed to make certain they do not include activities that maximally load the patellofemoral joint, such as stair climbing (other than discussed above) or deep squats. If the hamstring muscles are tight, hamstring stretching should be initiated. Slow stretches, as shown in Figure 14–17, are recommended.

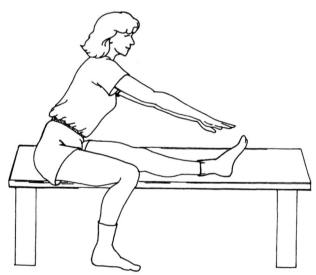

Figure 14–17. Hamstring stretch. For stretching the left hamstring and the right side of the back, slowly bend forward from the hips toward the foot of the left leg from a sitting position with the legs spread. Keep the head forward and the back straight. Hold the stretch for 20 seconds. With repetitions, the stretch will become easier. Repeat the stretch with the opposite leg.

Prognosis

Although the patellofemoral stress syndrome may be associated with significant pain, which temporarily incapacitates the athlete, this overuse syndrome is not typically associated with any permanent impairment. Unlike chronic patella subluxation or multiple patella dislocations, patellofemoral stress syndrome infrequently results in chondromalacia or frank patellofemoral arthritis.[9] Treating the athlete with patellofemoral stress syndrome may be frustrating, however, as symptoms may initially be quite refractory.

Patella Plica

Patella plica (also called synovial plica or patella shelf) is a normal developmental fold of tissue that sits retropatellarly. It is the embryonic remnant of the divisions in the knee.[13]

Symptoms

The remnant is normally thin and filmy, but following multiple episodes of minimal trauma or one severe acute traumatic episode to the patellofemoral joint, this fold of tissue can become thickened. When the patella rides over this thickened fold, it can cause an audible "pop" and associated pain. The pain may be reported by the athlete as being diffuse or as being definitely associated only with the "pop" and localized well along the medial side of the joint. She may feel a catching sensation as the patella tries to slide under the thickened fold.

Pain can be gradual in onset over days and weeks, as this tissue slowly thickens with multiple low levels of trauma, or it can be acute, especially if the athlete has performed a knee-intense activity and the plica has acutely been irritated and thickened.

On physical examination, the athlete may have a small effusion. She will feel tenderness over the medial parapatellar area over the location of the plica. Moreover, an au-dible "pop" or snap can be felt as the knee actively extends, and this sound is accompanied by pain. Occasionally, the "pop" can also be produced by passive knee extension.

Treatment

For the acutely symptomatic athlete, having her rest the knee in extension in a soft knee immobilizer for 5 to 10 days and prescribing a nonsteroidal anti-inflammatory agent such as aspirin may decrease inflammation and resolve the symptoms completely.

Treatment of the athlete with chronic pain from a symptomatic plica is more difficult. Rest and anti-inflammatory agents can be tried. Exercises to alter patella tracking may also be helpful. In rare cases, excision of the patella plica must be done to relieve symptoms.

Patella Pain: Summary

Patella pain is one of the most common musculoskeletal complaints in female athletes. It may result from repeated episodes of patella dislocation, from multiple patella subluxations, from patellofemoral stress syndrome, or from symptomatic patella plica. Diagnosis is made on history and physical examination. Altering patella tracking while decreasing acute inflammation is the basis of most treatment programs.

IMPINGEMENT SYNDROMES

Impingement syndromes result when soft tissues are repetitively traumatized between bony prominences. For example, shoulder impingement refers to irritation of bursa and rotator cuff tissue, which becomes trapped between the humeral head and acromion with shoulder elevation if the humeral head is not firmly held in the glenoid fossa. Impingement syndromes commonly occur about the ankle, the wrist, and the shoulder, and they are particularly common in women involved in gymnastics, racquet sports, swimming, throwing sports, ballet, diving, ice skating, and crew (see Table 14–1).

Ankle Impingement

Impingement of soft tissues about the ankle may occur with either repetitive marked dorsiflexion, such as that seen with landings in gymnastics, or repetitive marked plantar flexion, such as occurs in dance, gymnastics, and diving. Athletes with anterior capsular impingement complain of pain in the region just lateral to the anterior tibial tendon as it crosses the ankle. The pain is increased with dorsiflexion activities.

Posterior capsular pain may be harder to localize. The athlete describes her pain as posterior in the ankle, deep to the Achilles tendon. The pain is present when she rises to her toes, and in fact it may prevent her from achieving a forced plantar flexed position. On palpation of her peroneal tendons, Achilles tendon, and posterior tibial tendon, no tenderness is found.

Ankle radiographs of the athlete with soft tissue ankle impingement appear normal, but occasionally athletes may demonstrate bony abnormalities (beaking of the tibia and talus anteriorly, and hypertrophy of the talar process posteriorly) (Fig. 14–18).

Treatment of most athletes with ankle impingement syndromes is conservative. Oral and/or local administration of anti-inflammatory agents, ice massage, ultrasound, electrical stimulation, and other physical therapy modalities may help diminish the inflammatory response. Use of an anterior ankle pad, for anterior impingement, or a posterior pad to prevent hyperextension with posterior impingement may be helpful. The athlete should review her fundamentals, as alteration of technique may diminish symptoms; for example, "landing short" in gymnastics results in a hyperflexed position and may precipitate anterior capsulitis. In the rare athlete with excessive bony hypertrophy, surgical excision may be required.

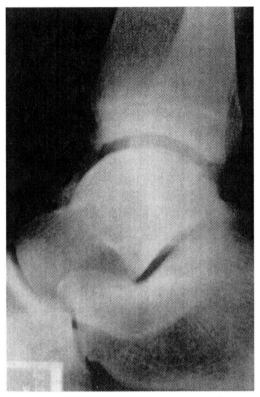

Figure 14–18. Beaking of the anterior talar-tibial surface, secondary to multiple flexor impingements.

Wrist Impingement

Impingement of the palmar capsule of the wrist is not as common as that of the dorsal capsule. Dorsal capsular impingement may develop acutely if an athlete falls on an outstretched hand or absorbs a sharp impact on the dorsiflexed hand, such as might occur in a tumbling routine in gymnastics, in a poor angle of contact with a volleyball, or in improper baton handoff in track.

The athlete with dorsal impingement will complain of pain diffusely along the dorsal wrist structures. The pain is made worse with forced dorsiflexion. A fracture of the radius or navicular must be considered in the differential diagnosis of any athlete presenting with a painful wrist. The pain of dorsal capsulitis will not be limited to the snuffbox, as with navicular fractures, and the pain is more distal (centered over the radial-carpal junction) than that seen with a nondisplaced radial fracture. Moreover, with capsular impingement, radiographs are normal.

Analgesic cream applied to the area of maximum tenderness and ice massage, as well as other physical therapy modalities, may be helpful in decreasing symptoms. After the acute pain subsides, strengthening exercises for the wrist extensors and flexors are recommended prior to returning to the sport. Chronic impingement pain—that is, pain that has been present at a low level of discomfort for several months—is more difficult to resolve than the pain of acute impingement. Similar treatment routines are used, however. Taping the wrist upon return to activity may be beneficial in the athlete with either an acute or a chronic wrist impingement.

Shoulder Impingement

Shoulder impingement is commonly seen in swimmers and in athletes participating in throwing and racquet sports. It is frequently associated with some element of anterior shoulder subluxation in young athletes. In the impingement syndrome, a weakened rotator cuff allows upward migration of the humeral head in the glenoid, causing compromise of the humeral-acromial space. As this space becomes compromised, the tissues contained therein, those of the subacromial bursa, and the rotator cuff itself can become traumatized and inflamed. With greater inflammation, there is greater mass of tissue, and therefore, a vicious cycle of pain, swelling, more pain, and more swelling is established. Shoulder impingement may be associated with bicipital tendinitis, since the biceps tendon lies in the subacromial space and can be irritated by the impingement process part of the syndrome.

The athlete with shoulder impingement complains of pain at the tip of the acromion or in the proximal arm. Frequently the pain radiates down the external rotators of the shoulder. Tenderness can be elicited if the examiner places one hand on the patient's acromion, holding it down while elevating the arm in either forward or side flexion,

mimicking the impingement process that occurs dynamically during sport. This maneuver is termed the "impingement sign" (Fig. 14-19).

No atrophy is generally found. The biceps tendon will be tender if it is involved in the impingement process. There is often tenderness over the acromioclavicular joint, especially if arthritis of this joint is present, as in the older patient who develops the impingement syndrome. Acromioclavicular arthritis is less common in the younger competitive athlete. Typically, external rotation strength is diminished over the opposite side, but abduction is possible.

Shoulder radiographs are usually normal in the young athletic individual with shoulder impingement. In the impingement syndrome of some athletes, one occasionally sees osteophytic spurring of the inferior surface of the acromion or sclerosis of the lateral aspect of the humeral head from repetitive trauma.[14]

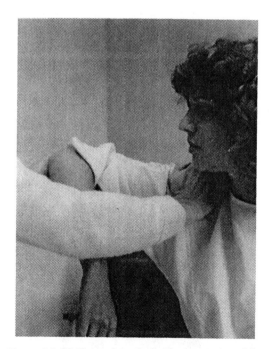

Figure 14-19. To produce the impingement sign of the shoulder, the examiner holds down the acromioclavicular area while elevating the extremity at the elbow in a pronated, abducted, and forwardly flexed position. If this maneuver reproduces the pain of impingement, it is called a positive impingement sign.

A treatment program for the athlete with an impingement syndrome may include temporarily avoiding any activity that requires the elbow to be raised above shoulder height, combined with physical therapy modalities and oral anti-inflammatory agents. After the initial inflammatory response subsides, exercises to strengthen the rotator cuff muscles, to reinstitute proper mechanics of the shoulder, are advised. Many different exercise routines can be used to strengthen the rotator cuff. The

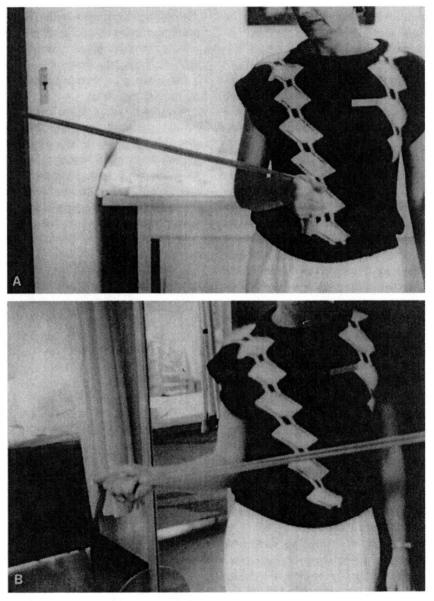

Figure 14–20. (*A*) Patient using rubber tubing to strengthen the internal rotators of the shoulder. Note that the elbow is held tightly to the side and the forearm is rotated internally to the abdomen, as the rubber tubing is affixed to the door. (*B*) Patient demonstrating use of rubber tubing to strengthen external rotators of the shoulder. Again, the elbow is held tight to the side and the forearm is rotated externally against the resistance of rubber tubing affixed to the door.

simple exercises using rubber tubing attached to a door (Fig. 14-20) were adapted from the program initiated by the Naval Academy.[15] The athlete should be advised to review technique with her trainer or coach, as frequently impingement is precipitated by an alteration in form. For example, in swimming, an increase in internal rotation of the arm at the shoulder may cause impingement of the tissues.

Chronic impingement syndromes are much more difficult to treat. Physical therapy modalities and oral anti-inflammatory agents can be tried. However, the key to improvement of symptoms is to reinstitute proper shoulder mechanics through a rotator-cuff–strengthening exercise program. The athlete should be advised that such a program will take anywhere from 4 to 6 weeks, so she should not become discouraged. Controversy exists as to the role of injected steroids to diminish symptoms. The decision to use these should depend on the assessment of each individual case.

OTHER COMMON CONDITIONS

Achilles Tendinitis

Achilles tendinitis is the result of damage to the fibers of the Achilles tendon or to its tendon sheath. It can be seen in sports requiring repetitive ankle flexion and extension (e.g., track, basketball, soccer). It also occurs in athletes who wear boots, such as skaters and skiers, from the irritation of the boot on the tendon.

Acute Achilles tendinitis is usually characterized by pain that is exacerbated when the patient actively plantar flexes or resists passive dorsiflexion of the foot. Chronic Achilles tendinitis usually results in severe pain on first rising in the morning, which lessens with activity. It also generally causes considerable pain at the start of a workout, which lessens as the workout progresses, unless the inflammation is severe and then the pain is persistent.

When asked to localize her pain, the athlete will touch either the tendon behind the ankle or its insertion into the superior posterior tip of the calcaneus. In acute tendinitis, the examiner can feel crepitation over the tendon as the athlete moves her foot from dorsiflexion to plantar flexion. The Achilles tendon may appear swollen when compared with the uninjured tendon. This swelling may be easier to assess if the patient stands facing away from the examiner or if she lies prone on the examining table.

Treatment

Rest is essential in the treatment of acute Achilles tendinitis. The athlete can substitute nonimpact load activities that require infrequent ankle motion (e.g., rowing machine, swimming) to maintain fitness. If walking is painful, crutches to assist ambulation, heel lifts to relax the Achilles tendon, or in very severe cases, cast immobilization, may be needed. Rarely, the athlete will require surgical release of the inflamed tendon sheath.

Oral anti-inflammatory agents, local anti-inflammatory creams, ice massage (rubbing the inflamed area with an ice cube), ultrasound, iontophoresis, or electrical stimulation can all be useful in decreasing acute inflammation. Steroid injections are not recommended because, if injected into the tendon itself rather than the tendon sheath, they may weaken the tendon.

Stretching an acutely injured tendon can delay healing, but once the acute inflammation has subsided, exercises to stretch as well as to strengthen the Achilles tendon are begun. Stretching can be done by standing on a slant board with the heel lower than the ball of the foot, by leaning against a wall (facing it) with the feet flat on the floor, or by using a towel under the ball of the foot to pull the foot gently into increasing dorsiflexion. Toe raises are an effective strengthening exercise.

After pain has completely disappeared with walking, stretching, and gently jogging, the athlete can gradually resume her running sport. Icing following activity for several months is recommended, and the athlete should always warm up well and stretch prior to sport.

Shin Splints

"Shin splints" may be used as a general term to refer to any pain between the tibial tubercle and the ankle that is not a stress fracture or compartment syndrome. However, many physicians use the term to refer specifically to pain along the anteromedial aspect of the tibia at the origin of the posterior tibial muscle (Fig. 14–21).

Running on hard surfaces, running in inappropriate shoes, having weak lower leg muscles, and improper stretching have all been blamed for causing shin splints. Running on hard surfaces or in noncushioned shoes may increase stress on the longitudinal arch of the foot and, hence, indirectly on the posterior tibial muscle and tendon that help support this arch.

Diagnosis of shin splints is made by history and physical examination. Pain may initially increase with activity, usually improves as the activity proceeds, and may return following activity. The pain of shin splints is localized to a 2- to 4-inch area on the anteromedial aspect of the tibia at the origin of the muscle. Radiographs usually are negative, but occasionally some diffuse periosteal reaction at the posterior tibial muscle origin can be seen.

Shin splints must be differentiated from a stress fracture of the tibia. The pain of a stress fracture increases with activity and is relieved with rest. The athlete with a stress fracture of the tibia will have a very discrete area of pain on palpation of the tibia (see below).

As with other overuse syndromes, shin splints can be treated with rest, local and/or oral anti-inflammatory agents, physical therapy modalities (e.g., ultrasound and electrical stimulation), and ice massage (more effective than an ice bag). Stretching and strengthening exercises for the posterior tibial muscle, as well as the associated toe flexor muscles, are recommended. Support of the tendons by arch supports or taping may be beneficial.

In patients with chronic shin splints, slow return to sports may be advocated despite the persistence of mild symptoms, as long as the possibility of a stress fracture has been eliminated. The athlete should be very careful to warm up sufficiently and perform adequate stretching prior to beginning activ-

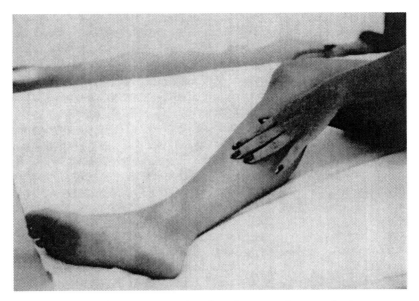

Figure 14–21. Patient with shin splints demonstrating area of pain.

ity. If an activity causes severe pain, it should be discontinued. The athlete may be able to substitute another activity (e.g., changing from running to biking) until her symptoms improve sufficiently to permit return to her preferred sport.

Stress Fractures

When the rate of bone breakdown from activity (a normal process) is greater than the rate of bone formation (repair), a stress fracture may result. Stress fractures have been reported to occur more often in female than in male athletes.[16] The reason for this increased incidence may be a lack of conditioning or improper training technique, rather than a true predisposition to injury. A woman who fails to condition slowly and sensibly for her sport does not give her bone ample time to increase in cortical thickness to meet the mechanical demands of the activity.

The most common location of stress fractures in women is the tibia;[17] also common are fractures of the fibula and metatarsals. Fractures of the pars interarticularis are a special type of stress fracture, as noted in the section on low back pain.

Some investigators have tried to relate the low estrogenic secondary amenorrhea seen occasionally in competitive female athletes to osteoporosis and a higher incidence of stress fractures.[18,19] However, the only area of diminished bone content in these women has been in the cancellous bone of the vertebral bodies;[20] no change in the density of cortical bone has been found. (See Chapter 5.) Most stress fractures occur just proximal to the metaphysis, in the areas of cortical bone. Therefore, the relationship of stress fractures to low estrogenic secondary amenorrhea is not clearly understood. More investigation needs to be done in this area.

Diagnosis

The pain of a stress fracture is typically restricted to a limited anatomic area. It is made worse with activity and may be relieved with rest. Radiographs are helpful in diagnosing stress fractures only if the pain has been present for a minimum of 2 to 3 weeks. Since stress fractures are really "microfractures," the fracture line itself is often not visible on the x-ray film. Radiographs do not demonstrate an abnormality until significant healing reaction of the periosteum (healing callus) is present.

To diagnose a stress fracture before a healing callus is visible radiographically, a bone scan can be done. This study will detect increased osteoblastic activity as soon as microfractures occur. Bone scans are particularly valuable in diagnosing intracapsular stress fractures, such as those of the femoral neck. In this location, bone has no periosteum. Hence, radiographs demonstrate no abnormality until intracortical healing takes place, and this takes longer than periosteal healing.

Treatment and Exercise

In treating stress fractures, the primary consideration is to decrease the mechanical stress on the bone to allow healing to occur. Neither cast immobilization nor operative stabilization is generally required. For stress fractures of the lower extremity, the athlete should use a cane or crutch until she can bear weight on the extremity without pain.

Swimming and bicycling can be started early in the treatment of stress fractures. These activities will maintain cardiovascular endurance and muscle tone, but are non–weight-bearing activities and therefore do not stress bones of the lower extremities in the same manner as running and walking. Psychologically, the athlete will fare much better if she can participate in some sporting activity during her treatment course.

Because stress fractures heal at variable rates, it is better to advance activity as pain resolves rather than to establish routine time intervals for activity adjustment. When no pain results from walking long distances unassisted by crutches or cane, running can be attempted.

Low Back Pain

Causes of low back pain have been listed as mechanical, neurologic, neoplastic, infectious, and metabolic. Mechanical causes, the most frequent in athletes, include nerve root impingement; repetitive microtrauma resulting in overuse syndromes such as tendinitis, fasciitis, and stress fractures; and some anatomic abnormalities. Most anatomic abnormalities, such as asymmetric lumbar or sacral facets, scoliosis, increased lumbar lordosis, and transitional vertebrae, do not usually result in back pain. However, unequal leg lengths (generally a difference of 1.5 cm or greater) may cause low back pain on a mechanical basis, especially in runners.

Athletes with mechanical low back pain may present with either an acute episode of severe low back pain, or with pain slowly increasing over several days or months. Pain associated with numbness or tingling of the lower extremities, or pain radiating from the back into the leg, implies nerve root impingement (neurologic back pain).

On physical examination, mild, moderate, or severe spasm of the paravertebral muscles may be found. Palpation of the low back region usually elicits pain. Reflexes, motor function, and sensation are normal in both lower extremities. Radiographs may be nor-

mal or show a lumbar list (curve) secondary to muscle spasm.

Most mechanical low back pain runs a 2- to 3-week course and is self-limited. If pain lasts longer despite the institution of conservative therapy with bed rest, muscle relaxants, anti-inflammatory agents, physical therapy modalities, and a graded exercise program, the athlete's symptoms deserve further evaluation to rule out the possibility of spondylolysis (a defect in the pars interarticularis, as in Fig. 14–22), spondylolisthesis (forward slipping of one vertebra on an adjacent vertebra, also in Fig. 14–22), large disk herniation, infection, neoplasm, or metabolic disease.

Spondylolysis

Female gymnasts have been found to have a greater incidence of spondylolysis or defects in the pars interarticularis than the general population.[21] Defects in the pars interarticularis in the athletic population present an intriguing diagnostic problem: Is this defect a stress fracture resulting from repetitive hyperextension and flexion activities of the area, or is it a developmental abnormality? The youngest reported pars defect occurred in a 3½-month-old child. An increased incidence of the defect is seen between the ages of 5½ and 6½; by age 7, 5% of all white children have been found to have a pars defect.[22] A familial predisposition for this defect has been reported.

If initial radiographs demonstrate a well-established pars defect indicative of an older injury, return to athletics can follow a period of rest. A strengthening program should be instituted prior to returning to activity. Bent-knee sit-ups, walking, and swimming all help to develop abdominal and paravertebral muscles.

Stress Fractures

In athletes with normal radiographs and persistent low back pain, the possibility of stress fracture must be entertained. A bone scan may be required to establish this diag-

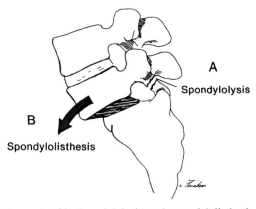

Figure 14–22. Spondylolysis and spondylolisthesis. (From Norkin CC and Levangie PK: Joint Structure and Function, ed 2. FA Davis, Philadelphia, 1992, p 164, with permission.)

nosis. If this is positive, resting from activities for a minimum of 3 to 4 months is recommended, and many physicians suggest immobilization in a spica or plastic orthosis.[23] Anti-inflammatory and muscle relaxing agents can be useful for symptomatic relief. A program of abdominal and back-strengthening exercises should be instituted prior to returning to athletics.

Spondylolisthesis

Spondylolisthesis occurring in association with spondylolysis is most common in females between the ages of 9 and 13 years. Unlike spondylolisthesis in the adult, which tends to remain stable, spondylolisthesis in children can increase in severity during the years of rapid growth. Children known to have spondylolisthesis who complain of back pain should be examined carefully to note any progression of their slip.

There is disagreement over whether athletes with mild spondylolisthesis should return to contact sports: some authorities have suggested that they can do so if they are protected by a brace. Although this may be acceptable in a football lineman, female gymnasts would find it difficult to compete in such a restrictive device.

Rarely, the athlete with spondylolisthesis may have persistent significant pain following a treatment program consisting of rest, anti-inflammatory agents, and using a brace. Fusions are occasionally performed in these recalcitrant cases. A few athletes have even returned to their sport following fusions for spondylolisthesis, but contact sports are generally not recommended in these athletes.

Herniated Lumbar Disk

Athletes with nonradicular back pain unresponsive to conservative measures or with radicular back pain should be evaluated for a possible herniated lumbar disk. In the athlete with radicular pain, careful neurologic examination may enable localization of the pain to a particular nerve root or disk

level. Initial treatment of the athlete with suspected disk herniation is similar to that for mechanical low back pain—rest and oral anti-inflammatory medications, followed by a program for strengthening paravertebral and abdominal muscles prior to a return to sport. Muscle relaxing agents and physical therapy modalities may be helpful in diminishing pain secondary to muscle spasm.

In the athlete whose pain is unresponsive to such treatment over 2 to 3 weeks, or who has increasing neurologic complaints (increased weakness, muscle atrophy, decreased sensation in the lower extremities, absent reflexes, etc.), further evaluation by computerized axial tomography (CAT) scan, magnetic resonance imaging, or myelogram should be done. If a ruptured disk is confirmed by these studies, surgical decompression of the ruptured disk may need to be done. However, less than 30% of myelogram-proven ruptured disks need operative intervention.[24] Most improve with conservative measures.

Vertebral Apophysitis

Another cause of back pain in the skeletally immature population is vertebral apophysitis, that is, irritation of the growth centers of the vertebral body. Inflammation is believed to result from traction on the apophysis (the growth center) from the anterior longitudinal ligament, as it is stretched in repetitive extension maneuvers that are a part of sports such as gymnastics, diving, and skating.

Rest often relieves symptoms, yet bony changes may persist. Prior to returning to sports, these youngsters should begin a strengthening and flexibility program for back and abdominal muscles. Symptoms determine when a child may resume full participation in sports.

Bunions

The abnormal prominence of the inner aspect of the first metatarsal head and resultant lateral displacement of the great toe is

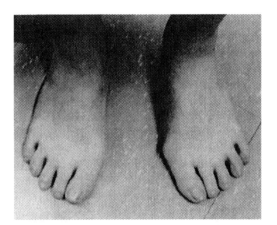

Figure 14-23. Young girl with bunions on metatarsus primus varus.

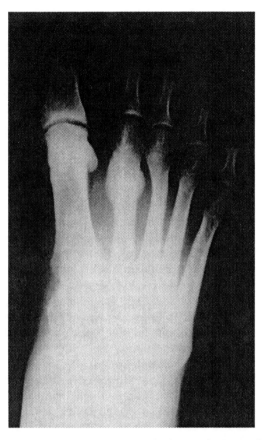

Figure 14-24. Runner who has had stress fractures of the second and third metatarsals following her bunionectomy procedure. The stress fracture of the second metatarsal is old and has a good healing reaction associated with it, whereas the stress fracture of the third metatarsal is new, and no healing reaction is yet seen.

termed a bunion. Bunions appear to be more common in women, and hence, they are more common among female athletes than among male athletes. Many women have inflammation of the bursa overlying the medial prominence or flare of the great toe metatarsal head associated with their metatarsus primus varus (Fig. 14-23), but this bursal enlargement also occurs without significant lateral displacement of the great toe. Shoe alteration and protective pads to reduce pressure over the metatarsal flare are often helpful in diminishing symptoms. The problem is more difficult when the athlete has not only bursitis but also degenerative changes in the metatarsophalangeal joint, a condition seen in athletes involved in kicking sports.

The athlete with a bunion must be careful when choosing shoes. She should look for shoes with a sufficiently wide forefoot, yet a narrow enough heel to prevent her foot from sliding forward in the shoe. With forward slippage, the first ray is forced into a valgus position and pressure is exerted on the medial metatarsal head.

If pain persists despite all conservative treatment, bunionectomy can be performed, but great care must be taken to avoid altering foot mechanics disadvantageously by such a surgical procedure. Figure 14-24 demonstrates multiple stress fractures of the middle metatarsals in a long-distance runner following a bunionectomy. Operative procedures should not be done purely for cosmetic reasons; they should be reserved for cases in which pain is unresponsive to conservative care.

Morton's Neuroma

Pain between the second and third metatarsal heads, or between the third and fourth metatarsal heads, made worse by transverse compression of the forefoot, generally results from inflammation and scarring about the interdigital nerve (i.e., Morton's neuroma). The patient may complain of numbness in the toes supplied by the compromised nerve. Swelling between the metatarsal heads at the site of the neuroma may also be noted.

The mechanism of development of this lesion is not clearly understood, but it appears to involve scarring of both the nerve and the vessel accompanying it.[25] It has been theorized that compression of the adjacent metatarsal heads creates repetitive trauma to these structures, producing the scarring.

In some cases, a metatarsal pad will alleviate symptoms. The athlete should be advised to wear wider shoes and place antiskid pads in her shoes to prevent forward migration of her foot in the shoe, causing transverse compression of the metatarsal heads. Local injection into this area may be helpful in decreasing or resolving symptoms.

If all these measures fail, excision of the neuroma may be performed, but the athlete should be warned that postoperative swelling of the foot can persist for 3 to 4 weeks following the procedure. She should plan resection of the neuroma for an appropriate time in her competitive season to permit an adequate recovery.

SUMMARY

Over the last several decades, there has been an increasing awareness of women's sports injuries. With the advent of better conditioning programs for women, the rate of sports injuries has diminished. When an injury does occur, prompt diagnosis and treatment of the injury is needed to minimize the time lost from sport.

Guidelines for the athlete's return to exercise after orthopedic injury or surgery are discussed in greater detail in Appendix A.

REFERENCES

1. Albohm M: Equal but separate—insuring safety in athletics. JNATA 13:131, 1978.
2. Anderson J: Women's sports and fitness programs at the U.S. Military Academy. Phys Sportsmed 7(4):72, 1979.
3. Eisenbert I, and Allen W: Injuries in a women's varsity athletic program. Phys Sportsmed 6(3):112, 1978.
4. Clarke K, and Buckley W: Women's injuries in collegiate sports. Am J Sports Med 8:187, 1980.
5. Whiteside P: Men's and women's injuries in comparable sports. Phys Sportsmed 8(3):130, 1980.
6. Gillette J, and Haycock C: What kinds of injuries occur in women's athletics? 18th Conference on the Medical Aspects of Sports, American Medical Association, 1977, p 18.
7. Shiveley RA, Grana WA, and Ellis D: High school sports injuries. Phys Sportsmed 9(8):46, 1981.
8. DeHaven K: Athletic injuries: Comparison by age, sport, and gender. Am J Sports Med 14:218, 1986.
9. Hunter L, Andrews J, Clancy W, et al: Common orthopaedic problems of the female athlete. American Academy of Orthopaedic Surgeons Instructional Course Lecture, Vol 31, 1982, p 126.
10. Hunter LY: Women's athletics: The orthopedic surgeon's viewpoint. Clin Sports Med 3:809, 1984.
11. Turba JE: Formal extensor mechanism reconstruction. Clin Sports Med 8:297, 1989.
12. Palumbo PM: Dynamic patellar brace: A new orthosis in the management of patellofemoral disorder. Am J Sports Med 9:45, 1981.
13. Boland A: Soft tissue injuries of the knee. In Nicholas J, and Hershman E (eds): The Lower Extremity and Spine in Sports Medicine. CV Mosby, St Louis, 1986, p 938.
14. Cone R, Resnick D, and Danzig L: Shoulder impingement syndrome: Radiographic evaluation. Radiology 150:29, 1984.
15. Regan K, and Underwood L: Surgical tubing for rehabilitating the shoulder and ankle. Phys Sportsmed 9(1):144, 1981.
16. Micheli L: Injuries to female athletes. Surgical Rounds 2:44, 1979.
17. Protzman R, and Griffis C: Stress fractures in men and women undergoing military training. J Bone Joint Surg 59:825, 1977.
18. Caldwell F: Light-boned and lean athletes: Does the penalty outweigh the reward? Phys Sportsmed 12(9):139, 1984.
19. Mitchell D: Case presentation. In Bulletin of the Department of Gynecology and Obstetrics, Emory University School of Medicine, 6:74, 1984.
20. Lutter J: Mixed messages about osteoporosis

in female athletes. Phys Sportsmed 11(9):154, 1983.

21. Jackson D, Wiltse L, and Cirincrone R: Spondylolysis in the female gymnast. Clin Orthop 117:68, 1976.

22. Hoshina H: Spondylolysis in athletes. Phys Sportsmed 8(8):75, 1980.

23. Micheli L: Low back pain in the adolescent: Differential diagnosis. Am J Sports Med 7:362, 1979.

24. Jackson D, and Wiltse L: Low back pain in young athletes. Phys Sportsmed 2:53, 1974.

25. Bossley C, and Cairney P: The intermetatarsophalangeal bursa: Its significance in Morton's metatarsalgia. J Bone Joint Surg 62B:184, 1980.

CHAPTER 15

Medical Conditions Arising during Sports

ARTHUR J. SIEGEL, M.D.

THE PHYSIOLOGY OF ATHLETES

CARDIAC CHANGES WITH
  EXERCISE AND TRAINING: RISKS
  AND BENEFITS
Primary and Secondary Prevention
  of Heart Disease Through Exercise

EXERCISE AND CANCER RISK

HAZARDS OF EXERCISE
Heat Stress
Hematologic Effects: Iron Status and
  Anemia
"Runner's Diarrhea"
Effects on the Urinary Tract
Exercise-Induced Asthma

Exercise-Induced Anaphylaxis
Exercise-Induced Urticaria

PSEUDOSYNDROMES IN
  ATHLETES
Pseudoanemia ("Runner's Anemia")
"Athletic Pseudonephritis"
Serum Enzyme Abnormalities:
  Muscle Injury and Pseudohepatitis
Pseudomyocarditis

SCREENING THE ATHLETE FOR
  MEDICAL CLEARANCE

CAUTION: WHEN NOT TO
  EXERCISE

The 1990s promise to be a dynamic step forward in women's health, with recognition of gender disparities in health care[1] and a clear mandate from the National Institutes of Health to close the gap through research on women's health.[2] A new NIH program is called CHOICES:

Cancer
Heart disease
Osteoporosis
Interventions and
Community
Evaluation
Studies

This program, committed to improving health outcomes in women, carries a strong mandate to examine the gender-specific health benefits of exercise as endorsed by the U.S. Preventive Services Task Force for the general population.[3]

261

The purpose of this chapter is to consider gender-focused medical conditions arising during sports and to place these considerations in the forward-looking context of the role of exercise in improving women's health.

THE PHYSIOLOGY OF ATHLETES

Things are not always what they appear to be. Athletes acquire an altered physiology from training, and as a result of those changes, basic laboratory tests that are abnormal for nonathletes may be normal for athletes. The medical literature is full of descriptions of medical conditions or illnesses in athletes that have subsequently been shown to be physiologic or normal responses to exercise. For example, athletic nephritis and athlete's anemia have been appropriately reclassified as pseudosyndromes. A physician who is unfamiliar with laboratory data in athletes may diagnose disease when none exists.

The following case history illustrates the complexities of medical conditions that may arise through intense sports activity:

A 21-year-old woman was brought to the emergency room scantily clad and comatose, having been found, unresponsive, by the roadside. Her blood pressure was 68/40, pulse 36 bpm and regular, respirations 8 and unlabored, temperature 96°F. Examination showed no evidence of head injury or other trauma. The chest was clear. The heart was markedly enlarged with an LV lift and pansystolic murmur with an S3 gallop. Abdominal examination was unremarkable. The extremities showed the appearance of muscle wasting with scant subcutaneous tissue and a height/weight ratio below the fifth percentile. Laboratory data included a hematocrit value of 30%, a urinalysis positive for protein and trace amounts of blood, and hyaline casts present in the sediment. Serum creatinine was borderline elevated at 1.7, liver and cardiac enzymes were two to three times normal, with a CPK 10 times normal. Chest radiograph showed marked cardio-

megaly without congestive heart failure. The ECG showed a first-degree AV block with voltage criteria for LVH, ST-segment changes consistent with early repolarization or acute ischemia.

This case illustrates the challenging differential that may arise during the acute evaluation of individuals—athletes or otherwise—with abnormal clinical examinations and laboratory data. Although this scenario might well fit an individual with an advanced stage of a debilitating illness (even AIDS), it is also entirely compatible with a nondisease state and might easily fit the description of an elite female marathon runner enjoying a nap after competition! The inability to arouse this patient with appropriate stimulation, or a marked elevation of body temperature, or both, might raise the possibility of severe heat injury or even heat stroke.

This sample case illustrates the importance of a working knowledge of the effects of endurance training on exercise physiology, to assess specific conditions that may arise in athletes during sport, as well as to differentiate true clinical problems from changes in laboratory data that may not indicate any underlying illness or dysfunction. A number of pseudosyndromes have been recognized in athletes, from the athletic heart syndrome to pseudonephritis, pseudoanemia, and pseudohepatitis. These are examples of abnormal laboratory findings that may result from strenuous training and not be connected to any underlying organ dysfunction.[4,5]

These pseudosyndromes must be differentiated from a range of medical complications that may arise in the athlete during prolonged strenuous exercise or competition, especially due to overexertion states. After briefly discussing some medical benefits conferred by exercise, this chapter will examine both aspects of medical conditions arising during sports: true exercise-related illnesses, conditions, or risks; and the spectrum of pseudosyndromes or apparent disorders that may arise as a result of altered physiology through training.

CARDIAC CHANGES WITH EXERCISE AND TRAINING: RISKS AND BENEFITS

Electrocardiographic changes in trained individuals include a variety of rhythm and conduction disturbances, as well as depolarization changes, that in other clinical settings would be characteristic of various diseases.[6] The heart, as studied by echocardiography, shows changes in both chamber size and myocardial mass, which vary with type of training. Endurance-trained athletes tend to have dilated chambers with a minor degree of increase in left ventricular wall thickness, resembling the volume-overload pattern seen in valvular regurgitation. In contrast, isometric or strength training induces a greater increase in wall thickness and total myocardial mass without chamber dilatation, as is seen in valvular aortic stenosis. Work hypertrophy, as documented by these studies, is associated with supernormal left ventricular performance during exercise, and, like the arrhythmias that may coexist, it is usually benign in nature. It is generally felt that asymptomatic athletes with documented myocardial hypertrophy and abnormal electrocardiograms do not require provocative or invasive cardiovascular testing prior to training or competition. In the absence of chest pain or syncope, bradyarrhythmias or even low grades of heart block and ventricular irritability need not be pursued as they would in symptomatic patients with suspected heart conditions. The sole caveat concerns the rare occurrence of sudden cardiac death in young athletes during sport, which is discussed in Chapter 16.

Primary and Secondary Prevention of Heart Disease Through Exercise

According to the American Heart Association, nearly half of the 500,000 people who die annually of heart attacks in the United States are women. Four recent studies of coronary artery disease in women point to basic similarities between men and women in the characteristics of disease and their response to preventive measures. For instance, atherosclerotic plaques found in women have similar compositions to those of men,[7] and daily aspirin use promotes primary prevention in women as well as in men.[8,9] Nevertheless, a gender bias in access to health care has been identified[10,11] and might be called "sex, lies, and balloon angioplasty." Attention to the need for gender-neutral diagnosis and treatment is growing.

While the incidence of coronary heart disease is low in women, compared with men, diseases of the circulatory system account for roughly two thirds of all deaths among women in the United States. The incidence of mild myocardial infarction or death from coronary heart disease in premenopausal women is below 1 in 10,000 per year. A large number of cardiovascular deaths occur in women after age 75, but cardiovascular deaths also account for one third of all deaths from age 65 to 74. Death rates from cardiovascular disease in women are 40% lower than in men for persons between 35 and 64 years of age, and the relative mortality rate for women falls to 25% of male levels for ages 35 to 44.[12] Nevertheless, cardiovascular death rates may be increasing in women, especially during the postmenopausal period, perhaps related to increases in the numbers of women who have smoked cigarettes throughout their lives. Although smoking-adjusted rates for coronary heart disease in women under 45 years of age have not increased in the United States, Framingham data from other studies indicate an increase in coronary disease in postmenopausal women, with a risk profile similar to that observed in men. Risk factors for coronary artery disease in women include the standard triad of hypertension, hypercholesterolemia, and cigarette smoking. Regular exercise produces a beneficial effect on such a risk profile, reducing resting blood pressure, increasing the "good" or HDL cholesterol, and creating a positive incentive to stop smoking.

As has been shown for men, cardiac risk reduction in women is closely tied to exercise. Diet programs for weight reduction should be augmented by exercise in order to increase HDL cholesterol levels.[13] The importance of moderate exercise in a weight-reduction program was demonstrated using brisk walking and light jogging designed to attain 60% to 80% of the maximal heart rate for 25 minutes three times per week. Thus, the new guidelines endorsed by the American College of Sports Medicine indicate that an aerobic effect linked directly to an improvement in cholesterol profiles may result from less intense exercise than had been advocated previously. The more conservative CDC recommendations are similar but do not specify intensity levels.

The second risk factor for coronary artery disease is hypertension, which also has been shown to improve with the addition of an exercise program.[14] In addition, exercise has been found beneficial in patients with non–insulin-dependent diabetes mellitus, in whom coronary artery disease is accelerated by approximately a decade.[15]

Exercise training also improves quit rates in women participating in smoking cessation programs.[16] The adverse effect of smoking may be greater in women than in men.[17] Young women now have high smoking rates, and a combination of smoking cessation with exercise may be mutually reinforcing. Women who stop smoking may experience minor weight gain, including increased body fat, but lean body mass increases as a benefit of exercise.[18,19] In addition, the enjoyment of improved exercise performance is an extra incentive to avoid smoking and to pursue a prudent, low-fat diet. When needed, transdermal nicotine may improve the effectiveness of smoking cessation programs.[20,21]

Finally, postmenopausal estrogens have been shown by careful studies to proong life and reduce coronary artery disease mortality.[22,23] On the other hand, anabolic steroids are atherogenic and hazardous.[24]

EXERCISE AND CANCER RISK

A great volume of literature supports the beneficial effects of exercise in the primary and secondary prevention of coronary artery disease, but few data exist on specific relationships between exercise and cancer. A recent study from the Journal of the National Cancer Institute reports a relationship between increased physical activity and decreased risk of colon cancer.[25] Such a relationship does not prove causality or a protective relationship, however.

Low-dose postmenopausal estrogen replacement does not appear to increase the risk of breast cancer,[26] and it does improve the safety of exercise by preventing osteoporosis and reducing coronary heart disease.

HAZARDS OF EXERCISE

Heat Stress

Adaptation of the athlete to environmental stresses such as heat, cold, or altitude depends on specific physiologic responses, which may be different in women. Aerobic exercise involves the generation of internal heat through performance of muscular work. As the core temperature rises, an increased amount of cardiac output is delivered to the skin so that heat can be dissipated in the form of sweating. Heat is lost principally through evaporation of sweat from the body surface, which cools off the individual at the price of losing vital circulating fluids. Prolonged strenuous exercise invariably leads to dehydration, which may then lead to fatigue, confusion, lethargy, and persistent excessive body temperature. Advanced states of heat exhaustion from exercise may lead to coma and even cardiac arrhythmias and sudden death. These rare and extreme hazards can be avoided by adequate knowledge of the steps that prevent dehydration and hyperthermia during exercise.

The capacity to dissipate body heat generated during prolonged strenuous exercise depends on both internal and environmental factors. The capacity for heat acclimatization depends on an increase in the rate of sweat generation for the level of exertion and a lower sodium content. As judged by such changes, heat-acclimatized men and women show similar adaptive patterns. After acclimatization, women's heart rates and rectal temperatures in hot and humid conditions at rest and after activity are the same of those of men.[27] Lower sweat rates in women are required to maintain comparable body temperatures, suggesting an improved efficiency in heat-release mechanisms. Acclimatization to hot weather is facilitated by underlying fitness capacity, but still requires 7 to 10 days for optimal adaptation. It should be accomplished gradually, starting at 50% maximum effort and increasing 5% to 10% daily. Competitive athletes and recreational runners alike, men or women, must respect the limitations of internal (adaptive) and external (climatic) stresses.

An increased risk for heat exhaustion might be hypothesized in women during the second half of the menstrual cycle, from elevations in basal body temperature owing to progesterone effects. However, increased susceptibility to heat injury during the luteal phase has not been demonstrated in the scientific literature. Wells[28] studied the heat responses of women at different stages in their menstrual cycle in hot-dry and neutral environments. Sweat rates and evaporative heat loss did not vary through the menstrual cycle.

Drinkwater and colleagues[29] studied heat adaptation in female marathon runners and showed a relationship between physical fitness as measured by $\dot{V}o_2max$ and resistance to heat injury. Female runners with high $\dot{V}o_2max$ (49 mL·kg^{-1}·min^{-1} vs. 39 mL·kg^{-1}·min^{-1}) had lower heart rates, lower skin and rectal temperatures, and quicker onset of sweating compared with less-conditioned individuals. These findings are similar to patterns in men, and they con-

firm a resistance to heat-stress injury from physical conditioning. Nevertheless, a high level of physical fitness will not protect an athlete from heat exhaustion or potentially fatal heat stroke, which may accompany overexertion in a given level of training. Considerations for women are almost identical to those in men for heat-intolerance susceptibility.

The guidelines for prevention of heat injury as outlined by the American College of Sports Medicine should be considered, whether racing or out for a recreational jog.[30] The first tenet of prevention is adequate hydration before exercise. This is best done by consuming 8 to 10 ounces of water 10 to 20 minutes before beginning a strenuous workout. The warm-up phase of exercise allows the muscles and tendons to adapt to the biomechanics of exercise while the blood flow increases to exercising muscle. As body temperature rises, the sweating mechanism kicks into place, with the perception of "second wind." Prolonged exercise should involve taking breaks to consume additional water and, when appropriate, moistening the body surface with sponging or spraying to assist in the cooling process. Such measures provide a form of "external sweating," which helps to dissipate heat through evaporation without needing to use internal fluid resources as the sole source of water for evaporation.

Sweating involves the loss of more water than sodium and chloride in comparison to their concentrations in blood. As a result, serum levels of sodium rise continuously during exercise. For this reason, salt supplements are undesirable prior to or during strenuous exercise, and in events lasting less than 2 to 3 hours individuals should rely on the use of water alone as the optimal repletion fluid in the prevention of heat injury. Potassium supplements are likewise unnecessary for participants in events lasting less than 3 hours. Exclusive and *excessive* water intake during prolonged events such as an ultramarathon, however, may lead to hyponatremia or low sodium levels.

Appropriate dress during exercise is another important component to the prevention of heat stress. This involves dressing in light and loose-fitting clothing during hot-weather exercise, especially on humid days when the sweating mechanism is less efficient. In addition, exercising in full sunlight increases the risk, but using a hat for protection from radiant energy in sunlight will help to protect the athlete from dehydration.

Finally, individuals should use extreme caution when they sit in saunas or hot tubs after exercising. They should immediately leave if they feel the least bit dizzy, weak, or faint. All people are dehydrated after exer-cising, and saunas and hot tubs can cause considerable additional fluid loss, even in the absence of visible sweating.

Educating runners about heat acclimatization, prehydration, and control of exercise intensity during training and racing should result in less frequent heat injury. Emergency care when such complications do arise should prevent the fatalities that still occur from the medical consequences of severe exertional heat stroke. Physicians should encourage heat-injury precautions, encouraging races to be run at cooler times of the day and canceled when wet-bulb temperatures exceed 28.0°C. Drinking 10 to 12

Table 15–1. MEDICAL ADVICE TO RUNNERS

Training

If possible, try to acclimatize yourself to heat if the race if is to be run in hot weather. Try to run at least 36 to 50 miles a week in training runs and take occasional longer runs. If you cannot comfortably run 15 miles 1 month before the marathon, you may have trouble running the race safely. Cut back mileage several days before the race to avoid exhaustion on race day.

Diet

Eat what you feel comfortable with. Extreme changes, such as carbohydrate loading, may affect you adversely. A slight increase in vitamin C and salt intake may be beneficial, especially in hot-weather races. Decreasing protein intake and substituting carbohydrates several days before the race may increase your stores of muscle glycogen.

Clothing

Wear light-colored clothing to protect against heat and, if possible, wear mesh clothing on a hot day. Natural fibers such as cotton will chafe less than synthetics. On a warm day, if you are comfortably warm at the starting line, you are probably overdressed.

Fluids

Drink early and often. Try to drink 1 pint of water 10 minutes before you run and at least half a cup of water every 15 minutes thereafter. Wetting the skin with hose sprays or sponges can bring temporary comfort but is no substitute for drinking. You are adequately hydrated before a race if your urine is a pale straw color. Since dehydration can actually blunt your thirst mechanism, don't let thirst be your guide for drinking. If you are not used to electrolyte-glucose drinks, you may want to avoid them during the race.

Running the Race

Begin slowly. On humid days, when the temperature is 75°F or greater, slow your pace by 45 to 60 s/mile. If you experience persistent localized pain, seek medical help. The signs of heat exhaustion are headache, tingling or pins and needles in the arms, back, and extremities, fatigue, a weak pulse, cool, moist skin, profuse sweating, and cold chills. The signs of heatstroke are headache, convulsions, altered behavior or mental state, red-hot skin, and absence of sweating. If you feel any of those symptoms, seek medical help or at least slow down or walk. Race officials will be instructed to remove you from the course if you appear to be at risk of injuring yourself. If you have a pre-existing injury or medical condition that could endanger your health, do not run.

Finish Line

Get out of the sun. Drink fluids. If you don't feel well or feel faint, seek medical help. Get into dry clothes as quickly as possible.

Source: From Editorial Staff: Marathon medicine. Emerg Med 17(16):89, 1985, with permission.

ounces of cold fluids, either diluted commercial drinks or fruit juice diluted with 2 to 3 parts cold water, is recommended to replenish fluid and potassium losses (see Chapter 6). Athletes should not wait to become thirsty, since 2 to 4 lb of fluid loss may occur before thirst becomes intense. Warm fluids should not be consumed, as they are absorbed more slowly than cold fluids. Commercial drinks are high in sugar and may cause abdominal cramps if not diluted. Cotton socks to absorb sweat, and white or light-colored clothing to reflect the sun's rays are also recommended. These preventive strategies are summarized in Table 15–1. The best prevention, though, is an informed runner who knows her limits.

The best treatment of heat injury is immediate rapid cooling performed on-site and without delay. In an Australian study,[31] the mean time it took to cool patients who had rectal temperatures $\geq 41.5°C$ was 37 minutes. No runners experienced the severe sequelae of heat stroke with this rapid-cooling approach. If treatment is delayed, major medical complications including fulminant rhabdomyolysis, acute renal failure requiring dialysis, hepatic necrosis, and disseminated intravascular coagulation can occur, although infrequently.[32,33] Common heat injuries and their treatment are seen in Table 15–2.

Hematologic Effects: Iron Status and Anemia

Obligatory iron loss through menstruation creates a potential risk for iron depletion and, if mild or subclinical, secondary anemia. Studies in apparently normal, healthy college-age women document the depletion of total body iron stores (by examination of stained bone marrow aspirates) in up to 25% of subjects.[34] Rates of iron deficiency among apparently healthy college athletes may be somewhat higher, as reported in one blood study.[35]

Confusion is likely to arise between true iron-deficiency anemia and the so-called pseudoanemia, or "runner's anemia," of en-

durance training, which is discussed in greater detail later in the chapter. A differentiation of true anemia (an absolute decrease in red cell mass) from pseudoanemia (a relative or dilutional decrease in hemoglobin value) cannot be made from measurement of the hemoglobin and hematocrit determinations alone. The clarification of true iron-deficiency anemia versus "pseudoanemia" in female athletes requires the direct measurement of body iron stores. This can be done by measurement of serum iron and iron-binding capacity or serum ferritin levels, which are normal in the case of the "pseudoanemia" but low in the case of true iron deficiency.[5] This differential is shown in Table 15–3.

In addition to menstrual losses, women face the additional possibility of ongoing iron loss during endurance training through additional body fluids such as sweat, urine, and feces. A significant loss of stores may occur over time if not accompanied by a balanced intake of iron in the diet. Recent studies have shown that some long-distance runners develop guaiac-positive stools during long-distance training and competition, which revert to normal within 72 hours.[36] Runners with anemia and guaiac-positive stools deserve a systematic medical investigation to rule out an intrinsic bowel problem unrelated to the exercise training.

The possible causes of blood loss include intestinal ischemia, stress gastritis, drug-induced lesions, and loss of blood from preexisting lesions. Another possible cause of iron loss is hematuria, as discussed in a later section. All these disorders may add to the burden of iron depletion in the athlete and create a true iron-deficient state.

The diagnosis of iron-deficiency anemia in women or men requires specific measurement of the serum iron parameters as noted previously. Low values for serum iron with a reciprocally increased serum iron binding capacity or a low serum ferritin level, or both, indicate the depletion of total body iron stores and the need for specific supplementation. Treatment should consist of 300 mg of ferrous sulfate given once or twice

Table 15–2. COMMON RACE INJURIES AND THEIR TREATMENT

Heat Cramps

A mild response to heat stress.

Treatment

If unaccompanied by serious complications, treat with rest, oral fluids, cooling down, stretching, ice and massage, and muscle massage.

Heat Exhaustion

A serious situation in which hypovolemia develops as a result of excessive fluid loss. The rectal temperature may range between 100 and 105°F or higher. The runner experiences lassitude or dizziness, nausea, headache, and muscle weakness. Although the runner is probably volume-depleted, sweating should be evident.

Treatment

For mild cases, treat the same as for heat cramps. For serious cases, including those with hypotension, persistent headache and vomiting, or altered mental states, initiate IV fluid resuscitation, cool vigorously (with an ice-water bath, for example), and consider transport to an emergency facility.

Heatstroke

Often characterized by motor disturbances, such as ataxia, and severe nervous system disturbances, such as confusion, delirium, or coma. Circulatory collapse and hypotension are possible. Rectal temperature usually exceeds 105°F but may be lower after a period of collapse and cooling. The skin is usually warm but the victim may not sweat, although sweating usually occurs in the initial stages.

Treatment

Cool the runner immediately with hosing or fanning and ice applied to major arteries such as the carotid, axillary, femoral, and popliteal. If rectal temperature monitoring is possible, place the patient in an ice-water bath. Massage her extremities, raise her legs, place her in the shade, and begin volume replacement with 1 to 2 liters of half-normal saline, although more may be required. Transport immediately to a medical facility.

Hypothermia, Exposure

Rare and most likely to occur in underdressed runners during cold-weather runs who either don't run fast enough to generate adequate heat or exhaust themselves early.

Treatment

Runners with a rectal temperature of 96.8°F or lower should be stripped of wet clothing, given warm clothing, and wrapped in blankets. If the runner is not shivering, she may be hypoglycemic. Give slightly sweet drinks. Monitor rectal temperature in those whose temperature is 91.2°F or lower.

Hypoglycemia

May present as sweating, tremor, mental confusion, and combativeness.

Treatment

Rest and sugar or electrolyte glucose drinks.

Hypovolemic Collapse

Seen most often in hot-weather races at the finish line, especially in runners who drink little or no liquid during the race. Hypotension, caused by diminished vasoconstriction, can lead to syncope. Runner's pulse will be weak and runner may be faint, cyanosed, or vomiting. It can occur as late as half an hour after the runner finishes the race if fluid intake is insufficient and will be worse if she's vomiting or has diarrhea.

Treatment

Take rectal temperature; have patient rest with legs raised; hydrate intravenously initially, then orally. Hypovolemia is usually self-limiting.

Source: Modified from Editorial Staff: Marathon medicine. Emerg Med 17(16):82, 1985, with permission.

daily for at least a year. Patients should be rechecked after that time to establish the return of serum iron stores to the normal range. Persistent abnormalities may de- serve further clinical investigation for sources of iron loss (menses, renal losses, gastrointestinal losses) if compliance with the treatment has been established.

Table 15-3. LABORATORY DIFFERENTIATION OF TRUE ANEMIA VERSUS PSEUDOANEMIA

	Pseudoanemia	True Anemia
Hemoglobin/ hematocrit	Decreased	Decreased
Red cell mass	Normal	Decreased
Plasma volume	Increased	Normal
Total blood volume	Increased	Normal
Iron/iron-binding capacity (IBC)	Normal	Decreased
Ferritin	Normal	Decreased

Source: From Siegel AJ,[5] with permission.

It is reasonable to suggest routine iron supplementation for female athletes undergoing intense training, just as is recommended for pregnant women, because both conditions increase iron requirements. Routine iron supplementation, however, does not yield demonstrable benefits for the athlete with adequate iron stores.

Even in the absence of anemia, a decrease in body iron stores may cause a diminished exercise performance or capacity, related to the role of iron in the tissue cytochrome and myoglobin systems. Recent reports have highlighted the importance of identifying borderline iron-deficiency states in athletes, even in the absence of anemia, through measurement of serum ferritin levels. Low serum ferritin levels indicate a need for treatment, even in the presence of normal serum iron levels. However, normal ferritin levels may not always exclude iron deficiency. Acute inflammation, such as can be caused by infection or injury from heavy training, can transiently raise serum ferritin levels to normal range. Therefore, when iron deficiency is strongly suspected, ferritin levels should be assessed after the athlete has recovered from any febrile illness or stopped training for 2 or 3 days. Symptoms of fatigue and declining performance may be identical in "overtraining" and in marginal iron-deficiency states. Clinical observations suggest that repletion of diminished iron stores may reverse these symptoms and improve exercise performance.[37]

"Runner's Diarrhea"

More common than gastrointestinal bleeding is the rather frequent occurrence of runner's diarrhea, which is an expression of increased bowel motility akin to the irritable bowel syndrome seen with emotional stress in a large number of individuals. Manifestations range from minor abdominal cramping to severe, watery diarrhea during prolonged strenuous exercise, which can interfere with performance and is intensified by the stress of competition. This condition, sometimes termed "runner's trots," is often successfully treated with precompetition doses of antispasmodic agents.[38]

Effects on the Urinary Tract

As discussed in the subsequent section on "athletic pseudonephritis," many apparent urinary abnormalities in athletes are transient, benign conditions, although more serious complications can sometimes arise. A positive Hemastix reaction without detectable blood on microscopic analysis of urine is suggestive of myoglobinuria. This reaction may be quite common, if not universal, in marathon runners after peak efforts, resulting from transient rhabdomyolysis during extended physical exertion.[39] Elevations of serum creatine kinase up to 30 times normal have been noted in marathon runners without perceived urinary symptoms or evidence of injury. Other studies have shown transitory decrements in creatinine clearance following marathon competition, which may be prerenal or related to volume depletion rather than due to tubular injury.[40]

Whereas exertional rhabdomyolysis is common, acute renal failure is extremely rare.[33] It has been reported in patients with sickle cell trait, who are at increased risk of renal tubular necrosis following rhabdomyolysis, which may then proceed to other complications such as disseminated intravascular clotting.

Heat stress, prolonged strenuous exercise, muscle injury, and urinary abnormalities are interrelated. It is crucial for physi-

Table 15–4. DIFFERENTIAL DIAGNOSIS FOR ABNORMAL TEST RESULTS

Laboratory Findings	Clinical Condition	Exercise-Induced Findings
Low hemoglobin, low hematocrit	Anemia (true iron deficiency)	Pseudoanemia (see Table 15–3)
Abnormal urinalysis (hematuria, proteinuria)	Renal disease	Transient changes
Positive test for GI bleeding	Intrinsic gastrointestinal pathology	Transient finding due to maximal exercise
Abnormal liver enzymes: lactic acid dehydrogenase (LDH), serum glutamic oxaloacetic transaminase (SGOT)	Hepatic inflammation (true hepatitis)	Transient muscle injury accompanied by release of enzymes from skeletal muscle that are also present in liver tissue (pseudohepatitis)
Elevation of total creatine kinase and the MB isoenzyme	Myocardial disease	Chronic skeletal muscle injury or exercise-induced rhabdomyolysis

Note: The pseudosyndromes listed above (last column) are more common in rigorously training endurance athletes than in beginners.
Source: From Siegel AJ,[5] with permission.

cians to identify runners with acute hypovolemia occurring in heat-stress injury so that they can institute the rapid rehydration that will prevent attendant renal injury. Cases of acute renal failure following severe dehydration in marathon runners have been reported, although such injury is clinically preventable.[33] There is no evidence that permanent or progressive renal injury results from prolonged strenuous training, as done by long-distance runners. Reported acute increases in serum creatinine levels are readily reversible with rest and rehydration. Progressive renal damage from recurrent low-grade rhabdomyolysis and myoglobinuria is a theoretical possibility but has not been demonstrated to date. Again, prevention is the best treatment, and runners should be encouraged to take fluids liberally during and immediately after strenuous physical effort. The differential diagnostic features of urinary sediment changes and other diagnostic tests are shown in Table 15–4. Prevention and treatment are summarized in Tables 15–1 and 15–2.

Exercise-Induced Asthma

Exercise-induced asthma (EIA) is a relatively common, readily diagnosable and treatable form of reversible bronchospasm.[41] It occurs with high frequency in individuals with an allergic or asthmatic background, in whom exercise provokes or increases symptoms. Bronchospasm also occurs in subjects who do not have a clinical history of overt asthma, in whom symptoms may be unappreciated or subclinical until the additional work of breathing during exercise is imposed. The frequency with which such reactions are detected depends upon the sensitivity of measurements used, as well as on the type of exercise.

The typical course of symptoms is a slow onset of bronchospasm as one starts exercising, reaching a peak in 6 to 8 minutes. Symptoms often stabilize or subside if exercise is continued, and some of these individuals can exercise through their attacks after some initial difficulty. The postexercise rebound is well described, as difficulty may return or intensify after cessation of activity. Figure 15–1 shows the typical pattern of observed pulmonary function parameters with the relationship to time in healthy subjects and in those with EIA. The four parameters of lung function shown reflect the impairment during and after exertion. Simple spirometry with a measure of the timed or 1-second vital capacity is adequate to confirm suspected clinical cases in most instances.

Exercise-induced asthma causes the same bronchial smooth-muscle contraction that results from allergen-triggered asthmatic

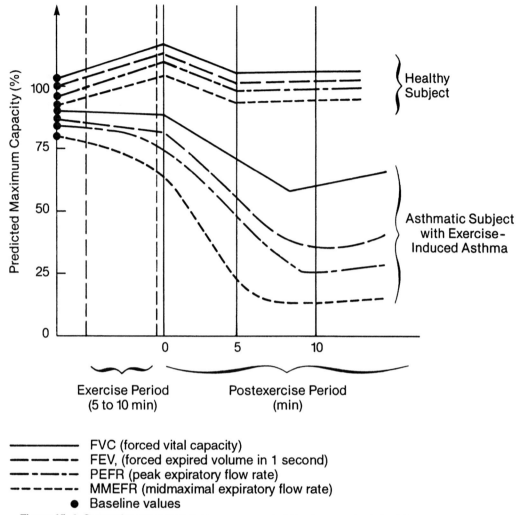

Figure 15–1. Comparison of spirometric measurements following exercise in healthy subjects and in patients with exercise-induced asthma. (Adapted from Gerhard H, and Schachter FN: Exercise-induced asthma. Postgrad Med 67(3):93, 1980, with permission.)

response. Recent investigations, however, reveal that EIA is not triggered by an allergic response, but rather by reactions of large and small airways to changes in humidity during cold-air breathing. McFadden and Ingram[41] have shown that the magnitude of the bronchoconstrictive response to a fixed exercise task or to a fixed level of ventilation depends on the temperature and/or water content of the inspired air. Lower air temperatures and lower humidity favor the obstructive response, which does not occur in susceptible subjects when inspired air is fully saturated with water at body temperature. Airway cooling from heat loss during high ventilatory work is the specific precipitant. These findings explain why corticosteroids are ineffective in treating exercise-induced asthma, whereas warming of inspired air through a face mask can be effective.

A wide range of treatments is available for patients with EIA, including warming of inspired air in cold weather as a preventive measure, and use of specific pharmacologic agents employed in the treatment of traditional asthma. Those treatments approved

Table 15–5. ANTIASTHMATIC MEDICATIONS APPROVED BY THE INTERNATIONAL OLYMPIC COMMITTEE FOR THE OLYMPIC GAMES*

Medication	Aerosol	Oral
Theophylline	NA	Yes
Cromolyn sodium	Yes	NA
Albuterol	Yes	Yes
Terbutaline sulfate	Yes	Yes
Corticosteroid	Yes	Yes

*Drug Commission of IOC requires name of athlete, country, drug, and dosage.

Source: From Eisenstadt WS, Nicholas SS, Velick G, et al: The Physician and Sportsmedicine 12(12):100, 1984, with permission.

by the International Olympic Committee for the Olympic Games are listed in Table 15–5. These agents can be taken as pre-exercise doses to block the onset of or to minimize bronchoconstriction. A warm-up period is often useful in reducing EIA, but inhalation of a bronchodilator just prior to peak exercise is highly beneficial. Sympathomimetics are disallowed in some competitive situations, so that alternatives such as cromolyn sodium must be used. Cromolyn is not a bronchodilator and is most effective when administered 30 minutes prior to peak effort. Physicians must be aware of these special circumstances as well as of the range of treatments available to the recreational athlete.

Persons susceptible to exercise-induced asthma should be encouraged to participate in sports and exercise, which may have a beneficial effect on general physical conditioning and preservation of lung function. The adequately informed primary care physician can enhance the capability of patients to lead full and active lives despite the need for specific treatment.

Exercise-Induced Anaphylaxis

Individuals with a history of allergic reactions such as childhood eczema, seasonal rhinitis, or even asthma are prone to a second exercise-related reaction that begins with diffuse itching and may result in generalized hives or urticaria. Such symptoms may occur after years or decades of being allergy-free and may be limited to minor discomfort. The reaction can, however, progress to generalized angioedema, including facial swelling and laryngeal spasm, with compromise of the upper airways. This reaction was reported in a group of young athletes after a variety of sports and may be unpredictable in occurrence and severity for any individual.[42] Some authors have suggested that exposure to a specific allergen such as shellfish, to which the individual is subclinically sensitized, may then combine with exercise to trigger the allergic response. Exercise causes mast cells to release vasoactive mediators similar to those in cold-induced urticaria, in which histamine is released in the skin after cold exposure. Susceptibility is not related to training or expertise, and exercise-induced anaphylaxis has been reported in national champions and in world record holders.[43] Management can entail preventive measures such as the administration of mild antihistamines or perhaps cromolyn sodium prior to exercise. However, these treatments are only partially effective at best and do not completely prevent the reaction. Such pretreatment may be necessary for individuals only at times of peak risk, since the urticarial response may occur only seasonally, when allergic predisposition is heightened. Just as a shellfish-allergic patient avoids eating shellfish, avoiding specific foods prior to exercise may control or eliminate the allergic response in these individuals.

The pathogenesis of exercise-induced anaphylaxis is identical to immunologic-mediated anaphylaxis, even though the trigger is physical rather than allergic.[42] Effector mast cells fire to release histamine, the slow-reacting substance of anaphylaxis, bradykinins, and other mediators, which then cause the angioedema. Facial swelling is an indication for specific emergency measures, such as the intramuscular administration of 8 mg of dexamethasone or the subcutaneous administration of aqueous epinephrine 1:1000, 0.1 to 0.3 mL, along with the insertion of an IV tube for fluid administration.

Hypotension may develop from generalized, increased vascular permeability, which may require stabilization with fluids and vaso-pressive drugs. Dopamine (400 mg) and D5W (500 mL), given intravenously at an appropriate rate, may sustain blood pressure in the face of circulatory collapse. While potentially life-threatening, exercise-induced anaphylaxis has not yet resulted in a reported fatality. Patients who have had this reaction, as well as individuals with known bee-sting sensitivity (hymenoptera), should have epinephrine available for administration if severe allergic manifestations develop.

Exercise-Induced Urticaria

In the spectrum of allergic reactions to exercise, some individuals may develop blotchy red rashes, sometimes with itching, during a workout. This is called exercise-induced hives or urticaria, and it results from histamine release in the skin owing to rapid superficial temperature changes. Like exercise-induced asthma, exercise-induced urticaria may occur more readily with temperature provocation, either cold or warm. Local symptoms of cold urticaria are redness, itching, wheals, or edema in the skin, not the subcutaneous swelling seen in anaphylaxis, as described previously. Systemic symptoms and circulatory collapse do not occur.

This condition is benign and can be handled with reassurance to the athlete. Low doses of antihistamines may diminish symptoms and may be prescribed if the side effect of drowsiness is not more bothersome than the itching.

PSEUDOSYNDROMES IN ATHLETES

Pseudoanemia ("Runner's Anemia")

As previously mentioned, athletes may show a low hemoglobin concentration without actually suffering from depleted iron stores. Systematic observations have documented a drop in hemoglobin, hematocrit, and red blood cell count at the end of a 9-week training program in previously sedentary college women.[37] Values may fall to low-normal or within abnormal ranges during progressive training, with a return to baseline upon resumption of sedentary status. "Pseudoanemia" also occurs in male athletes, owing to hemodilution from an increase in plasma volume. Studies of red cell mass in athletic pseudoanemia show normal or high values, with low hemoglobin parameters resulting from an expanded plasma volume. The specific measurement of body iron stores, or its reflection in normal values for serum iron and iron-binding capacity or ferritin levels, establishes this dilutional cause of a low hemoglobin concentration.

"Athletic Pseudonephritis"

The occurrence of exercise-related urinary abnormalities has been extensively reviewed in the literature and in medical-specialty books, with the term "athletic pseudonephritis" applied to conditions associated with abnormal urinary sediments.[40,44] Severe volume depletion and dehydration can, indeed, lead to proteinuria and hematuria with the presence of formed elements such as proteinaceous casts. A prospective study of 50 male physician marathon runners showed that microscopic hematuria occurred in 18% in initial postrace urinalyses, but cleared within 24 to 48 hours.[45]

Exercise-related hematuria appears to be a frequent and self-limited benign condition that does not warrant extensive invasive work-up. Gross hematuria occurred in only 1 out of 50 subjects and must be considered a complication of nontraumatic sports such as running. A work-up of a series of patients with so-called 10,000-meter hematuria identified bladder trauma as the cause of this hematuria.[46] Other studies suggest that the bleeding may come from the kidneys. Concomitant bladder or renal pathology cannot be summarily excluded after gross hematuria related to exercise; therefore, it is reasonable to suggest intravenous pyelography and cystoscopy to exclude specific causes.

Serum Enzyme Abnormalities: Muscle Injury and Pseudohepatitis

Prolonged strenuous exercise may be associated with transient elevations of skeletal muscle enzymes, which are also present in hepatocytes or liver cells. Serum levels of glutamic-oxalo-acetic transaminase and lactic dehydrogenase are routinely used as screening tests for hepatic dysfunction, and elevated levels of these enzymes may frequently be assumed to represent hepatitis in runners. Measurement of specific serum enzymes such as creatine kinase can resolve this dilemma, so that elevations of creatine kinase and these other enzymes indicate transient muscle injury rather than liver disease in the endurance-trained athlete. Several recent studies indicate that athletes may have enzyme elevations two to three times the upper limits of normal compared with age-matched and sex-matched sedentary individuals (see Table 15–4). These values may increase tenfold after racing, because of transient exertional rhabdomyolysis.[39] These findings are often accompanied by muscle soreness in the athlete and indicate the need for rest and maintenance of hydration. Specific clinical symptoms such as persistent headache, nausea, vomiting, or flank pain should lead to the investigation of impaired renal function or other complications, as noted in the prior sections.

One avenue for excluding liver disease in a runner with abnormal enzyme profiles is to measure liver-specific "enzymes" such as alanine aminotransferase and γ-glutamyl transpeptidase. Some transient increases in these liver-specific proteins have been documented in marathon runners after racing, indicating possible release from hepatocytes due to indirect trauma or decreased hepatic blood flow.[47] Persistence of abnormal liver function tests might warrant measurement of serum hepatitis markers to exclude chronic hepatitis, but need not lead to invasive testing such as a liver biopsy. Many runners have been referred to specialists for consideration of this procedure on the basis of the muscle injury parameters, as described earlier. Such invasive testing is usually unnecessary and should be avoided.

With reference to the biliary tract, it should be noted that some individuals have a genetic condition (Gilbert's disease) in which bilirubin conjugation may be impaired under physiologic stress such as strenuous exercise, infections, or prolonged fasting. Such individuals may develop an increase primarily in unconjugated serum bilirubin and may appear mildly jaundiced. This condition is benign and asymptomatic, and can be detected by somewhat elevated levels of unconjugated bilirubin in the face of otherwise normal liver enzymes. This elevation of unconjugated bilirubin is usually transient, whereas liver disease usually leads to persistent elevations of unconjugated bilirubin in the face of elevated liver enzymes. These findings are in contrast to those in patients with chronic hemolytic anemias, in whom pigment gallstones may be formed because of an increased biliary excretion of breakdown products of hemolysis, leading to significant elevations of direct bilirubin. Pigment gallstones have been reported in long-distance runners and attributed to runner's hemolysis, although this must be a very rare and unusual occurrence.[48]

Pseudomyocarditis

In addition to the abnormalities in total creatine kinase that indicate transient muscle injury, as noted earlier, chronic endurance sports participation may lead to transient elevations of the MB isoenzyme or heart-specific fraction of creatine kinase in serum.[49] Such elevations may at times be quantitatively similar to findings in patients with a variety of heart diseases such as cardiomyopathy, myocarditis, or injury secondary to ischemic heart disease.

Large increases in the serum total creatine kinase and CK-MB activities may be found in both men and women after competition. Cardiac isoenzymes are present in trained skeletal muscle, perhaps on the basis of chronic muscle fiber injury and repair.[50] Studies using heart scan techniques fail to reveal any underlying heart injury in these individuals. Abnormal elevations of serum CK-MB in an otherwise asymptomatic female athlete without cardiorespiratory symptoms can be reasonably attributed to an exercise-induced injury to skeletal muscle and not to a myocardial source (see Table 15–4).

SCREENING THE ATHLETE FOR MEDICAL CLEARANCE

With an estimated 25 to 50 million young women engaging in sports activity, some basic concepts of medical clearance prior to sports participation justifiably arise. A sports-related questionnaire for athletes provides an opportunity for health screening with the purpose of identifying predisposing medical conditions that might lead to complications during sports participation. A sample questionnaire is included in Appendix 15–1, which addresses the major factors of sports injury as complications for young athletes and also screens for pre-existing medical conditions, medication allergies, and other possible complications. Such a medical checklist is useful in preventing problems during training and competition, such as exercise-induced asthma, anaphylaxis, and other conditions discussed in this chapter. This gives the physician an opportunity to screen for areas of major concern such as possible familial heart disease, and also to practice prevention with regard to conditions such as sports-related anemia and oligomenorrhea, which commonly arise. A sample physical examination form for recording findings is given in Appendix 15–2, and a list of medical conditions disqualifying an individual for sports participation as provided through guidelines of the American Medical Association is found in

Appendix 15–3. This focuses on acute conditions that should be evaluated prior to competitive sports participation. These sample materials are useful for identifying pre-existing medical conditions that may influence or affect sports participation, and they help prepare the athlete for safer training and participation.

CAUTION: WHEN NOT TO EXERCISE

While the preceding sections emphasize the health benefits of exercise, the question remains of how much and how soon. Chest pain, dyspnea, or syncopal episodes should be contraindications to exercise until the causes are established and relieved, and serious medical conditions are excluded. Illnesses such as diabetes, ischemic heart disease, and arthritis may in fact be ameliorated by appropriate low levels of exercise. Safe limits can be established through cardiovascular assessment, including exercise testing in such cases. Cardiac, pulmonary, and musculoskeletal diseases may make exercise difficult, but patients respond positively to exercise training, with improved levels of function. Old age itself is not a contraindication to regular exercise, which in fact facilitates balanced nutrition and cardiovascular health.[51] In addition, physical activity correlates with a reduced risk of depression in healthy adults of all ages.[52]

After musculoskeletal injury, orthopedic surgery, and even general surgery, a graduated return to exercise and training is necessary. The intensity and duration of workouts should be decreased to start, with training progressively increased at increments of no more than 10% per week. A gradual return to exercise intensity promotes smooth recovery and reduces risk of reinjury or clinical setback.

Similarly, athletes must adjust to the realities of medical illness, including the impact on exercise capacity of minor illnesses such as viral syndromes, flulike illnesses, and especially respiratory infections. Athletes must take time off from training during febrile illness, as acute illness places stress on all organ system reserves and exercise would pose the danger of prolonging the illness and incurring additional injury. Many viral illnesses are systemic; that is, all organ systems are subject to transient viral exposure. Exercise at such times can be hazardous and even lead to arrhythmias and collapse during workouts or competition. As a working guideline, I emphasize to athletes the importance of rest as well as stress in training, and point out the necessity of allowing the body to recover from intercurrent illness in order to make future training safe and productive.

Appendix A gives greater detail on exercise following an infection.

SUMMARY

This chapter has addressed various medical conditions that may arise in sports-active women and that present clinical dilemmas to the office practitioner. On the one hand, athletes may develop abnormal clinical or laboratory findings that represent physiologic adjustments to training and are not indications of underlying illness. On the other hand, athletes do place themselves at risk for developing problems such as transient hematuria, gastrointestinal bleeding, anemia, and heat injury, which require specific monitoring to rule out non–exercise-related conditions.

Careful assessment of the individual athlete, together with a background fund of information, will enable the practicing physician to provide reassurance when appropriate and to respond to underlying clinical problems as they may arise.

The knowledgeable physician can assist the sports-active patient in enhancing her athletic goals while reducing concern over sports-related symptoms or conditions. When dealing with athletes, the physician should monitor and prescribe exercise as a coach, who must counsel sound principles of moderation and consistency over time. In this fashion, the physician can promote health-enhancing levels of exercise for inactive patients, and facilitate long-range planning for athletes who are likely to experience overuse injury through an imbalance of stress over rest and recovery. Whether the goal is an improvement in cardiorespiratory fitness from recreational exercise or competition from structured sports participation, moderation remains an important preventive and rehabilitative prescription.

REFERENCES

1. Council on Ethical and Judicial Affairs, American Medical Association: Gender disparities in clinical decision making. JAMA 226:559, 1991.
2. Healy B: Women's health, public welfare. JAMA 226:566, 1991.
3. Harris SS, Caspersen CJ, DeFriese GH, et al: Physical activity counseling for healthy adults as a primary preventive intervention in the clinical setting: Report for the US Preventive Services Task Force. JAMA 261:3588, 1989.
4. Bunch TW: Blood test abnormalities in runners. Mayo Clin Proc 55:113, 1980.
5. Siegel AJ: Understanding abnormal lab values in the female athlete. Contemp Obstet Gynecol 25:73, 1985.
6. Huston TP, Puffer JC, and Rodney WM: The athletic heart syndrome. N Engl J Med 313:24, 1985.
7. Dollar AL, Kragel AH, Fernicola DJ, et al: Composition of atherosclerotic plaques in coronary arteries in women <40 years of age with fatal coronary artery disease and implications for plaque reversibility. Am J Cardiol 67:1223, 1991.
8. Manson JE, Stampfer MJ, Colditz GA, et al: A prospective study of aspirin use and primary prevention of cardiovascular disease in women. JAMA 266:521, 1991.
9. Appel LJ, and Bush T: Preventing heart disease in women: Another role for aspirin? (Editorial). JAMA 266:565, 1991.
10. Steingart RM, Packer M, Hamm P, et al: Sex differences in the management of coronary artery disease. N Engl J Med 325:226, 1991.
11. Ayanian JZ, and Epstein AM: Differences in

the use of procedures between women and men hospitalized for coronary heart disease. N Engl J Med 325:221, 1991.

12. Gordon T: Cardiovascular risk factors in women. Pract Cardiol 5:137, 1974.

13. Wood PD, Stepanick ML, Williams PT, et al: The effects on plasma lipoproteins of a prudent weight-reducing diet, with or without exercise, in overweight men and women. N Engl J Med 325:461, 1991.

14. Somers VK, Conway J, Johnston J, et al: Effects of endurance training on baroreflex sensitivity and blood pressure in borderline hypertension. Lancet 337:1363, 1991.

15. Helmrich SP, Ragland DR, Leung RW, et al: Physical activity and reduced occurrence of non–insulin-dependent diabetes mellitus. N Engl J Med 325:147, 1991.

16. Marcus BH, Albrecht AE, Niaura RS, et al: Usefulness of physical exercise for maintaining smoking cessation in women. Am J Cardiol 68:406, 1991.

17. Chen Y, Home SL, Dosman JA: Increased susceptibility to lung dysfunction in female smokers. Am Rev Respir Dis 143:1224, 1991.

18. Williamson DF, Madans J, Anda RF, et al: Smoking cessation and severity of weight gain in a national cohort. N Engl J Med 324:739, 1991.

19. Moffatt RJ, and Owens SG: Cessation from cigarette smoking: Changes in body weight, body composition, resting metabolism, and energy consumption. Metabolism 40:465, 1991.

20. Daughton DM, Heatley SA, Prendergast JJ, et al: Effect of transdermal nicotine delivery as an adjunct to low-intervention smoking cessation therapy: A randomized, placebo-controlled, double-blind study. Arch Intern Med 151:749, 1991.

21. Hurt RD, Lauger GG, Offord KP, et al: Nicotine-replacement therapy with use of a transdermal nicotine patch: A randomized double-blind placebo-controlled trial. Mayo Clin Proc 65:1529, 1990.

22. Egeland GM, Kuller LH, Matthews RA, et al: Hormone replacement therapy and lipoprotein changes during early menopause. Obstet Gynecol 76:776, 1990.

23. Sullivan JM, Vander Zwaag R, Hughes JP, et al: Estrogen replacement and coronary artery disease: Effect on survival in postmenopausal women. Arch Intern Med 150:2557, 1990.

24. Glazer G: Atherogenic effects of anabolic steroids on serum lipid levels—a literature review. Arch Intern Med 151:1925, 1991.

25. Lee IM, Paffenbarger RS, Hsieh C, et al: Physical activity and risk of developing colorectal cancer among college alumni. J Natl Cancer Inst 83:1324, 1991.

26. Dupont WD, and Page DL: Menopausal estrogen replacement and breast cancer. Arch Intern Med 151:67, 1991.

27. Wyndham CH, Morrison JF, and Williams CG: Heat reactions of male and female caucasians. J Appl Physiol 20:357, 1965.

28. Wells CL: Sexual differences in heat stress response. Phys Sportsmed 5(9):78, 1977.

29. Drinkwater BL, Kupprat JC, Denton JE, et al: Heat tolerance of female distance runners. Ann NY Acad Sci 301:777, 1977.

30. Statement of the American College of Sports Medicine: Prevention of heat injuries during distance running. J Sports Med 9(7):105, 1976.

31. Sutton JR: Heatstroke from running. JAMA 243:1896, 1980.

32. Koppes GM, Daly JJ, Coltman CA, et al: Exertion-induced rhabdomyolysis with acute renal failure and disseminated intravascular coagulation in sickle cell trait. Am J Med 63:313, 1977.

33. Stewart PJ, and Posen GA: Case report: Acute renal failure following a marathon. Phys Sportsmed 8(4):61, 1980.

34. Scott DE, and Pritchard JA: Iron deficiency in healthy young college women. JAMA 199:147, 1967.

35. Steenkamp I, Fuller C, Graves J, et al: Marathon running fails to influence RBC survival rates in iron-repleted women. Phys Sportsmed 14(5):89, 1986.

36. McMahon LJ, Ryan MJ, Larson D, et al: Occult gastrointestinal blood loss in marathon runners. Ann Intern Med 100:846, 1984.

37. Martin DE, Vroon DH, May DF, et al: Physiological changes in elite male distance runners training for Olympic competition. Phys Sportsmed 14(1):152, 1986.

38. Priebe WM, and Priebe J: Runners' diarrhea (RD): Prevalence and clinical symptomatology. Am J Gastroenterol 79:827, 1984.

39. Siegel AJ, Silverman LM, and Lopez RE: Creatine kinase elevations in marathon runners, relationship to training and competition. Yale J Biol Med 53:275, 1980.

40. Poortsmans JR: Exercise and renal function. Sports Med 1:125, 1984.

41. McFadden ER, and Ingram RH: Exercise-induced asthma. Seminars in Medicine of the Beth Israel Hospital, Boston 301:763, 1979.

42. Sheffer AL, and Austen KF: New exercise-induced anaphylactic syndrome identified. Mod Med 1:96, 1981.

43. Siegel AJ: Exercise induced anaphylaxis. Phys Sportsmed 8(1):55, 1980.

44. Gardner KD Jr: Athletic pseudonephritis al-

teration of urine sediment by athletic competition. JAMA 161:613, 1956.

45. Siegel AJ, Hennekens CH, Solomon HS, et al: Exercise-related hematuria findings in a group of marathon runners. JAMA 241:391, 1979.

46. Blacklock NS: Bladder trauma in the long distance runner. 10,000 metres hematuria. Br J Urol 49:129, 1977.

47. Apple FS, and Rogers MA: Serum and muscle alanine aminotransferase activities in marathon runners. JAMA 252:626, 1984.

48. Leslie BR, and Sanders NW: Runner's hemolysis and pigment gallstones. N Engl J Med 313:1230, 1985.

49. Siegel AJ, Silverman LM, and Holman BL: Elevated creatine kinase MB isoenzyme levels in marathon runners. JAMA 246:1049, 1981.

50. Siegel AJ, Silverman LM, and Evans WJ: Elevated skeletal muscle creatine kinase MB isoenzyme levels in marathon runners. JAMA 250:2835, 1983.

51. Evans WJ, and Meredith CN: Exercise and nutrition in the elderly. In Munro HM and Danford DE (eds): Nutrition, Aging, and the Elderly. Plenum, New York, p 89.

52. Camacho TC, Roberts RE, Lazarus NB, et al: Physical activity and depression: Evidence from the Alameda County Study. Am J Epidemiol 134:220, 1991.

APPENDIX 15-1

Sport Candidate's Questionnaire

Name _____ Age _____ Date of birth _____

School _____ Grade _____ Sex _____

Athlete's address _____ Tel. No. _____

Parent's name & address _____ Tel. No. _____

Regular physician _____ Tel. No. _____

Medical History	Yes	No	Past or Present Please Circle Item(s) in ( )
1.	—	—	Discuss with a doctor a (health problem, injury, diet)?
2.	—	—	Discuss with a doctor (emotional problem, stress management)?
3.	—	—	Any close family member with (diabetes, migraines, asthma, heart trouble, high blood pressure)?
4.	—	—	Any family member who died suddenly under age 50, excluding accidents?
5.	—	—	Any (illnesses lasting more than 1 wk, chronic or recurrent illness)?
6.	—	—	Any (hospitalizations or surgery)?
7.	—	—	Any (injuries or illnesses) requiring treatment by a doctor?
8.	—	—	Any allergies (hay fever, hives, asthma, bee sting, or drug allergies)?
9.	—	—	Any medications taken regularly or within last 6 mo?
10.	—	—	Any neck injury?
11.	—	—	Any (concussions, skull fracture, loss of memory or consciousness, convulsions or epilepsy, headaches)?
12.	—	—	Any (eyeglasses, contact lenses, decreased vision, or temporary loss of vision)?
13.	—	—	Any (hearing loss, perforated eardrum, recurrent ear infections)?
14.	—	—	Any (broken nose, nosebleeds, dentures, braces, bridges, tooth caps)?
15.	—	—	Have you ever fainted *during* exercise?

Sport Candidate's Questionnaire—*Continued*

Medical History	*Yes*	*No*	*Past or Present* Please Circle Item(s) in ( )
16.	—	—	Any (heart trouble, murmur, arrhythmias, chest pain, high blood pressure)?
17.	—	—	Do you (smoke, drink alcohol, take drugs)?
18.	—	—	Any (pneumonia, tuberculosis, chronic cough)?
19.	—	—	Any loss of, or serious injury to (eye, testicle, kidney, lung)?
20.	—	—	Girls, any menstrual problems? Age at first menstrual period _____
21.	—	—	Any (hernias, kidney problems, ulcer, heartburn, bowel problems, hepatitis)?
22.	—	—	Any (diabetes, thyroid disorders, anemia, abnormal bleeding)?
23.	—	—	Any knee injury (sprain, fracture, dislocation, surgery, chronic pain)?
24.	—	—	Any ankle injury (sprain, fracture, dislocation, surgery, chronic pain)?
25.	—	—	Any bone (fracture, infection, deformity)?
26.	—	—	Any (injuries, sprains, dislocations, surgery) in (shoulder, wrist, finger, or any other joint)?
27.	—	—	Any skin disorders (recurrent rash, fungal infection, boils, athlete's foot)?
28.	—	—	Any injury not mentioned? _____
29.	—	—	Any (heat exhaustion, heat stroke)?
30.	—	—	Any reasons why you were unable to participate in the past or should not be able to in the future? _____

31. Date of last tetanus booster ____ _____

Explain Any Questions Answered With "Yes" Below

(please be as *specific* as possible: dates, treating physician, list medications, residual problems, etc.)

_____

_____

_____

Signature of student athlete _____ Date _____

Signature of parent or physician _____ Date _____

Source: From Gregg JR, and Spindler KP: Screening school-age athletes. Drug Therapy, September 1985, p 75, with permission.

Appendix 15–2

Physical Examination Form

Name _____ Age _____ Date of birth _____

School _____ Grade _____

Height (in) _____ Weight (lb) _____ Pulse _____ BP (sitting, right arm) _____

Vision (acuity) R __/__ L __/__ Check one: __ normal without glasses __ normal with glasses

_____ abnormal without glasses _____ abnormal with glasses

OK	*Circle in ( ) if Abnormality Present or Normal Condition Absent*	*Comments*	*Initials*
1. _____	Dental (dental prosthesis, severe caries)	_____	_____
2. _____	Skin, scalp, lymphatics (active infection, acne, rashes, adenopathy)	_____	_____
3. _____	Eyes/fundi (vision-color, depth, peripheral; pupils, extraocular movements, fundi)	_____	_____
4. _____	Ears, nose, throat (hearing, tympanic membranes, nasal septum, tonsils, throat)	_____	_____
5. _____	Neck (soft tissue) (adenopathy, thyroid, carotid pulses)	_____	_____
6. _____	Cardiovascular (PMI, pulses [femoral-branchial], rhythm, murmurs)	_____	_____
7. _____	Chest and lung (breath sounds, shape, excursion)	_____	_____
8. _____	Abdomen (hepatosplenomegaly, masses, costovertebral angle tenderness)	_____	_____
9. _____	Genitalia-hernia (scrotal contents, inguinal region)	_____	_____
10. _____	Sexual maturity (Tanner staging)	_____	_____
11. _____	Neurologic (sensation, deep-tendon reflexes, mental status)	_____	_____
12. _____	Orthopedic (all for active range of motion and strength besides information in parentheses)	_____	_____
_____	a. Cervical spine/back (scoliosis)	_____	_____
_____	b. Shoulders (symmetry)	_____	_____
_____	c. Arm/elbow/wrist/hand	_____	_____
_____	d. Hip/foot (passive range of motion hip, foot stance with weight bearing)	_____	_____
_____	e. Knee (ligamentous stability)	_____	_____
_____	f. Ankle (ligamentous stability)	_____	_____
_____	g. Flexibility	_____	_____
_____	h. % Body fat (specify method)	_____	_____
13. _____	Laboratory tests		

Hg _____ g/dl Hct _____ %

Transferrin saturation _____ %

Urinalysis _____

Other _____

14. _____ Review by team physician

_____ a. No athletic participation

_____ b. Limited participation, e.g., _____

_____ c. Clearance withheld until: _____

_____ d. Full unlimited participation

15. Comment/Advice: _____

_____

_____

16. Team physician's signature _____ Date _____

Source: From Gregg JR, and Spindler KP: Screening school-age athletes. Drug Therapy, September 1985, p 77, with permission.

Appendix 15–3

Disqualifying Conditions (Indicated by an X) for Sports Participation, by Type of Sport

Condition	Collision*	Contact†	Noncontact‡	Others§
General				
Acute infection (respiratory, genitourinary, infectious mononucleosis, hepatitis, active rheumatic fever, active tuberculosis)	X	X	X	X
Obvious physical immaturity in comparison with other competitors in group	X	X		
Hemorrhagic disease (hemophilia, purpura, other serious bleeding tendencies)	X	X	X	
Diabetes, inadequately controlled	X	X	X	X
Diabetes controlled	‖	‖	‖	‖
Jaundice	X	X	X	X
Ears				
Absence or loss of function of one eye	X	X		
Respiratory System				
Tuberculosis (active or symptomatic)	X	X	X	X
Severe pulmonary insufficiency	X	X	X	X
Cardiovascular System				
Mitral stenosis, aortic stenosis, aortic insufficiency, coarctation of aorta, cyanotic heart disease, recent carditis of any cause	X	X	X	X
Hypertension, organic	X	X	X	X
Previous heart surgery for congenital or acquired heart disease	¶	¶	¶	¶
Liver				
Enlargement	X	X		

*Football, rugby, hockey, lacrosse, etc.
†Baseball, soccer, basketball, wrestling, etc.
‡Cross-country, track, tennis, crew, swimming, etc.
§Bowling, golf, archery, field events, etc.
‖No exclusions necessary.
¶Each patient should be judged individually in conjunction with cardiologist and surgeon.
Source: From Blum RW: Preparticipation evaluation of the adolescent athlete. Postgrad Med 78:2, 52–55, 1985, with permission.

CHAPTER 16

Cardiovascular Issues

PAMELA S. DOUGLAS, M.D.

AEROBIC CAPACITY

CARDIAC FUNCTION IN
RESPONSE TO EXERCISE

EXERCISE
ELECTROCARDIOGRAPHIC
TESTING

EXERCISE LIMITATIONS IN HEART
DISEASE
Mitral Valve Prolapse
Anorexia Nervosa
Sudden Death
Other Forms of Heart Disease

$\mathbf{A}$s participation in both competitive and noncompetitive sports increases, the numbers of female athletes, of athletes with known forms of heart disease, and of older athletes more likely to have occult heart disease, also increases. In general, the cardiovascular responses to exercise are similar in both sexes, both in healthy individuals and in those with heart disease. However, physiologic and pathologic differences do exist between the sexes and are important in the evaluation and treatment of the exercising woman.

Exercise of any type or intensity requires increased oxygen delivery to working tissue. This is accomplished through peripheral mechanisms, which include the differential perfusion of vascular beds and increased oxygen extraction by muscle, and through central or cardiac mechanisms, chiefly an increase in cardiac output. Thus, maximal exercise, or maximal oxygen uptake, is determined by maximal increases in the peripheral arteriovenous O_2 difference, and by cardiac output and its components, stroke volume and heart rate.

AEROBIC CAPACITY

In the average sedentary woman, maximum aerobic workload is 15% to 30% lower than in the average sedentary man,[1,2] even when corrected for body size. This may be due to a number of factors. Women normally possess a lower total oxygen-carrying capacity of blood, owing to lower blood volume, fewer red blood cells, and lower hemoglobin content. Women also have smaller hearts, even when corrected for body size, with smaller stroke volumes and therefore higher heart rates for a given cardiac output or oxygen uptake. Finally, women generally possess a higher percentage of adipose tissue and a lower percentage of working muscle than do men. These differences combine to produce, on average, a lower maximal level of work or aerobic capacity in women.

In part, these "physiologic" differences may also be explained by considering that, on the average, men are more active than women and therefore maintain a more trained state, particularly as women tend to become relatively more sedentary after puberty. Several factors support this hypothesis. Training programs produce similar increases in aerobic capacity in both sexes, even when older individuals are examined.[2–4] Maximal oxygen uptake in individual highly trained female athletes can approach and equal that of similarly trained males.[5] Finally, there is little difference in exercise capacity between boys and girls under the age of 12.[1]

Regardless of cause, recognition of the lower maximal aerobic capacity and higher heart rates during submaximal exercise in women as compared with men is essential to the accurate interpretation of exercise results in women. Sex-specific standards have been developed for maximal aerobic capacity, as well as nomograms for the calculation, in women, of maximal capacity from submaximal heart rate and oxygen uptake values. Exercise performance in women cannot be adequately evaluated without reference to such standards.

CARDIAC FUNCTION IN RESPONSE TO EXERCISE

In addition to differences in aerobic capacity, the normal cardiac response to exercise in women may be different than in men.[6] The most widely used diagnostic test for the evaluation of left ventricular function during exercise is the gated blood pool scan. This test involves the use of radiolabeled red blood cells (using technetium) to determine ejection fraction, or the percentage of blood within the left ventricular chamber that is ejected with each heart beat, at rest and at maximal exercise. Normal individuals

have been defined as those able to increase their ejection fraction by at least five percentage points during exercise.[7] Persons with a lesser increase, or even a decrease, are felt to have a component of myocardial dysfunction, or at the least, impaired cardiac reserve. Higginbotham and associates[8] studied healthy, sedentary adults and found that the generally accepted "normal" increase in left ventricular ejection fraction during exercise occurred only in men and not in women. Of the 16 women studied, only 7 increased their ejection fraction by five points or more (compared with 14 of 15 men), and the average ejection fraction was unchanged (63% at rest compared with 64% at peak exercise). In contrast, the average ejection fraction in men increased from 62% to 77% (Fig. 16–1).

In addition, the mechanisms used to increase cardiac output during exercise appeared different in men than in women. In men, end-diastolic left ventricular size did not change, whereas end-systolic size decreased, leading to increases in stroke volume and ejection fraction. In contrast, women achieved a similar increase in stroke volume by increasing end-diastolic size while end-systolic size remained unchanged. Thus, women appeared to dilate their left ventricles, or increase preload, whereas men increased ventricular shortening. The physiologic basis for these different mechanisms of achieving the same end—increasing cardiac output and therefore oxygen supply to muscle—is unknown, as is its significance for preserved health or training.

These findings have important clinical implications. If good health is defined by the healthy male pattern of response, the remainder of the population, or women who normally respond differently, may be falsely diagnosed as unwell. Since exercise gated blood pool scanning is commonly used to measure the cardiac functional response to exercise and is recommended as a diagnostic test for the evaluation of a variety of cardiac complaints, the problem is potentially a large one. At special risk for misdiagnosis

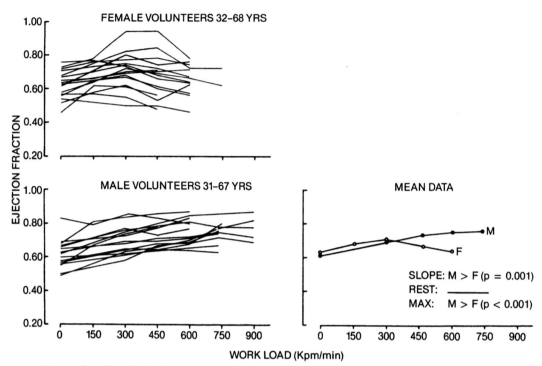

Figure 16–1. Ejection fraction responses during exercise in which the workload was increased every 3 minutes. Progressive individual data are shown for women *(top left)* and men *(bottom left)*. Mean submaximal and maximal group data are plotted on the right as mean data ± standard deviation for normal female (F) and male (M) volunteers. Significant intergroup differences are shown for the slope of the response, as well as for data from subjects at rest and during maximal exercise. (From Higginbotham et al.,[8] with permission.)

as having impaired cardiac function is the healthy woman, whether sedentary or active, undergoing evaluation of cardiac function. In a similar manner, a woman with mild known cardiac disease may be classified as having more severe impairment than is actually the case, owing to use of the male response as a normal reference standard.

In contrast to aerobic capacity and the functional response to exercise, other aspects of cardiac-related exercise physiology appear to show few differences between men and women. Aging affects aerobic capacity of healthy individuals of both sexes similarly, causing a decline in maximal oxygen uptake. This results from a decrease in both the maximal achievable heart rate and the mechanical performance of the myocardium, as well as limitations in the functioning of other organ systems (Fig. 16–2).

Blood pressure is little changed in the normal person following either isotonic or isometric exercise training. There is some evidence that both systolic and diastolic pressures may be reduced by training in individuals with hypertension; however, these effects are small and not known to differ between the sexes.[9]

The hearts of both men and women appear to adapt similarly to exercise training.[1,2] This has been documented in studies of women pursuing typically female-dominated sports such as field hockey and dance,[10,11] as well as those pursuing jogging, swimming, and triathlon trainings.[12–14] Weight training or isometric exercise appears to produce cardiovascular effects similar to those of aerobic, dynamic exercise.[15] A detailed discussion of the structural cardiac changes associated with dynamic and

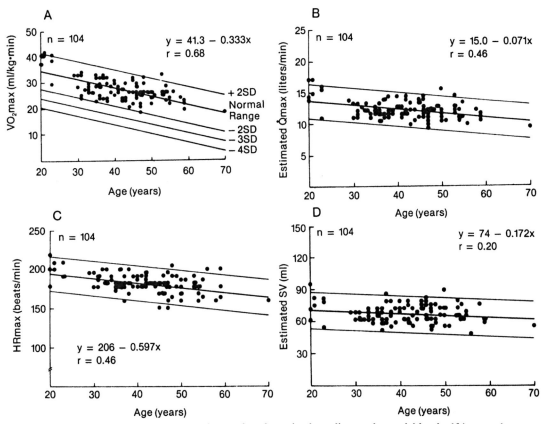

Figure 16–2. Derived values for observed and maximal cardiovascular variables in 104 normal, healthy women. (*A*) Observed age- and weight-adjusted value of maximal oxygen uptake ($\dot{V}O_2$max). The regression line is shown and the normal range indicated by ±2 standard deviations (SD). The standard deviation for oxygen uptake is 3.59 mL·kg^{-1}·min^{-1}). (*B*) Estimated age-adjusted values of maximal cardiac output are $\dot{Q}$max. The standard deviation for cardiac output is 1.35 L·min^{-1}. (*C*) Observed age-adjusted values of maximal heart rate (HRmax). The standard deviation for heart rate is 14 beats per minute. (*D*) Estimated age-adjusted values of maximal stroke volume (SV). The standard deviation for stroke volume is 8 mL. (From Hossack et al.,[6] with permission.)

resistive exercise training is beyond the scope of this chapter and has been well reviewed.[14] At present, no differences between the sexes have been found in the extent or incidence of cardiac adaptations to exercise.

Female athletes develop clinical findings of left ventricular hypertrophy, including an enlarged heart on chest radiograph, increased left and right ventricular cavity sizes and wall thicknesses on echocardiography, and increased voltage on ECG, reflecting an increased myocardial mass.[16] Following weight training, the cardiac chambers tend to remain normal-sized and the walls become hypertrophied. Athletes of

both sexes develop cardiac arrhythmias with training, probably because of alterations of vagal tone and catecholamine metabolism. Although sinus bradycardia is most common, low-grade atrioventricular block, premature atrial or ventricular contractions, and repolarization abnormalities are also seen.[14] Highly trained aerobic athletes also demonstrate a greater prevalence of multivalvular regurgitation.[17]

Since many of these adaptive changes may also signify the presence of true heart disease, it is important to recognize that for women, as well as men, physical training may lead to physiologic structural and elec-

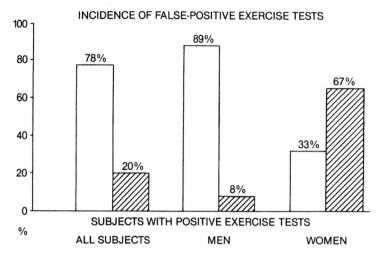

Figure 16–3. The marked difference in the incidence of false-positive test results between men and women is statistically significant (p < 0.001, regardless of coronary anatomy). Hatched bars indicate the percentage of positive exercise test results associated with normal coronary arteries or less than 50% stenosis (false-positive results). Open bars indicate the percentage of positive tests associated with 75% or greater coronary stenosis (true-positive results). Overall, 60 of 77 subjects (78%) had both positive exercise tests and significant coronary disease. In men, 55 of 62 (89%) had true-positive test results, whereas only 5 of 15 women (33%) did. This difference is statistically significant (p < 0.001). (From Sketch et al.,[18] with permission.)

EXERCISE ELECTROCARDIOGRAPHIC TESTING

The most common form of heart disease in the United States today is coronary atherosclerosis. Coronary stenoses limit the delivery of adequate amounts of oxygen to the heart, a problem often not noted until oxygen demands are increased by exercise. Thus, monitoring of electrocardiographic recordings capable of detecting cardiac ischemia during a controlled exercise protocol is the most widely used diagnostic procedure for the detection of coronary disease. In men, regardless of symptoms, such exercise testing is an excellent screening test, with few false-positive results. In contrast, in women, the incidence of false-positive test results (appearance of electrocardiographic changes characteristic of myocardial ischemia leading to a diagnosis of coronary disease in its absence) is quite high, perhaps as high as two thirds of all positive tests (Fig. 16–3).[18,19]

Several factors partially explain this difference. The most important of these is the age-related difference in the prevalence of heart disease between men and women. In general, the effect of disease prevalence in the population studied has a great impact upon the accuracy and usefulness of any given diagnostic test. This is termed Bayes' theorem and is highly applicable to the comparability of exercise testing results in men and women.[20] Because coronary disease is relatively less likely in a younger middle-aged woman, any given positive test result is more likely to be a false rather than a true result. Thus, the diagnostic utility of exercise testing for coronary artery disease in women is lower than for men. To eliminate the Bayesian factor, Barolsky and co-workers[21] studied the utility of exercise testing in groups of men and women with similar disease prevalences. This markedly improved the validity of test results, although women still had a higher incidence of false-positive test results.

Another reason for the high rate of false-positive test results is the higher incidence in women of other characteristics that are associated with nondiagnostic results.[22,23] These characteristics include atypical chest pain, resting electrocardiographic abnormalities including nonspecific ST- and T-wave changes, and ingestion of medications such as digoxin and anxiolytics. Since these characteristics appear more commonly in women than in men, test results are more frequently confounding in women.

Several alternative strategies have been proposed to render exercise testing more useful in women. These include more stringent use of probability analysis,[24] alternate or additional electrocardiographic lead placement,[25] consideration of R-wave amplitude as well as ST-segment changes,[26] and use of thallium-201 myocardial scintigraphy with exercise testing.[19,27] The addition of isotope imaging does markedly improve the specificity of exercise testing; however, the false-positive rate is still higher for women than for men. In part, this may be due to attenuation of tracer signal resulting from overlying breast tissue.[27,28] In addition, thallium scanning is costly, time consuming, and requires radiation exposure and the availability of special equipment and trained personnel.

The different sensitivity and specificity of exercise testing in women has important clinical implications. In diagnostic exercise testing performed to define and classify preexisting complaints, women with chest pain due to noncardiac causes are far more likely to be wrongly diagnosed as having coronary disease than anemia. This is obviously an undesirable event and, in addition to causing a great deal of patient anxiety, may lead to taking unnecessary medications and/or undergoing additional testing, which is more expensive and may endanger health. In contrast, a negative test result is a good indication of the absence of heart disease. Exercise testing performed to ensure that a training program may be undertaken safely is at even greater risk of producing a false suspicion of cardiac disease. The high false-positive rate of exercise testing in women makes it a very poor screening test for cardiovascular disease in women, regardless of symptoms. Unfortunately, no better alternative screening or diagnostic test exists for women, nor is the remarkably low predictive accuracy of exercise testing in women fully understood.

EXERCISE LIMITATIONS IN HEART DISEASE

The effects of exercise in those with heart disease appear to be similar in both men and women. However, since little attention has been focused on the potential differences between men and women, it is possible that such differences do exist but have been overlooked. It is known that women in general have a worse prognosis following myocardial infarction[29] and a higher mortality and lower immediate success rate following coronary artery bypass grafting[30] than men have. Whether this dichotomy extends to other forms of therapy, such as exercise training, is unknown. A low level of physical fitness, as measured by treadmill testing, is a powerful risk factor for coronary heart disease and cardiac death in women, as it is in men.[31] Longitudinal studies of exercise intervention have shown some benefit in cardiac risk factors such as lipid profiles, blood pressure, obesity, and diabetes mellitus, although the effect is generally smaller in women than in men.[32]

In men, the use of exercise in the treatment of known coronary heart disease, or for rehabilitation following myocardial infarction or revascularization surgery, is of established value in hastening recovery and improving the quality of life in the short term; longer-term benefits such as reduction of recurrence or improved long-term survival are more difficult to prove. Rehabilitative programs for those with nonischemic heart disease are more controversial. However, the effectiveness of exercise regimens in the primary and secondary treatment of any form of heart disease has not been examined in adequate numbers of women; their effectiveness can only be extrapolated from studies performed in men. Possible sex-related differences have not been explored.

Mitral Valve Prolapse

In contrast to most forms of either congenital or acquired heart disease, mitral valve prolapse occurs with greater frequency in women than in men. For this reason, information regarding cardiac function and exercise in this disease process may be more likely to represent the female than the male circumstance. Mitral valve prolapse is a generally benign syndrome characterized by a broad variety of cardiac findings, which may include some or all of the following: midsystolic, nonejection click; late systolic murmur; echocardiographic or cineangiographic evidence of systolic billowing of the mitral valve leaflets into the left atrium; thickened mitral valve; atypical chest pain; palpitations; dizziness; abnormal electrocardiogram; atrial or ventricular arrhythmia; systemic emboli; mitral regurgitation; Marfan's syndrome; syncope; and sudden death.[33]

The question of myocardial involvement in mitral valve prolapse has been raised by documentation of left ventricular segmental contraction abnormalities, and by its association with chest pain and ventricular arrhythmias. This has led to the examination of global function using rest and exercise ejection fractions as measured by gated blood pool scanning.[34–36] As might be expected, owing to the preponderance of women with the disease, patients with mitral valve prolapse have an "abnormal" failure to increase ejection fraction in response to exercise. This has been taken to be suggestive of a "cardiomyopathic process"[34] and renders difficult the accurate diagnosis of the etiology of chest pain (ischemic versus nonischemic).[35,36] However, as noted previously, normal healthy females also may fail to increase their ejection fraction with exercise; therefore, it is difficult to label the behavior of those with mitral valve prolapse as indicative of myocardial pathology.

In the overwhelming majority of cases, mitral valve prolapse is a benign, isolated auscultatory or echocardiographic finding that has no known influence on exercise performance or the advisability of pursuing competitive or recreational sports. This view is supported by the rarity of complications documented during exercise. It must

be kept in mind, however, that the natural history of the disorder is not well known and its clinical significance remains somewhat controversial. The American College of Cardiology has recommended that a small subset of patients with mitral valve prolapse limit competitive participation to low-intensity sports such as bowling and golf.[37] These patients include those with a history of syncope, a family history of sudden death due to mitral valve prolapse, chest pain worsened by exercise, repetitive ventricular ectopy or sustained supraventricular tachycardia (especially if worsened by exercise), moderate or severe mitral regurgitation, and dilatation of the ascending aorta (associated with Marfan's syndrome). It was recommended that no restrictions be placed on those with any or all other manifestations of the mitral valve prolapse syndrome.

Anorexia Nervosa

Another disorder primarily afflicting women and thought to affect cardiac performance is anorexia nervosa, which is discussed in Chapter 17. Previous studies of starvation have demonstrated decreased heart size, blood pressure, and heart rate, which may not be reversible with refeeding. A recent study[38] has shown that cardiac function is preserved and that the observed changes in cardiac architecture, load, and function are appropriate responses to decreased blood pressure. These parameters, as well as exercise performance, return to normal with weight gain. Thus, the observed cardiac abnormalities should not in themselves represent limitations to exercise.

Sudden Death

The risk factors predisposing to unexpected sudden death in women and the prevalence of coronary artery disease in such patients are somewhat different from those in men.[39] Data from the Framingham Heart Study showed that age and, marginally, cholesterol were risk factors in both sexes. In addition, hematocrit, vital capacity, and glucose were significantly related to the incidence of sudden death in women only. In men, additional risk factors for sudden death were those associated with coronary disease, including systolic blood pressure, obesity, smoking, and electrocardiographic evidence of left ventricular hypertrophy.

Although the significance of these findings for the exercising woman is unknown, several other forms of heart disease are clearly associated with sudden death during exercise. As far as is known, relative risks for men and women relate to the prevalence of these cardiac illnesses; the consequences or severity of each disease process do not differ in men and women, and female patients should observe the same restrictions.

Chief among cardiac diseases causing sudden death in young people during exercise is hypertrophic cardiomyopathy. This disease is idiopathic, genetically transmitted, and characterized by a thickened left ventricle with normal chamber size. Because cardiac adaptation to exercise may produce a similar picture, differentiating between physiologic and pathologic hypertrophy may be difficult and may depend on identification of other pathologic features such as asymmetric septal hypertrophy and systolic anterior motion of the mitral valve. Any athlete suspected of having this disorder should be fully evaluated by a cardiovascular specialist. The American College of Cardiology recommends that patients with this disease should never participate in high-intensity competitive sports, regardless of disease severity.[37] Those with marked hypertrophy, significant left ventricular outflow tract obstruction, arrhythmias, or a family history of sudden death or syncope should not participate in any form of athletic endeavors.

Other Forms of Heart Disease

Consideration of the exercise limitations imposed by each form of heart disease is beyond the scope of this review. In addition, there is no evidence available to indicate differences in disease processes, other than those discussed previously, that would suggest different exercise limitations in men and women. The reader is referred to the Task Force on Cardiovascular Abnormalities in the Athlete and its recommendations regarding eligibility for competition.[40] This conference, which was sponsored by the American College of Cardiology and by the National Heart, Lung and Blood Institute, compiled an up-to-date, comprehensive summary of both resistive and dynamic exercise limitations in all forms of congenital and acquired heart disease. It must be stressed that any person with known or suspected heart disease, regardless of sex, should undergo a full cardiovascular evaluation before undertaking exercise training or sports competition. These recommendations apply equally to male and female athletes.

SUMMARY

In conclusion, although many aspects of the female cardiac response to exercise appear similar to the male response, many other aspects have not been fully examined with respect to differences between the sexes. In areas that have been studied, a number of important differences exist. Because many of these differences must be kept in mind for the correct interpretation of diagnostic cardiac exercise testing performed in women, an appreciation of the normal female response is vital. These differences are just as important to keep in mind in examining the female athlete as they are in examining the sedentary woman. Much research remains to be done before a complete examination can be made of all the unique aspects of cardiovascular problems in the exercising woman.

REFERENCES

1. Åstrand I: Aerobic work capacity in men and women with special reference to age. Acta Physiol Scand 49:169, 1960.

2. Åstrand PO: Human physical fitness with special reference to sex and age. Physiol Rev 36:307, 1956.

3. Adams GM, and de Vries HA: Physiologic effects of an exercise training regimen upon women aged 52 to 79. J Gerontol 28:50, 1973.

4. Wessel JA, Small DA, Van Huss WD, et al: Age and physiological responses to exercise in women 20–69 years of age. J Gerontol 23:269, 1968.

5. O'Toole ML, Hiller WDB, Douglas PS, et al: Cardiovascular responses to prolonged cycling and running. Med Sci Sports Exerc 17:219, 1985.

6. Hossack KF, Kusumi F, and Bruce RA: Approximate normal standards of maximal cardiac output during upright exercise in women. Am J Cardiol 47:1080, 1981.

7. Borer JS, Bacharach SL, Green MV, et al: Real-time radionuclide cineangiography in the non-invasive evaluation of global and regional left ventricular function at rest and during exercise in patients with coronary artery disease. N Engl J Med 296:839, 1977.

8. Higginbotham MB, Morris KG, Coleman E, et al: Sex-related differences in the normal cardiac response to upright exercise. Circulation 70:357, 1984.

9. Seals DR, and Hagberg JM: The effect of exercise training on human hypertension: A review. Med Sci Sports Exerc 16:207, 1984.

10. Cohen JL, Gupta PK, Lichstein E, et al: The heart of a dancer: Noninvasive cardiac evaluation of professional ballet dancers. Am J Cardiol 45:959, 1980.

11. Zeldis SM, Morganroth J, and Rubler S: Cardiac hypertrophy in response to dynamic conditioning in female athletes. J Appl Physiol 44:849, 1978.

12. Douglas PS, O'Toole ML, Hiller WDB, et al: Left ventricular structure and function by echocardiography in ultraendurance athletes. Am J Cardiol 58:805, 1986.

13. Douglas PS, Hiller WDB, O'Toole ML, et al: Left ventricular structure and function in ultraendurance athletes. Med Sci Sports Exerc 17:203, 1985.

14. Huston TP, Puffer JC, and Rodney WM: The athletic heart syndrome. N Engl J Med 313:24, 1985.

15. Stone MH, and Wilson GD: Resistive training and selected effects. In Goldberg L, and Elliot DL (eds): The Medical Clinics of North America. WB Saunders, Philadelphia, 1985.

16. Douglas PS, O'Toole ML, Hiller DB, et al: Electrocardiographic diagnosis of exercise-induced left ventricular hypertrophy. Am Heart J 116:784, 1988.

17. Douglas PS, Berman GO, O'Toole ML, et al: Prevalence of multivalvular regurgitation in athletes. Am J Cardiol 64:209, 1989.

18. Sketch MH, Mohiuddin SM, Lynch JD, et al: Significant sex differences in the correlation of electrocardiographic exercise testing and coronary arteriograms. Am J Cardiol 36:169, 1975.

19. McCarthy D: Stress electrocardiography in women. Int J Cardiol 5:727, 1984.

20. Patterson RE, Eng C, and Horowitz SF: Practical diagnosis of coronary artery disease: A Bayes' theorem nomogram to correlate clinical data with noninvasive exercise tests. Am J Cardiol 53:252, 1984.

21. Barolsky SM, Gilbert CA, Faruqui A, et al: Differences in electrocardiographic response to exercise in women and men: A non-Bayesian factor. Circulation 60:1021, 1979.

22. Linhart JW, Laws JG, and Satinsky JD: Maximum treadmill exercise electrocardiography in female patients. Circulation 50:1173, 1974.

23. Detry JMR, Kapita BM, Cosyns J, et al: Diagnostic value of history and maximal exercise electrocardiography in men and women suspected of coronary heart disease. Circulation 56:756, 1977.

24. Melin JA, Wins W, Vanbutsele RJ, et al: Alternative diagnostic strategies for coronary artery disease in women: Demonstration of the usefulness and efficiency of probability analysis. Circulation 71:535, 1985.

25. Guiteras P, Chaitman BR, Waters DD, et al: Diagnostic accuracy of exercise ECG lead systems in clinical subsets of women. Circulation 65:1465, 1982.

26. Ilsley C, Canepa-Anson R, Westgate C, et al: Influence of R wave analysis upon diagnostic accuracy of exercise testing in women. Br Heart J 48:161, 1982.

27. Friedman TD, Greene AC, Iskandrian AS, et al: Exercise thallium-201 myocardial scintigraphy in women: Correlation with coronary arteriography. Am J Cardiol 49:1632, 1982.

28. Stolzenberg J, and Kaminsky J: Overlying breast as cause of false-positive thallium scans. Clin Nucl Med 3:229, 1978.

29. Puletti M, Sunseri L, Curione M, et al: Acute myocardial infarction: Sex-related differences in prognosis. Am Heart J 108:63, 1984.

30. Fisher LD, Kennedy JW, Davis KB, et al: Association of sex, physical size, and operative mortality after coronary artery bypass in the coronary artery surgery study (CASS). Thorac Cardiovasc Surg 84:334, 1982.

31. Blair SN, Kohl HW, Paffenbarger RS, et al: Physical fitness and all-cause mortality: A prospective study of healthy men and women. JAMA 262:2395, 1989.

32. Lokey EA, and Tran ZV: Effects of exercise

training on serum lipid and lipoprotein concentrations in women: A meta-analysis. Int J Sports Med 10:424, 1989.

33. Jeresaty RM: Mitral valve prolapse-click syndrome. Prog Cardiovasc Dis 15:623, 1973.

34. Gottdiener JS, Borer JS, Bacharach SL, et al: Left ventricular function in mitral valve prolapse: Assessment with radionuclide cineangiography. Am J Cardiol 47:7, 1981.

35. Newman GE, Gibbons RJ, and Jones RH: Cardiac function during rest and exercise in patients with mitral valve prolapse. Am J Cardiol 47:14, 1981.

36. Ahmad M, and Haibach H: Left ventricular function in patients with mitral valve prolapse: A radionuclide evaluation. Clin Nucl Med 7:562, 1982.

37. Maron EJ, Gaffney FA, Jeresaty RM, et al: Task force III: Hypertrophic cardiomyopa-

thy, other myopericardial diseases and mitral valve prolapse. J Am Coll Cardiol 6:1215, 1985.

38. St. John Sutton MG, Plappert T, Crosby L, et al: Effects of reduced left ventricular mass on chamber architecture, load, and function: A study of anorexia nervosa. Circulation 72(S):991, 1985.

39. Schatzkin A, Cupples LA, Heeren T, et al: The epidemiology of sudden unexpected death: Risk factors for men and women in the Framingham Heart Study. Am Heart J 107:1300, 1984.

40. Mitchell JH, Maron BJ, and Epstein SE: 16th Bethesda Conference: Cardiovascular abnormalities in the athlete: recommendations regarding eligibility for competition. J Am Coll Cardiol 6:1186, 1985.

CHAPTER 17

Eating Disorders

JACK L. KATZ, M.D.

Two striking developments in recent decades have made the topic of eating disorders germane to any scientific work on women and exercise. The first is the enormous increase in dedicated athletic participation by women. What traditionally had been almost exclusively the domain of men has now become a flourishing and important aspect of living for a substantial number of women in industrialized societies. The second is the dramatic rise in the incidence of eating disorders, specifically anorexia nervosa (AN) and bulimia nervosa (BN). As these syndromes are primarily disorders of women (90% to 95% of all cases), and as issues related to weight, food intake, and physical activity are central both to eating disorders and to athletics, it is not surprising that the topic of eating disorders is relevant to this book's mission of examining the physiologic, medical, and psychologic ramifications of exercise in women.

While this chapter will review in detail the nature, theories of etiology, and approaches to treatment of the eating disorders, it will also seek to address those concerns that are particularly related to exercise. For example,

1 Is sustained, strenuous exercising, especially by women, a risk factor for the development of an eating disorder?
2 Are women with a vulnerability to eating disorders drawn to serious athletic activity as a way of dealing with that vulnerability?

3 Do anorexia nervosa and intense athletic involvement share common underlying psychologic themes and conflicts?

4 What are the physical risks to the exercising woman with a known eating disorder?

EPIDEMIOLOGY

As indicated earlier, since the 1960s, there has been a remarkable increase in the incidence of the eating disorders that goes beyond heightened diagnostic acuity.[1] Surveys of the lifetime prevalence of AN in women have generally yielded a figure of about 1%,[1,2] while representative figures for BN fall around 4%.[3] Thus, perhaps almost 5% of women in industrialized societies can be expected to develop an eating disorder at some time during their life.

Clearly, these are not trivial figures, and they have prompted various speculations about the sources of this alarming increase in frequency. The most common proposals are that the media's emphasis on thinness as a culturally desirable physical characteristic has prompted more widespread dieting than ever before, and that the increasingly complex and demanding roles of women in our society have created particular stress and conflict for them around issues of identity and control, which are being played out by excessive attention to appearance.[4] However, we should also note that, perhaps because of better nutrition or subtle evolutionary trends, female adolescents are experiencing menarche and puberty earlier than ever before. Thus, they are encountering biologic and psychosocial stresses at an earlier age than previously. If today's parents are also more self-absorbed than were those of prior generations, their children's earlier exposure to these stresses is being met by less, rather than more, nurturance and support, and food may then take on particular symbolic importance.[5]

Finally, although AN and BN can occur in males and can also occur in persons living in noic background being the critical variable, achievement orientation of the families may be the more relevant common denominator.

nonindustrialized societies, they have a particular affinity for females growing up in industrialized cultures. Earlier writings suggested that white, upper-middle-class girls were at particular risk, but more recent reports suggest that minority groups are now also vulnerable.[6] Rather than socioeconomic background being the critical variable, achievement orientation of the families may be the more relevant common denominator.

SETTING AND ONSET

Anorexia Nervosa

Although there are perhaps "typical" circumstances associated with the onset of AN, it must be emphasized that a substantial minority of patients present histories that can deviate conspicuously from the usual stereotypic scenario.

Classically, the impending anorectic individual is in her teens, most likely approaching either 14 or 18 years of age (i.e., about to make a significant transition in her schooling). She has seemingly been a well-functioning girl, who indeed is often described by her parents as having been "perfect . . . never a problem." She is highly conscientious about her schoolwork, appears to have friends, and is usually well organized. But beneath this veneer of health, there is often found a girl with low self-esteem, one who is compulsive in her style, works excessively conscientiously to maintain her grades (i.e., is an "overachiever"), and is overly dependent in her relationships. She is also, more often than not, slightly overweight, has a "sweet tooth," and has grown up in a family that is weight conscious or diet conscious (e.g., because someone is diabetic).

Usually, but not always, a psychosocial stressor can be identified which correlates chronologically with the onset of consciously initiated dieting (although the connection between the dieting and the stressor may not be consciously made by the individual). Common triggering events are a loss (e.g., parental death or divorce), a blow to self-esteem (e.g., a failed first heterosexual relationship), or a separation (e.g., a vacation abroad, beginning college). Of course, some of these circumstances are intrinsic to adolescence and, while indeed stressful, are hardly unique to the life histories of anorectic girls.

Like most American female adolescents and adults who are embarking on a diet, the person at risk for AN makes the conscious decision to reduce or even virtually eliminate fats and carbohydrates. What makes her different from her peers, though, is the intensity of her drive to lose weight, her stoic pleasure in enduring hunger pains, and her increasing preoccupation with achieving thinness at the expense of all other goals.

Initially, there is a sense of exhilaration, a "high," which may be consequent to a newly found sense of mastery or to the accolades she begins to receive from peers and adults for her willpower and her improving figure. But it is also conceivable that this phenomenon is mediated by a rise in the body's endorphin level. Such a rise has been shown to occur, at least initially, in conjunction with two aspects of the unfolding AN: decreased food intake[7] and increased physical activity.[8] It has even been speculated that an unconscious attempt to recapture this initial, possibly endorphin-mediated, high drives the anorectic into her ever-downward spiral.

However, as indicated at the outset of this section, exceptions to this textbook picture abound. Not all future sufferers of AN are bright overachievers with compulsive styles, and not all begin their dieting in association with a psychosocial stressor. Some may actually follow the lead of a girlfriend in embarking on a diet; others may have initially lost weight as a consequence of a bona fide medical illness (most commonly, perhaps, infectious mononucleosis); still others begin to lose weight because of a real loss of appetite associated with a state of depression; and not all anorectic women are initially overweight or come from weight- or food-preoccupied families.

The possible role of intense athletic activity (e.g., long-distance running) in the pathogenesis of anorexia nervosa will be discussed in a later section.

Bulimia Nervosa

The setting, precipitating events, and onset for AN have been described with rather impressive agreement, including the acknowledgment of exceptions to the usual pathogenetic formulations, but BN remains a somewhat more difficult disorder to elucidate.

However, we have come to recognize at least two forms of bulimia nervosa, which literally means "nervous ox-hunger." In one, what starts out as fairly typical AN evolves into BN over a course of time, typically 1 to 2 years. Thus, after weight has been driven down, and in the presence of ongoing rigid and severe dieting, the anorectic individual may one day, to her shock and horror, suddenly embark on an uncontrollable binge. Not infrequently, two circumstances coincide to facilitate the appearance of the binge: an upsetting experience producing a dysphoric state (depression, anger, or anxiety) and the availability in abundance of "forbidden" foods (typically carbohydrates). The vulnerability to the binge may be further enhanced if the food is available in private (e.g., in one's own apartment or after everyone else has retired for the evening). After the binge, there is considerable disgust, shame, and guilt, followed by firm resolve not only never to permit this to happen again but also to diet even more rigorously to compensate for the weight presumably gained from the binge. However, with increasing frequency, the binges recur, until ultimately the binging may become a more conspicuous part of the clinical picture than the dieting.

In the other form, the individual becomes a binger without having ever passed through the emaciated, officially diagnosed phase of AN. However, the initial circumstances and the emotional states are probably the same in both forms. Although nonanorectic bulimic women may have never been substantially underweight, most, if not all, have been chronic dieters whose weights have fluctuated frequently and substantially. Thus, chronic dieting with unstable weight appears to be a risk factor for BN in non-anorectic persons as well.

CLINICAL FEATURE

While the etiology of the eating disorders remains controversial, as we shall discuss in a later section, the phenomenology of AN and BN has been impressively delineated over the past two decades, and a rich, coherent, and reliable clinical picture of these syndromes is now available. Both eating disorders can be regarded as syndromes characterized by an admixture of psychologic, behavioral, and biologic disturbances.

Anorexia Nervosa

Core Features

Self-imposed, Rigidly Enforced Dietary Restriction. Classically, this is viewed as being at the heart of AN. Thus, in the face of growing hunger and progressive weight loss, the anorectic individual consciously and deliberately elects to pursue a sustained course of restricted food intake. As previously noted, carbohydrates and fats are increasingly avoided; while protein is "permitted," many anorectics go on to become exclusive vegetarians. Rituals in the preparation and consumption of food are also characteristic. Obviously, such dieting must be differentiated from true anorexia, that is, real loss of appetite, which can occur with certain medical illnesses or affective disorders. However, as noted earlier, some patients actually give a history of having lost weight in conjunction with medical illness or depression, only to have the process catapult them into consciously pursued dieting with weight loss and, ultimately, full-blown AN. One dilemma for parents, of course, is to know when the dieting that is ubiquitous

among western female adolescents has gone beyond the bounds of "normal." The presence of the features that follow will help answer that question, but early prediction of which dieting adolescent will go on to develop an actual eating disorder is a perplexing challenge for even the most expert in the field.

Substantial Weight Loss. With progression of the dieting, this is the symptom that typically calls attention to the illness. The *Diagnostic and Statistical Manual of Mental Disorders,* third edition revised (DSM-III-R),[9] specifies a weight loss to at least 15% below expected body weight (including projected weight for a still-growing adolescent), but the diagnosis of AN should be made with the full clinical picture in view, rather than solely via mechanical reliance on a designated percentage of weight loss.[10]

Morbid Concern with Losing Control over Eating and Becoming Fat. A fear of loss of control is central to the psychology of AN. It is concretized around the dual concern that food intake and weight will become uncontrollable. Thus, the anorectic woman believes that she cannot be "thin enough," much less "too thin," because there is always the lurking threat that someday the floodgates will open and her insatiable appetite will spring forth to produce not only a gain in weight but a body of "humongous" dimensions.

Obsessional Preoccupation with Food. Given the fear of loss of control over eating and weight, it is not surprising that the anorectic's central preoccupation is with food. One might, however, view this repetitive, morbid dwelling on past, present, and future diet in either biologic terms (i.e., as a reflection of starvation's physiologic effects on central nervous system function and consequently on appetite and related cognition) or psychodynamic terms (i.e., as a reflection of an unconscious conflicted wish or impulse that underlies the conscious preoccupation). In either case, the important fact is that, increasingly, the anorectic individual devotes her time to fantasies and plans about buying, cooking, and eating various foods; this obsession progressively impinges on all other aspects of her existence.

Distorted Body Image. Facilitating the descent into AN is the impaired capacity of its victims to gauge accurately their physical dimensions. While normal female adolescents generally see themselves as somewhat larger than they really are (and perhaps this is one reason for the vulnerability of females for developing eating disorders), anorectic patients markedly overestimate their bodily dimensions—as established by objective studies with distorting lenses, calipers, and so on.[11] Clinically, the 70-lb anorectic adult will continue to talk about the need to lose some poundage here or there, despite her obvious emaciation. Paradoxically, this tendency appears to intensify with progression of the emaciation, thereby further confounding attempts at treatment.

Amenorrhea. Close to 100% of women who meet the above criteria will experience a loss of menses (or not achieve menarche if the illness begins prepubertally and goes untreated). DSM-III-R specifies that at least three menstrual cycles (exclusive of hormone administration) should be missed for amenorrhea to be diagnosed in a previously regularly menstruating female. Obviously, there is no analogous feature in men (although sperm count does drop significantly). Interestingly, not only does amenorrhea usually occur relatively early in the course of AN, but, in approximately 25% to 35% of anorectic women, it actually appears to occur prior to any significant weight loss (although usually after dieting has begun). Furthermore, menses may take many months to resume after weight restoration; AN has also developed in women after stopping oral contraceptives. It is because of aberrations such as these in hypothalamic-pituitary-ovarian axis function that endocrinologists have had a long-standing interest in AN.[12]

Common Features

High Level of Physical Activity. A dramatic and highly prevalent symptom is the striking level of physical activity that accompanies the excessive dieting. While many anorectic women were physically active people prior to the onset of their eating disorder, their exercising takes on an increasingly frenetic quality as the syndrome unfolds.[13] Like the dieting, the physical activity (most commonly running, calisthenics, swimming) becomes ritualized and rigid. When starvation begins to be serious, the hyperactivity will usually give way to weakness and lethargy, indicating the need for urgent medical care; however, the extreme denial characteristic of these patients may permit exercising to continue, sometimes even in the face of advanced emaciation.

Insomnia. Although often overlooked in the early literature on AN, difficulty in both falling asleep and sleeping soundly is a common complaint.[14] It is not clear whether this symptom is a consequence of malnourishment, anxiety, mood disturbance, excessive exercise, or some other aspect of the syndrome, but it is sufficiently distressing so that many anorectic patients will find themselves becoming increasingly dependent on sedatives, particularly benzodiazepines, to attain satisfactory sleep.

Cold Intolerance. Conceivably as a result of diminished adipose tissue peripherally and more likely as a consequence of starvation's effect on hypothalamically mediated thermoregulation centrally, AN commonly elicits significant cold intolerance. This symptom, compounded by the psychologic defense of denial, accounts for the dress typical of anorectic women, namely, multiple layers of sweaters or sweatshirts, which both keep them warm and hide their emaciation.

Use of Emetics, Cathartics, Diuretics, and Other Chemical Agents. In addition to their excessive restriction of food intake, many anorectic women will employ various external agents to prevent weight gain. Thus, some will induce vomiting (particularly the bulimic subgroup) by mechanical means (inserting a finger, toothbrush handle, or appliance cord into the throat to trigger the gag reflex) or chemical means (usually with syrup of ipecac). Some will use enemas or laxatives to "clean out" their gastrointestinal system (leading to chronic constipation eventually). And still others will illicitly take diuretics to minimize the contribution of body fluids to their weight, thyroid hormone to increase metabolic rate, or amphetamines to suppress appetite.[15]

Ritualistic Involvement with Food-Related Activities. Paradoxically, the very object that is dreaded, namely food, is often central not only to the anorectic individual's thoughts but also to her behavior. Thus, those with AN appear to derive vicarious (and probably sadistic) pleasure from watching others eat what they have cooked or baked for them. They are often involved in preparing exotic dishes and commonly display various rituals when they eat. Women with both AN and BN frequently also hoard and steal food, and a substantial number of patients with eating disorders actually work as waitresses.

Difficulty in Recognizing Satiation. Despite its formal name, and contrary to some of the earlier writings, AN is not a "nervous loss of appetite" and its victims do experience hunger pains (at least before the disease has entered the chronic phase). However, they are subject to real difficulty in experiencing (or, more likely, interpreting) sensations of satiation. They will often complain of being unable to know whether they are full or still hungry after eating a meal.

Drug Abuse. About one quarter of all eating-disorder patients (almost all of whom are anorectic-bulimic or just bulimic) give prior or concurrent histories of drug abuse, typically with sedatives and/or with stimulants (which, of course, may also serve as anorexogenics). Cocaine use is common, but heroin use is rare. These patients, who frequently also carry a diagnosis of "borderline personality," appear vulnerable to drug abuse by virtue of their emotional lability, impulsive tendencies, and general anxiety, as well as their specific panic over possibly losing control of their weight.[16]

Depressive Symptomatology. Although it is the symptomatology surrounding food, eating, and weight that usually brings the individual with an eating disorder to professional attention, at some point in their life perhaps fully half of all patients with eating disorders manifest episodes of depressive symptomatology that meet the criteria for a formal diagnosis of affective disorder.[17] Thus, they may feel dejected, guilty, pessimistic, and hopeless; sleep poorly; have difficulty concentrating; and even entertain suicidal thoughts. Whether such states are a consequence of starvation,[18] reflect a genuine co-morbid affective disorder, are part of the affective lability characteristic of a borderline personality disorder, or are simply reactive to the disruptions in normal living and interpersonal relations invariably produced by an eating disorder remains a controversial issue.[17] Vegetative signs (e.g., appetite loss and weight decline, insomnia, decreased libido, constipation) are particularly difficult to assess in the presence of an eating disorder; moreover anhedonia, loss of reactivity to the environment, motor retardation, and diurnal mood variation (i.e., the classic features of melancholia) are characteristically not evident.

Obsessional Features. Between 25% and 50% of all anorectic patients manifest behavioral and cognitive patterns typical of obsessive-compulsive disorder.[19] Thus, eating and exercise rituals, compulsive hand washing or checking, obsessive ruminations, excessive perfectionism, and so forth, are common. Most of these individuals give histories of similar tendencies prior to the onset of the eating disorder, but it should also be noted that starvation studies in normal volunteers have established that obsessive-compulsive, as well as affective, disturbances can be a common consequence of starvation.[18]

Bulimia Nervosa

As described earlier, BN will evolve either in the context of established AN or independently of it, but typically in one who has frequently dieted and experienced weight fluctuations. Characteristically, the binge takes place in private, usually during the evening hours, and involves the consumption of huge quantities of food (often thousands of calories in the same sitting). The binge foods are commonly those that are most assiduously avoided during the rest of the bulimic's day, namely carbohydrate-rich items, but virtually any morsel of food in the house is a potential target of the binge. Typically, the binge terminates in self-induced vomiting. Although most bulimic women vomit, however, not all do, and vomiting should *not* be considered a prerequisite for the diagnosis of BN. Some individuals simply exhaust themselves from the binge and eventually settle into a troubled sleep; others will try to compensate by using laxatives or enemas, as well as by dieting excessively between binges.

The binge, which may occur anywhere from several times per 24-hour period to several times per month (at least twice per week for at least 3 months, according to DSM-III-R[9]), elicits enormous personal shame. Not only are patients disgusted with themselves, but they are also initially unwilling to discuss their symptoms with anyone else. (This may account for the paucity of references to bulimia in the literature until the past two decades, when it began to "come out of the closet.") More importantly, each binge triggers off an ever-greater resolve to diet, and this only intensifies the fast-feast cycle. As with the anorectic patient's eating, the bulimic patient's binge can become ritualized. Thus, the time, setting, and type of food become increasingly important and fixed. However, in those bulimic persons who vomit, the vomiting can take on its own significance, eliciting reinforcement from the physical relief it provides for the abdominal discomfort, emotional relief for the concern and guilt about having consumed so many calories, and perhaps psychologic relief via symbolic resolution of unconscious conflicts about such matters as sex, pregnancy, and relationship with parents. As DSM-III-R notes,[9] a persistent overconcern with body shape and weight is not confined to restricting (i.e., nonbulimic) anorectic women but is also characteristic of normal-weight bulimic women.

BIOLOGY OF EATING DISORDERS

While the psychologic and behavioral features of the eating disorders obviously produce a dramatic clinical picture, it is commonly the ensuing impaired physiology that brings the afflicted individual to medical attention. The biology of AN is essentially the biology of starvation, whereas the biology of bulimia is principally a reflection of the physiologic derangements produced by chronic vomiting and/or laxative/diuretic abuse, as well as by the violent swings in food consumption.

Physical Sequelae

The physical consequences of the eating disorders are summarized in Table 17-1. It should be noted that the not uncommon combination of AN and BN in the same individual creates the possibility of findings from both disorders being present simultaneously in that person. Moreover, even in the normal-weight bulimic woman, the frequent interbinge dieting and postbinge vomiting can produce physical effects similar to those seen in the pure restricting anorectic woman; for example, while osteoporosis is well known to occur in women with AN, it has now also been documented in women

Table 17-1. POTENTIAL PHYSICAL FINDINGS IN EATING DISORDERS

Anorexia Nervosa

Emaciation
Dry skin
Lanugo (fine downy hair)
Loss of scalp hair and brittle nails
Cold extremities with impaired temperature regulation
Hypotension
Bradycardia
Cardiac rhythm disturbances
Edema

Bulimia Nervosa

Tooth decay
Salivary gland enlargement
Calluses on hands
Facial and other petechial hemorrhages
Cardiac rhythm disturbances

with BN,[20] reflecting both decreased estrogen and increased cortisol production.[21]

The degree of emaciation in AN will obviously depend on the net caloric balance between the limited food intake and the typically excessive exercise expenditure; in BN, weight will reflect the balance among binging, vomiting, possible cathartic use, possible substance and medication abuse, possible excessive exercising, interbinge dieting, and so on, so that the individual might be below, at, or above ideal body weight. The possibility of deception about weight by patients with AN (whether by outright lying, adding weights to one's body or clothing, or filling oneself up with water) should always be borne in mind by the examining physician.

The diminished sympathetic tone consequent to starvation in AN is associated with bradycardia and lowered blood pressure. But what has also become evident is that more serious cardiac complications of starvation—such as rhythm disturbances, mitral valve prolapse, and congestive heart failure—are not rare.[22] The perils of continued intensive exercise as AN progresses are evident in light of these potential cardiac problems.

The salivary gland enlargement seen with binging and vomiting, while of a benign nature (sialoadenosis), can combine with the not infrequently seen edema in eating disorders to reinforce the patient's conviction that she is fat and must thus further intensify her dieting efforts. The tooth decay in BN is a direct consequence of gastric juices bathing tooth enamel during repeated vomiting, while calluses on the hands are produced by the patient repeatedly sticking her fingers down her throat to elicit the gag reflex. Petechial hemorrhages can occur in the face, cornea, or soft palate following an extreme episode of binging and vomiting.

Radiologic, ECG, and EEG Abnormalities

In addition to osteoporosis, several other physical and physiologic changes can occur

Table 17-2. POTENTIAL RADIOLOGIC, ELECTROCARDIOGRAM, AND ELECTROENCEPHALOGRAM FINDINGS IN EATING DISORDERS

Anorexia Nervosa and Bulimia Nervosa

Osteoporosis on x-ray
Diminished gastric emptying on fluoroscopy
Cerebral atrophy and ventricular enlargement on CAT scan or MRI
Conduction, wave, and rhythm changes on electrocardiogram
Nonspecific spike abnormalities on electroencephalogram

in both anorectic and bulimic women, and are discernible with special procedures (Table 17-2). For instance, cerebral atrophy and ventricular enlargement in the brain have been reported in patients with either AN[23] or BN,[24] and presumably are consequent to malnutrition and reversible. Delayed gastric emptying can also occur in both groups, possibly consequent to such gastric insults as inadequate bulk intake, repeated vomiting, or bizarre diets. Electrolyte imbalance from vomiting, particularly hypokalemia, can produce significant, even fatal, abnormalities in cardiac function, and thus an electrocardiogram should be obtained for all vomiters; moreover, the frequently abused emetic, syrup of ipecac, can produce a serious cardiomyopathy.[25] Finally, about 25% of all eating-disorder patients demonstrate nonspecific abnormalities on electroencephalography, usually unilateral or bilateral spikes in the temporal-occipital region; the basis for this finding is not known, but such EEG abnormalities are what prompted one of the earliest pharmacotherapy trials in this field, using phenytoin.[26]

Laboratory Findings

The typical laboratory abnormalities in AN and BN are presented in Table 17-3. (Endocrine abnormalities are treated separately.)

A moderate anemia is not unusual in AN. Hematocrit values under 35% and hemoglo-

Table 17–3. POTENTIAL LABORATORY
FINDINGS IN EATING DISORDERS

Anorexia Nervosa

Anemia and leukopenia
Partial diabetes insipidus
Glucose tolerance abnormalities
Abnormal liver function tests
Elevated serum cholesterol, carotene, and uric acid
    levels
Depressed serum or urinary zinc, magnesium, and
    copper levels

Bulimia Nervosa

Evidence of dehydration (e.g., elevated BUN)
Hypokalemia, hypochloremia, and metabolic alkalosis
    (but possible metabolic acidosis in laxative abuse)
Elevated serum amylase
Glucose tolerance abnormalities

bin levels under 11.0 g/dL are common, and
a panleukopenia also is not rare. The excretion of large amounts of dilute urine, reflecting partial diabetes insipidus, can appear if
starvation becomes severe and chronic
enough to affect hypothalamic function,
renal function, or both. Diabetes mellitus-
like changes in glucose tolerance test results
will also begin to appear with long-term
avoidance of carbohydrates: fasting blood
sugar falls to relatively low levels (less than
70 mg/100 mL), an excessive and sustained
rise is noted after glucose load (greater than
180 mg/100 mL), and a "rebound" hypoglycemia (less than 50 mg/100 mL) may appear
as a delayed but excessive insulin outpour-
ing then occurs. Patients will often claim
that their "problem" is "hypoglycemia,"
while physicians may actually propose the
presence of diabetes, but these glucose abnormalities are the consequence, not the
cause, of the chronic starvation and erratic
carbohydrate consumption. Interestingly,
despite being at seemingly normal weight,
bulimic individuals can also have a low
serum glucose level[27] and can show a lower-
than-expected rise on intravenous glucose
challenge (which paradoxically can set off
subjective cravings for carbohydrates).[28]
These findings presumably reflect the
highly chaotic, nonnutritional dietary intake

of bulimic women, despite their adequate
net caloric state.

Vomiting is particularly pernicious because of its possible effects on electrolyte
balance. The low potassium level and metabolic alkalosis it produces can lead to cardiac arrhythmias and even to cardiac arrest
and death. Vomiting may also lead to dehydration, which can then confuse the interpretation of electrolyte values by producing
spuriously high figures.

Other laboratory abnormalities in AN can
include an elevated level of plasma carotene, in part due to the high carrot consumption characteristic of anorectic patients (because of the low calorie value of carrots) but
possibly also related to low thyroid (particularly T_3) values; hypoproteinemia and liver
enzyme abnormalities in severe and chronic
cases (although characteristically uncommon in earlier cases); and hypercholesterolemia, perhaps also secondary to low T_3
values. The serum uric acid level may rise,
and the serum or urinary zinc, magnesium,
and copper levels can decline.

Moderately elevated serum amylase levels occur in at least 25% of bulimic patients
consequent to excessive salivary gland activity in response to the frequent binging.
Fractionating the serum amylase, however,
will prevent overlooking a pancreatitis,
which can also occur in BN and may be the
source of the elevation.[29]

Endocrine Abnormalities:
Hypothalamic Implications

Because of the consistent and often early
occurrence of amenorrhea in patients with
AN, the endocrinology of AN has undergone
substantial investigation. As shown in Table
17–4, the characteristic endocrine abnormalities have now been well delineated.
When taken as a group, these findings
strongly suggest that hypothalamic function
is impaired in those with AN.[30,31] This possibility is further reinforced by the previously
noted abnormalities in temperature regulation and urine concentrating ability commonly seen with AN.

Table 17-4. POTENTIAL ENDOCRINE
FINDINGS IN ANOREXIA NERVOSA

Hypothalamic-Pituitary-Gonadal Axis Abnormalities

- Depressed plasma and urinary concentrations of gonadotropins (LH and FSH) in the face of depressed concentrations of estrogens and androgens
- Immature circadian LH secretory pattern
- Absence of monthly cycling in LH secretion
- Deficient LH "feedback" response to administered clomiphene citrate or ethinyl estradiol
- Usually deficient LH response to administered releasing hormone (LHRH), although correctable by daily "priming" with LHRH.

Hypothalamic-Pituitary-Adrenal Axis Abnormalities

- Elevated concentrations of plasma and urinary cortisol (but usually with maintenance of normal circadian rhythm)
- Diminished cortisol suppression by dexamethasone administration
- Elevated cortisol production rate (despite the elevated plasma level of cortisol)

Growth Hormone (GH) Abnormalities

- High-normal or slightly elevated concentrations of plasma GH
- Impaired GH response to induced hyperglycemia and hypoglycemia, L-DOPA, and TRH

Hypothalamic-Pituitary-Thyroid Axis Abnormalities

- Low normal concentration of plasma T_4 and distinctly low T_3
- Low or low normal concentration of plasma TSH (despite low T_3 and possibly low T_4 levels)
- Normal (or delayed but correctable with priming) TSH response to administered TRH

titive behavior, thus creating a vicious circle.[32]

While these endocrine aberrancies have been well documented in most women with AN, hypothalamic-pituitary-gonadal/adrenal abnormalities are also not infrequently present in women with BN.[33] Such findings again serve to remind us that bulimic women of totally normal weight do not eat normally and are often malnourished despite their seemingly normal appearance.

DIAGNOSIS, COURSE, AND PROGNOSIS OF THE EATING DISORDERS

In its typical presentation, and given the considerably enhanced sophistication in recent years of both professionals and lay persons in this area, the diagnosis of AN will pose little problem. Although several medical and psychiatric conditions are also associated with weight loss (Table 17-5), the anorectic patient's characteristic adolescent age, otherwise good physical health, and obvious pleasure in her increasingly skeletonlike appearance should elicit little diagnostic confusion. Problems can arise from the following confounding sources: deception about true weight or other symp-

We assume that this hypothalamic dysfunction is a consequence of the starvation and extreme weight loss in patients with AN. However, other variables conceivably play a role, such as the bizarre dietary intake (i.e., malnutrition as distinct from calorie insufficiency), psychologic factors (such as anxiety or depression), impaired sleep-wake patterns, and even excessive exercise. Although there is no firm evidence that the hypothalamic dysfunction precedes AN, it is conceivable that AN can adversely affect hypothalamic function and thereby secondarily impair hypothalamic control of appe-

Table 17-5. DIFFERENTIAL DIAGNOSIS
FOR ANOREXIA NERVOSA

Psychiatric Conditions

- Depression
- Mania
- Schizophrenia (paranoid)

Medical Conditions

- Malignancy
- Hypothalamic tumor
- Diabetes, hyperthyroidism, other endocrinopathies
- Infectious diseases (infectious mononucleosis, tuberculosis, etc.)
- Gastrointestinal disorders (malabsorption syndromes, regional enteritis, ulcerative colitis, etc.)
- Chronic alcoholism or other substance abuse

toms by the patient, later age of onset (an increasing number of cases now appear to be starting in the third, fourth, and even fifth decades of life), or the simultaneous presence of some other weight-losing condition to which the physician totally attributes the emaciation (e.g., substance abuse). Clearly, alertness to these possibilities is indicated when a person is suspected of having an eating disorder but does not quite fit the typical mold. Bulimia nervosa, of course, might be missed because of the usually normal weight of its sufferers, but, unlike women with AN, women with BN who consult a physician usually do so of their own accord and are thus more committed to discussing their difficulties honestly.

One of the extraordinary aspects of the eating disorders is that the outcome is so variable and unpredictable. At one end of the spectrum, probably a significant number of teenage girls "flirt" with AN, some perhaps even crossing over the border, only to respond to their parents' or physician's guidance or to their own good sense, and return to more normal eating and weight. At the other end are the 5% to 10% of patients who will die of direct complications of their eating disorder. The causes of death are cardiovascular collapse or cardiac arrest (particularly due to electrolyte imbalance from vomiting or cardiac toxicity from abuse of syrup of ipecac), overwhelming sepsis (due to compromised immune function secondary to starvation), or suicide.

Between these extremes, various courses and outcomes are possible: a single full-blown episode, recurring discrete episodes, or chronic disorder. The appearance of bulimia in AN is usually regarded as a particularly ominous prognostic sign because of its known likelihood to become associated with chronicity, although, paradoxically, it may somewhat alleviate the emaciation problem.[34] Moreover, as we shall discuss farther on, the frequent presence of co-morbid conditions can further complicate the course and prognosis of both AN and BN.

Minuchin and co-workers have claimed a better than 85% cure rate with their form of family therapy,[35] but most workers in the field report less successful results.[11,34,36] A consensus might be that about 40% of all treated eating-disordered patients recover, about 30% show moderate but not definitive improvement, and about 30% run a chronically debilitating course (in which group will be found the 5% to 10% who die of the illness). Clearly, the eating disorders should not be considered benign conditions.

CO-MORBIDITY

One of the more important developments of the past decade of clinical research in the eating disorders has been the documentation that there is substantial psychiatric co-morbidity with AN and BN. Whether these conditions are antecedents, concomitants, or consequences of the eating disorders, or whether they share similar etiologic or predisposing factors, is not clear, but it is now well established that at least four areas of psychopathology occur in eating disorder patients with an incidence beyond what chance alone would predict. The areas are depressive disorders, anxiety (including obsessive-compulsive) disorders, substance abuse, and personality (particularly borderline) disorders. While the incidence of the co-morbidity will vary with the category of psychopathology, the type of eating disorder (AN versus BN), and the setting in which incidence is being determined (inpatient versus outpatient versus community survey), it is probably safe to say that up to 75% of all eating-disorder patients will manifest at least one of these areas of co-morbidity.[19,37]

The presence of such co-morbidity has several ramifications. First, it is incumbent upon the treating physician to be alert to the presence of these other conditions. Second, it is likely that a concomitant psychiatric disorder will have an adverse influence on the course of the eating disorder. Finally, the diagnosed presence of a co-morbid condition means that the treatment plan will have to be comprehensive enough to include provision for both the eating disorder and the co-morbid disorder(s).[38]

THEORIES OF ETIOLOGY

The wide range of symptoms and signs found in the eating disorders has elicited an equally broad array of proposals to "explain" them. Yet, as our experience and sophistication with these syndromes have increased, we are becoming more cautious about accepting simple etiologic formulations.

Perhaps the first significant contribution historically to our understanding of eating-disordered individuals, particularly those with restricting AN, was made by Hilde Bruch,[39] who moved away from a symbolic-libidinal-conflictual framework—for example, seeing AN as a defense against an underlying wish for oral impregnation—toward more of an ego psychology framework. For Bruch,[40] AN came to represent a desperate attempt by the vulnerable adolescent to achieve a sense of identity and mastery independent from that of her overbearing and intrusive parents (particularly mother). She speculated that the mother's insensitivity to physiologic and emotional cues provided by the infant resulted in the developing child's experiencing deficiencies and confusion in identifying affective and visceral experiences and thus in gaining a reliable sense of self. This would lead to a basic sense of ineffectiveness, perplexity over bodily sensations, and disturbances in body image. In the context of the developmental transition of puberty and adolescence—producing such stresses as bodily changes, separation, heterosexual encounters, increased independence and responsibility, and scholastic demands—the anorexia-vulnerable person, who senses a family need for high achievement but who has little confidence in her capacity to be successful, presumably turns increasingly toward her own body as the one area in her life that she might truly control. Moreover, her thinness not only re-establishes a sense

of mastery and effectiveness but also helps to define her as someone special; that is, her unique appearance shores up her precarious self-image and meager sense of identity.

Because this scenario is played out in the context of the adolescent's family, however, subsequent investigators, such as Palazzoli[41] and Minuchin and co-workers,[35] have emphasized the importance of understanding and treating the family as a system. Thus, AN not only has significance for the diagnosed anorectic patient, but also reflects pathologic roles and relationships in the family. Minuchin's group identified four specific characteristics of such families: their members are excessively enmeshed in each other's affairs, severely mutually overprotective, rigid in their style of relating to each other and to the outer world, and unable to achieve appropriate resolution and closure on family conflicts. In this framework, AN represents an attempt on one level to achieve at least some "space" and autonomy within the family unit, while ensuring on another level that threats to the homeostasis of the family constellation—for example, by the designated patient's truly maturing and moving out on her own—are thwarted.

Still other themes have been emphasized by various writers: the need to keep the body in a state of biologic immaturity to avoid confronting sexual impulses and heterosexual relationships;[42] the response to a cultural milieu that promises women happiness and success if thinness can be attained;[4] and the symbolic attempt to rid the self of the bad mother—with whom the anorectic woman identifies her body—by literally starving it.[41] (The bulimic woman, on the other hand, might be attempting to regain mother by excessive eating or even by regurgitating back the lost object.[43])

Unfortunately, all of these formulations, whether intrapsychic, interpersonal, familial, or sociocultural, are based on observations made after the fact. Thus, inferences are offered about premorbid characteristics not only after AN has been diagnosed but also commonly after it has been present for months or years. The impact of such a pernicious condition on self-esteem, family dynamics, and perception of the environment cannot be readily determined; predisposing, precipitating, and perpetuating elements tend to become confused. Moreover, many of the common conflicts described (e.g., conflicts over separation, independence, and sexuality) are characteristic of normal adolescence as well, and the more pathologic features of self and family (e.g., feelings of emptiness and enmeshment) are common to other pathologic, but non-eating-disordered, conditions such as "borderline" and "psychosomatic" disorders.

For all these reasons, workers in the field have begun to move toward a "risk-factor" model for the eating disorders.[44,45] Rather than postulating a specific etiology, we have come to recognize that a variety of factors—cultural, familial, and individual—increase one's vulnerability to developing an eating disorder (Table 17-6). As the number and intensity of these risk factors increase, the vulnerability does as well. However, clearly not all persons with eating disorders need have exactly the same risk factors, and some persons with some risk factors might never develop a manifest eating disorder; protective individual and family characteristics, individual biologic differences, and serendipity in life events could serve to modify onset, course, and outcome.

Moreover, the sustaining effects of starvation and malnutrition in patients with AN should not be overlooked.[32] As dieting becomes prolonged, its impact on digestive capacity and function, endorphin levels, hypothalamic function, cognitive capacity, affective state, body image, menstrual regularity, response of peers, and so forth, may actually serve to reinforce further food avoidance, thereby creating an increasingly self-perpetuating, treatment-resistant situation.

Finally, whereas most of the focus in the eating-disorder literature has been on the etiology and pathogenesis of AN, we are now also beginning to understand more adequately the nature of the vulnerability for

Table 17-6. RISK FACTORS FOR THE DEVELOPMENT OF ANOREXIA NERVOSA

Cultural Risk Factors

- Westernized and contemporary culture
  - Equates thinness with both beauty and happiness
  - Emphasizes attention to self and body
  - Demands varied, and at times conflicting, roles of women
- Capable of readily disseminating cultural values and styles through visual media (e.g., movies, television, magazines)
- Has subcultures that particularly emphasize weight control (e.g., ballet, modeling, certain sports)
- Other?

Family Risk Factors

- Achievement-oriented
- Intrusive, enmeshing, overprotective, rigid, unable to resolve conflicts
- Frugal with support, nurturance, encouragement
- Overinvested in food, diet, weight, appearance, or physical fitness
- Known to have members with a formal history of eating disorder or affective disorder
- Other?

Individual Risk Factors

- Female
- Adolescent
- Slightly overweight
- Subject to feelings of ineffectiveness and low self-esteem
- Subject to conflicts and doubts about sense of personal identity and autonomy
- Subject to bodily perceptual disturbances (e.g., distorted body image, uncertain feelings of satiation after meals)
- Subject to overgeneralization and other cognitive distortions
- Subject to an obsessional style and conflicts about control
- History of childhood sexual abuse
- Other?

BN. While only a minority of bulimic women have a prior history of formally diagnosed AN, the overwhelming majority are chronic or intermittent dieters whose weight frequently fluctuates substantially.[3,46] On the biologic side, the loss of substantial weight (even if not to emaciated levels—e.g., an obese individual who diets to reach merely normal weight[47]), in the face of ongoing, severely restricted dietary intake, intensifies the drive to eat. On the psychologic side, this drive will most likely be responded to in excessive fashion (i.e., by binging) when the individual is also characterized by so-called borderline features (impulsivity, emotional instability, an all-or-nothing orientation to life, feelings of inner emptiness, and so on). Thus, it is the mesh between biologic and psychologic vulnerabilities that "loads the dice" for the emergence of BN.

TREATMENT

While the number of controlled studies on the efficacy of various treatment approaches to the eating disorders still remains relatively small, there has been a significant increase over the past two decades in such studies, as well as in empirical clinical experience in the management of AN and BN.[34,46,48] No sure-fire treatment for either condition has been found, but certain guidelines have begun to emerge.

Perhaps the most important principles in the treatment of the eating disorders are (1) the earlier the intervention, the greater is the likelihood of response; (2) the treatment approach should be tailored to the phase, severity, and setting of the disorder, and also to the unique characteristics of the individual patient; (3) multimodal treatment is more likely to be effective than unimodal treatment; and (4) open-mindedness and flexibility on the part of the therapist or treating team are crucial.

Whereas young adolescents who have just begun to diet excessively may respond to a good "educational" talk from a trusted pediatrician, individuals with more established cases of AN will require, at the very least, individual psychotherapy with a professional who has had experience working with eating-disordered patients. The therapy will typically focus progressively on concerns about control, self-esteem, and sense of identity; on recognizing and accepting bodily feelings and emotional states, and on facing the anxieties inherent in becoming an independent adult. The

therapist must be prepared to deal with educational issues (e.g., about food, calories, dieting), cognitive issues such as styles of thinking (e.g., all or none, overgeneralizing, personalizing), and psychodynamic issues (e.g., ambivalence toward parents, competitiveness with siblings, fantasies about one's body). Furthermore, the therapist must be supportive, reliable, and respectful, and must be prepared to address concrete issues concerning weight, while not permitting this to become the exclusive focus of therapy.

The critical place of the family as the battleground upon which an eating disorder evolves suggests that family therapy is at least as important as individual therapy, particularly in younger patients living with their families.[35,41] Family therapy will emphasize the workings of the family unit as a system and its need to be more flexible and less intrusive in response to perturbations produced by any of its members. Ideally, this will complement concurrent individual therapy.

Group therapy for the treatment of BN has elicited considerable interest in recent years.[46] Whereas nonbulimic anorectic women tend to say little in groups and actually can become competitive with each other over success in losing weight, bulimic women tend to be more open about their feelings in a group and also to benefit from being confronted about their secretive gorging and purging behaviors. Moreover, most therapy groups also incorporate cognitive-psychoeducational-behavioral elements, often in the context of a time-limited course of treatment, which can be effective in dealing with and aborting eating and thinking patterns that tend to perpetuate the starve-binge cycle.

While the aforementioned approaches are germane to the patient with relatively early AN or BN, as well as to the chronic but relatively stable patient, the importance of hospital treatment for the acutely starving anorectic individual or the severely bulimic person in electrolyte imbalance—or both, when they have lost control of their day-today life to the eating disorder—should not be minimized. Because restricting anorectic patients can lose weight precipitously, medical involvement should be a principal part of both the initial evaluation and subsequent outpatient treatment. Not only is the extent of weight loss important, but the rate must also be considered. Some chronic patients may be able to sustain a weight at 35% below their ideal after many years of AN, whereas a patient who has dropped to 25% below ideal in just a few months may represent an acute medical emergency. Clearly weight, electrolytes, blood chemistries, cardiac function, pulse, and blood pressure must be carefully examined to make a judgment about the need for hospital admission, but compulsive exercise, food-related rituals, or numerous daily binges that interfere with the patient's functioning or interpersonal relations are also indications for hospitalization.

The inpatient setting ideally would be a unit specifically geared for eating disorders. If necessary, however, a general medical or psychiatric floor can provide several important aspects of treatment. In addition to ongoing physiologic monitoring and supportive nursing, a hospital permits electrolyte correction with intravenous fluids, external restraints on binging and vomiting, application of a comprehensive behavior modification regimen to encourage weight gain, use of medications as indicated, and, in rare life-and-death circumstances, hyperalimentation (total parenteral nutrition) through an indwelling catheter in a subclavian vein. If the patient not only is severely emaciated but also categorically refuses to eat, feedings through a nasogastric tube also become an option.

A behavior modification approach assumes that the aberrant eating pattern, whatever its original determinants, has become a "habit" by the time that hospitalization becomes necessary. Thus, it might best be undone, like most habits, by the institution of an appropriate schedule of positive and negative reinforcers. Although common contingencies might include, for example, loss of visiting privileges or access to off-

unit activities, the most potent reinforcer—and one with obvious relevance to this book— may well involve access to exercise. The importance of exercise in the mental economy of most anorectic individuals has been demonstrated by Blinder, Freeman, and Stunkard.[49] Using a behavioral paradigm in which access to exercise was contingent on sufficient daily weight gain, they documented that significant and rapid improvement in weight could be attained during hospitalization.

Whether on an inpatient or outpatient basis, medication has also begun to be part of the therapeutic armamentarium. While the earlier literature mainly emphasized the use of chlorpromazine (Thorazine) in the acutely agitated, excessively exercising anorectic inpatient, the more recent emphasis has been on the use of antidepressants, particularly the monoamine oxidase inhibitors (MAOIs); the tricyclic antidepressants; and the serotonergic agent fluoxetine (Prozac), for the treatment of BN.[50] The rationale for their use has been the seeming overlap in clinical, familial, and laboratory features in bulimia and affective disorders, but this explanation remains controversial. Nevertheless, while controlled studies do suggest a statistically significant reduction in frequency of binges when these drugs are taken at therapeutic doses, a positive response is far from universal, and relapse both on and off medication is not uncommon.[51] Moreover, side effects are poorly tolerated, and bulimic patients who may binge on tyramine-containing foods are obviously not candidates for treatment with an MAOI. As noted earlier, the not-infrequent combination of EEG abnormalities and eating disorders has spurred interest in the application of anticonvulsants for binging, and both phenytoin (Dilantin) and carbamazepine (Tegretol) have been reported as helpful; however, controlled studies on efficacy have not been impressive.[51] Finally, lithium has also been reported to be beneficial in BN,[51a] but again without the benefit of controlled studies.

The only pharmacologic agent that has been shown to produce even a slight statistical advantage in treating restricting AN is cyproheptadine (Periactin), an antihistamine.[52] While the efficacy of this drug is hardly profound, it is worthy of mention for two reasons. First, its sedating effect can be helpful in dealing with the insomnia characteristic of AN. Second, its antiserotonergic properties seem to stimulate appetite, while fluoxetine, fenfluramine, and other serotonergic agents appear to damp down bulimic behavior.[52a]

It must, of course, be noted that the eating disorders become chronic conditions for many, if not most, of those afflicted with them. The therapist must often be prepared to engage in long-term treatment, to use multiple modalities (including hospitalization when indicated), and to be willing to settle for goals that emphasize minimizing morbidity rather than achieving full cure. Indeed, those patients and therapists who seek quick remedies are likely to meet only with frustration.

EXERCISE AND EATING DISORDERS

As indicated in the introduction to this chapter, the inclusion of substantial material on the eating disorders in a text devoted to women and exercise was prompted by several important concerns. Can vigorous exercise or athletic competition "cause," increase the risk for developing, or precipitate an eating disorder? Do people with a predisposition for an eating disorder commonly gravitate toward sports? Might physical activity in some fashion actually protect against the emergence of an eating disorder? Why is exercise so important to most persons who are anorectic? What impact does continuing to exercise have on the anorectic patient's attempt to regain weight with treatment? These and other questions are being asked with increasing frequency because of the growing number of women who are active athletically and the growing number of women who develop AN or BN.

While definitive answers to these questions are not available, our understanding of these issues has increased considerably over the past decade. For example, serious long-distance running triggering the emergence of classic AN has been described,[53] but this appeared to represent the precipitation of an eating disorder in persons who already had a strong predisposition for its development.

Indeed, with so many people running and exercising, we would be faced with an epidemic of AN or BN if such activities could actually "cause" an eating disorder. Nevertheless, the appearance of progressive weight loss, amenorrhea, and increasing preoccupation with calorie intake in a female athlete should alert the team physician or trainer to the possibility that the ordinarily high level of physical activity may be evolving into a manifest eating disorder. Possible biologic and psychologic mechanisms mediating this phenomenon have been proposed.[53]

The relationship between chronic extensive exercise and anorexia nervosa remains controversial. Eisler and Le Grange[54] have proposed four different models: (1) these are distinct phenomena which superficially resemble each other because the use of excessive exercise to work off calories is characteristic of AN, and athletes need to control weight to ensure maximum performance; (2) these are overlapping phenomena, with each increasing the risk for developing the other; (3) both phenomena are related in some fashion to a third variable (e.g., obsessive-compulsive tendencies or affective disorder), and thus occur together with more than chance frequency; (4) these are essentially variants of each other, with sexual, familial, developmental, and cultural factors accounting for why one or the other expression of the underlying basic vulnerability becomes manifest in a given individual.

Clearly, the last of these models is the most interesting and also the most provocative. Impetus for it came from a report by Yates and colleagues that appeared in the *New England Journal of Medicine*.[55] These authors reported that psychologic interviews of male obligatory runners (men who ran a minimum of 50 miles per week) revealed socioeconomic and personality characteristics strikingly similar to those reported in anorectic women. They speculated that obligatory running in men and AN in women both represent unconscious attempts to establish a more definitive sense of identity and effectiveness. Cultural values simply make it easier, they proposed, for men to use running and women, dieting. Moreover, they suggested that members of either sex who use running to solve problems of identity and effectiveness will be subject to depression and manifest eating disturbances when they cannot run (for example, if they have been injured); this possibility is consistent with case reports.[53]

In a recent book,[56] Yates has amplified these views. She proposes that at least some cases of eating disorders and some cases of compulsive exercising do not necessarily have their roots in psychopathology. Rather, they represent a striving for excellence, whether by dieting or exercising vigorously, but that, as the balance between caloric intake and expenditure begins to diminish, the ensuing physiologic deprivation elicits biologic mechanisms that serve to perpetuate the process. For example, acute exercise transiently damps down appetite, while loss of weight may produce decreased gastric capacity and feeling full quickly after relatively little intake; as appetite then progressively builds and becomes intense, the fear of utterly losing control becomes so anxiety-provoking that the exercising and dieting are further intensified by the performance/appearance-oriented individual. Pathologic runners also seem to have, in Dr. Yates' view, the same ambivalent feeling toward their body as AN patients, being prepared to inflict pain on it in order to conform to some preconceived ideal.

Nevertheless, the view that running is an analogue of AN has been questioned by Blumenthal and co-workers.[57] Using more precisely defined and quantitative psychologic assessment scales, they could not replicate the qualitative impressions of Yates and associates. Moreover, it has been argued that the weight loss and food aversions common to many serious athletes reflect the pressures and demands of the sport but should not be confused with the deep premorbid psychopathology of those with bona fide AN.[58]

Several more recent studies also raise questions about any underlying, fundamental (as opposed to a preciptating or perpetuating) relationship between extensive exercise (or competitive sports) and eating disorders. Owens and Slade,[59] for example, gave a questionnaire to 35 female marathon runners and found that, while their scores on the "Perfectionism" scale resembled those of anorectic patients, their "Dissatisfaction" scores were similar to those of normal control women and significantly lower than those of anorectic patients. Richert and Hummers[60] found no correlation between scores on the Eating Attitudes Test and hours devoted weekly to a variety of physical activities (e.g., swimming, bicycling), although, interestingly, hours spent jogging per week did show a significant correlation with EAT scores, perhaps lending some support to the thesis that runners represent a unique group among exercisers. On the other hand, Warren and co-workers,[61] looking at a variety of physical, behavioral, and attitudinal measures in a group of college athletes versus nonathletes, found no differences in varsity cross-country runners (unlike Richert and Hummers) or in a variety of other varsity athletes, but did find significantly more pathologic scores in varsity gymnasts.

That athletics might actually be protective against the emergence of an eating disorder remains a possibility. For example, a study of college women engaged in intramural sports between 1977 and 1982, when the incidence of AN was clearly increasing, found no evidence of low weight for height among the study subjects.[62] While women not vulnerable to AN might be attracted to college intramural sports, or eating disorders might be common among such women but be hidden by concomitant BN which maintains weight at a generally normal level, it is also conceivable that athletics contain physiologic or psychologic elements that are, in some manner, protective against the development of AN. Further support for such a thesis might be seen in a study of both abnormal eating attitudes and manifest AN in a large number of long-distance female runners.[63] While 14% revealed aberrant attitudes on the Eating Attitudes Test and the Eating Disorders Inventory, only 2.4% actually gave clinical evidence of having or possibly having had AN.

But are persons who are prone to eating disorders perhaps strongly "pulled" toward exercise and athletics? In addition to the previously mentioned report of relatively high percentages of female long-distance runners with elevated scores on eating attitude screening tests, it is well known that anorectic individuals are typically excessively active physically during the disorder's acute phase. Numerous hours are devoted daily to calisthenics, running, swimming, or other athletic activities; typically the exercising increasingly takes on a frenetic quality. This high level of physical activity might be seen as merely the expected manifestation of the conscious desire to work off as many calories as possible each day as part of the obsessional drive to attain supreme thinness. However, at least one report suggests that anorectic women are more active than their peers prior to the overt onset of the disorder, and that they continue to remain physically active even after apparent recovery from AN.[13] Furthermore, as noted earlier, the importance of physical activity for anorectic individuals is evident in the effectiveness of inpatient behavior modification programs that use access to physical activity as a reinforcer for weight gain.[49]

Presumably the truth rests somewhere in the middle of this debate. Those with conflicts over control and self-identity may seek solutions in exercise and sports competition, in dietary control, or possibly in both. Statistically, though, this group must certainly represent a very small percentage of the vast numbers, male and female, who engage in athletic activities. And among those who have manifest eating disorders, only a small percentage are likely to be involved in serious, competitive sports, given the vulnerability to pathologic fractures, cardiac

arrhythmias, loss of physical strength, dehydration, and electrolyte imbalance that characterizes these syndromes.

Once involved with athletic activity, some persons who are vulnerable to, but not yet manifesting, an eating disorder may actually discover a relatively healthy solution to some of their psychologic conflicts. On the other hand, other such individuals may find that the coincidental importance of weight for performance, the inevitable competitive defeats, the pressure to perform progressively more successfully, the disruption of training schedules by injuries, the obstacles to regular eating patterns periodically posed by the demands of the sport, the common discussions among athletes about weight and diet, and the impact of exercise on appetite[64] and on the body's endorphin system[8,65] only serve to intensify their predisposition.

Finally, for those individuals who are serious athletes and have developed AN, there are certain special considerations. Osteoporosis clearly puts the vigorous exerciser at risk for pathologic fractures, while the progressive emaciation will at some point compromise the quality of athletic performance (as must the growing preoccupation with calories and weight). Obviously, bulimic athletes are faced with particular cardiovascular peril, as they add dehydration and electrolyte imbalance from perspiring to that from vomiting. And the maintenance of a high level of physical activity can significantly compromise the effectiveness of therapeutic weight-regaining regimens, even in a hospital setting.[66]

EATING DISORDERS AND OTHER SPECIAL SUBCULTURES

The importance of the mesh between environmental demands and individual vulnerabilities is perhaps best demonstrated by the high prevalence of eating disorders among women in certain other subcultures.[67,68] These subcultures—such as ballet, acting, and modeling—are characterized by an *explicit* emphasis on the desirability of thinness. Thus, it is not surprising that many ballerinas, actresses, and models are underweight; yet, not all or even most have eating disorders.

There is evidence that sociocultural background can exert either a protective or a risk-enhancing influence even within such narrow subcultures. Thus, Hamilton and co-workers,[69] in a study of ballerinas in nine regional and national dance companies, found mean weight for the entire group to be 12% below ideal; however, no black American dancers reported having AN or BN, while 15% of the white American dancers admitted to having AN and 19% acknowledged the presence of BN. The anorectic ballerinas not only were thinner than their non-anorectic ballerina peers but also manifested generally greater psychopathology and were more likely to be dancers with the most competitive companies.

Finally, there is evidence that the presence of amenorrhea in ballerinas is mediated not by their extensive physical activity but by their inadequate nutritional intake.[70] This may well have implications for the amenorrhea common to other strenuous exercisers, such as long-distance runners. Hence, we again note a complex interaction of multiple variables, perhaps what we should expect in any exploration of human psychobiology.

SUMMARY

The eating disorders and participation in serious exercise have both become strikingly more common among women over the past two to three decades. Since both areas are characterized by concerns about weight, diet, and activity level, it is not surprising that questions about a possible relationship between them have also begun to emerge. Because AN and BN are not benign disorders, having behavioral, cognitive, emotional, and biologic consequences that can readily become debilitating and chronic, such concerns are hardly academic.

The available evidence relevant to these concerns, while still limited, suggests that a high level of physical exercise becomes a risk factor for the development of an eating disorder only when it occurs in an individual who has other predisposing risk factors, such as conflicts or doubts about sense of identity, self-esteem, and self-control. Extreme physical activity can also be a symptom of an already-emerging state of AN, but then the activity tends to be frenetic and the mental component involves the conscious desire to "burn off" calories, rather than a desire to experience the sheer fun of exercise or the gratification inherent in successful physical competition. It is conceivable that, for some athletes, female or male, extreme exercise can be a way of defending against certain conscious or unconscious conflicts, just as excessive dieting—or excessive stamp collecting, gambling, or drinking—might. For most women who now exercise regularly, however, particularly those whose exercise is not part of a subculture that explicitly attaches great status to thinness (such as ballet or modeling), the risk of developing an eating disorder does not appear to be enhanced, while the benefits of exercise to mental and physical well-being are undoubtedly substantial.

REFERENCES

1. Lucas AR, Beard CM, O'Fallon WM, and Kurland LT: 50 year trends in the incidence of anorexia nervosa in Rochester, Minn: A population-based study. Am J Psychiatry 148:917, 1991.
2. Crisp AH, Palmer RL, and Kalucy RA: How common is anorexia nervosa? A prevalence study. Br J Psychiatry 140:564, 1983.
3. Kendler KS, MacLean C, Neale M, et al: The genetic epidemiology of bulimia nervosa. Am J Psychiatry 148:1627, 1991.
4. Schwartz DM, Thompson MG, and Johnson CL: Anorexia nervosa and bulimia: The sociocultural context. Int J Eating Disorders 1(4):20, 1982.
5. Levenkron S: Treating and Overcoming Anorexia Nervosa. Charles Scribner's Sons, New York, 1982.
6. Smith JE, and Krejei J: Minorities join the majority: Eating disturbances among His-

panic and Native American youth. Int J Eating Disorders 10:179, 1991.

7. Kaye WH, Pickar D, Naber D, et al: Cerebrospinal fluid opioid activity in anorexia nervosa. Am J Psychiatry 139:643, 1982.

8. Appenzeller O: What makes us run. N Engl J Med 305:578, 1981.

9. Diagnostic and Statistical Manual of Mental Disorders, (3rd ed, revised). American Psychiatric Association, Washington, DC, 1987, p 65.

10. Askevold F: The diagnosis of anorexia nervosa. Int J Eating Disorders 2(4):39, 1983.

11. Garfinkel PE, and Garner DM: Anorexia Nervosa—A Multidimensional Perspective. Brenner/Mazel, New York, 1982.

12. Katz JL, and Weiner H: The aberrant reproductive endocrinology of anorexia nervosa. In Weiner H, Hofer MA, and Stunkard AJ (eds): Brain, Behavior, and Bodily Disease. Raven Press, New York, 1981, p 165.

13. Kron L, Katz JL, Gorzynski G, et al: Hyperactivity in anorexia nervosa: A fundamental clinical feature. Compr Psychiatry 19:433, 1978.

14. Lacey JH, Crisp AH, Kalucy RA, et al: Weight gain and the sleeping electroencephalogram: Study of 10 patients with anorexia nervosa. Br Med J 4:556, 1975.

15. Fornari V, Edleman R, and Katz JL: Medication manipulation in bulimia nervosa: An additional diagnostic criteria? Int J Eating Disorders 9:585, 1990.

16. Katz JL: Eating disorders: A primer for the substance abuse specialist (Part 2). J Substance Abuse Treatment 7:211, 1990.

17. Katz JL: Eating disorder and affective disorder: Relatives or merely chance acquaintances? Compr Psychiatry 28:220, 1987.

18. Keys A, Brozek J, Henschel A, et al: The Biology of Human Starvation. University of Minnesota Press, Minneapolis, 1950.

19. Fornari V, Kaplan M, Sandberg DE, et al: Depression and anxiety disorders in anorexia nervosa and bulimia nervosa. Int J Eating Disorders: 12:21, 1992.

20. Joyce JM, Warren DL, Humphries LL, et al: Osteoporosis in women with eating disorders: Comparison of physical parameters, exercise, and menstrual status with SPA and DPA evaluation. J Nucl Med 31:325, 1990.

21. Biller BMK, Saxe V, Herzog DB, et al: Mechanisms of osteoporosis in adult and adolescent women with anorexia nervosa. J Clin Endocrinol Metab 68:548, 1989.

22. Schocken DD, Holloway JD, and Powers PS: Weight loss and heart: Effects of anorexia nervosa and starvation. Arch Intern Med 149:877, 1989.

23. Dolan RJ, Mitchell J, and Wakeling A: Structural brain changes in patients with anorexia nervosa. Psychological Med 18:349, 1988.

24. Krieg JC, Lauer C, and Pirke KM: Structural brain abnormalities in patients with bulimia nervosa. Psychiatry Res 27:39, 1989.

25. Palmer EP, and Guay AT: Reversible myopathy secondary to abuse of ipecac in patients with eating disorders. N Engl J Med 313:457, 1986.

26. Green RS, and Rau JH: Treatment of compulsive eating disturbances with anticonvulsant medication. Am J Psychiatry 131:428, 1974.

27. Pirke KM, Pahl J, and Schweiger U: Metabolic and endocrine indices of starvation in bulimia: A comparison with anorexia nervosa. Psychiatry Res 14:13, 1985.

28. Blouin AG, Blouin JH, Braaten JT, et al: Physiological and psychological responses to a glucose challenge in bulimia. Int J Eating Disorders 10:285, 1991.

29. Kaplan AS: Hyperamylasemia and bulimia: A clinical review. Int J Eating Disorders 6:537, 1987.

30. Mecklenburg RS, Loriaux DL, and Thompson RH: Hypothalamic dysfunction in patients with anorexia nervosa. Medicine 52:147, 1974.

31. Katz JL, and Weiner H: A functional, anterior hypothalamic defect in primary anorexia nervosa? Psychosom Med 37:103, 1975.

32. Wortis J: Irreversible starvation. Biol Psychiatry 20:465, 1985.

33. Newman MM, and Halmi KA: The endocrinology of anorexia nervosa and bulimia nervosa. Endocrinol Metab Clin North Am 17:195, 1988.

34. Andersen AE: Practical Comprehensive Treatment of Anorexia Nervosa and Bulimia. The Johns Hopkins University Press, Baltimore, 1985.

35. Minuchin S, Rosman EL, and Baker L: Psychosomatic Families: Anorexia Nervosa in Context. Harvard University Press, Cambridge, 1978.

36. Herzog DB, Keller MB, Lavori PW, and Kacks NR: The course and outcome of bulimia nervosa. J Clin Psychiatry 52(Suppl):4, 1992.

37. Mitchell JE, Specker SM, and de Zwaan M: Co-morbidity and medical complications of bulimia nervosa. J Clin Psychiatry 52(Suppl):13, 1991.

38. Katz JL: Eating disorders and substance abuse. In Tasman A, Riba MB, and Yager J (eds): The American Psychiatric Press Review of Psychiatry, Vol 11. American Psychiatric Press, Washington, DC, 1992, p 436.

39. Waller JV, Kaufman MR, and Deutsch F: An-

orexia nervosa: Psychosomatic entity. Psychosom Med 2:3, 1940.

40. Bruch H: Eating Disorders: Obesity, Anorexia Nervosa, and the Person Within. Basic Books, New York, 1973.

41. Palazzoli MS: Anorexia nervosa. In Arieti S (ed): The World Biennial of Psychiatry and Psychotherapy, Vol 1. Basic Books, New York/London, 1970, p 197.

42. Abraham S, and Beaumont PJV: Varieties of psychosexual experience in patients with anorexia nervosa. Int J Eating Disorders 1(3):10, 1982.

43. Shulman D: A multitiered view of bulimia. Int J Eating Disorders 10:333, 1991.

44. Johnson C, Lewis C, and Hagman J: The syndrome of bulimia—Review and synthesis. Psychiatr Clin N America 7:247, 1984.

45. Katz JL: Some reflections on the nature of the eating disorders: On the need for humility. Int J Eating Disorders 4:617, 1985.

46. Johnson C, and Connors ME: The Etiology and Treatment of Bulimia Nervosa. Basic Books, New York, 1987.

47. Marcus MD, Wing RR, and Lamparski DM: Binge eating and dietary restraint in obese patients. Addictive Behav 10:163, 1985.

48. Garner DM, and Garfinkel PE (eds): Handbook of Psychotherapy for Anorexia Nervosa and Bulimia. Guilford Press, New York/London, 1985.

49. Blinder EJ, Freeman DMA, and Stunkard AJ: Behavior therapy of anorexia nervosa: Effectiveness of activity as a reinforcer of weight gain. Am J Psychiatry 126:1093, 1970.

50. Walsh BT: Psychopharmacologic treatment of bulimia nervosa. J Clin Psychiatry 52(Suppl):34, 1991.

51. Mitchell PB: The pharmacological management of bulimia nervosa: A critical review. Int J Eating Disorders 7(1):29, 1988.

51a. Hsu LKG: Treatment of bulimia with lithium. Am J Psychiatry 141:1260, 1984.

52. Halmi KA, Eckert E, LaDu TJ, and Cohen J: Anorexia nervosa—Treatment efficacy of cyproheptadine and amitriptyline. Arch Gen Psychiatry 43:177, 1986.

52a. Goldbloom DS: Serotonin in eating disorders. In Garfinkel PE, and Garner DM (eds): The Role of Drug Treatments for Eating Disorders. Brunner/Mazel, New York, 1987, p 124.

53. Katz JL: Long distance running, anorexia nervosa, and bulimia: A report of two cases. Compr Psychiatry 27:74, 1986.

54. Eisler I, and Le Grange D: Excessive exercise and anorexia nervosa. Int J Eating Disorders 9:377, 1990.

55. Yates A, Leehey K, and Shisslak CM: Running—An analogue of anorexia? N Engl J Med 308:251, 1983.

56. Yates A: Compulsive Exercise and the Eating Disorders: Toward an Integrated Theory of Activity. Brunner/Mazel, New York, 1991.

57. Blumenthal JA, O'Toole L, and Chang JL: Is running an analogue of anorexia nervosa? An empirical study of obligatory running and anorexia nervosa. JAMA 252:520, 1984.

58. Smith NJ: Excessive weight loss and food aversion in athletes simulating anorexia nervosa. Pediatrics 66:139, 1980.

59. Owens RB, and Slade PD: Running and anorexia nervosa: An empirical study. Int J Eating Disorders 6:771, 1987.

60. Richert AJ, and Hummers JA: Patterns of physical activity in college students at possible risk for eating disorder. Int J Eating Disorders 5:757, 1986.

61. Warren BJ, Stanton AL, and Blessing DL: Disordered eating patterns in competitive female athletes. Int J Eating Disorders 9:565, 1990.

62. Crago M, Yates A, Beutler LE, and Arimendi TG: Height-weight ratios among female athletes: Are collegiate athletics the precursors to an anorexic syndrome? Int J Eating Disorders 4(1):79, 1985.

63. Weight LM, and Noakes TD: Is running an analogue of anorexia? A survey of the incidence of eating disorders in female distance runners. Med Sci Sports Exerc 19:213, 1987.

64. Epling WJ, Pierce WD, and Stefan L: A theory of activity-based anorexia. Int J Eating Disorders 3(1):27, 1983.

65. Colt EWD, Wardlaw SL, and Frantz AG: The effect of running on plasma β-endorphin. Life Sci 28:1637, 1981.

66. Kaye WH, Gwirtsman HE, Obarzanck E, and George DT: Relative importance of calorie intake needed to gain weight and level of physical activity in anorexia nervosa. Am J Clin Nutr 47:989, 1988.

67. Druss RG, and Silverman JA: Body image and perfectionism of ballerinas: Comparison and contrast with anorexia nervosa. Gen Hosp Psychiatry 1:115, 1979.

68. Garner DM, and Garfinkel PE: Sociocultural factors in the development of anorexia nervosa. Psychol Med 10:647, 1980.

69. Hamilton LH, Brooks-Gunn J, and Warren MP: Sociocultural influences on eating disorders in professional female ballet dancers. Int J Eating Disorders 4:465, 1985.

70. Hamilton LH, Brooks-Gunn J, and Warren MP: Nutritional intake of female dancers: A reflection of eating problems. Int J Eating Disorders 5:925, 1986.

Exercise Following Injury, Surgery, or Infection

I. Exercise Following Breast Trauma or Surgery

CHRISTINE HAYCOCK, M.D.

MINOR TRAUMA

Patients who have minor abrasions or contusions do not require any time away from their athletic endeavors. Wearing a good supportive bra to minimize breast motion will suffice to keep them comfortable, along with a simple analgesic such as ibuprofen or aspirin.

MINOR SURGERY

Following minor surgery, such as a breast biopsy or excision of a small cyst, some limitation of upper arm use, especially throwing or lifting, is indicated for at least 3 to 5 days to allow good cosmetic wound healing. This is in addition to good breast support and analgesics.

If the excision has been deep or extensive, requiring a drain for more than 24 hours, then 5 to 7 days of limited upper arm use may be indicated. This is an individual decision that must be made by the operating surgeon.

If infection is present due to an infected hematoma, or develops postoperatively, then upper arm motion must be restricted until all evidence of infection is gone.

MASTECTOMY

Programs such as "Reach to Recovery," sponsored by the American Cancer Society, have shown the usefulness of exercise in the rehabilitation of the post-mastectomy patient. Fortunately, since radical mastectomics are now performed rarely, most patients do regain their full preoperative range of motion and strength in the ipsilateral arm.

The athlete would be encouraged to begin arm raising at about 4 to 5 days after mastectomy and gradually to increase the motion daily. This routine is true as a matter of fact for all such patients to prevent formation of scar tissue that would limit future motion. However, in an athlete, at about the 2-week point, I would encourage the use of weights, beginning with a pound and gradually increasing, to build back upper arm strength. Squeezing a ball or other device for this purpose is also indicated. A good supervised physical therapy regimen is strongly advocated.

There may be other limitations required for the mastectomy patient if she requires radiation therapy or chemotherapy. These would have to be individually determined, as no set rule is feasible. It would depend on such factors as the amount of radiation given, the duration of the treatment, and the effect on her skin. Certainly, mild exercise would probably be permissible.

REDUCTION OR AUGMENTATION MAMMOPLASTY

Patients who have reduction mammoplasty would be limited in the same manner as mastectomy patients. Exercise would be limited until healing is sufficient such that no drainage or raw areas exist; then the same regimen outlined for mastectomy patients could be followed.

Rehabilitation of the athlete following augmentation mammoplasty should include careful supervision by the plastic surgeon and a physical therapist, for physical and legal reasons. The type and size of the prosthesis used would play a role, especially if a silicone implant was used, since the rupture of such a device may have serious medical implications.

II. Exercise Following Obstetric/Gynecologic Surgery

MONA SHANGOLD, M.D.

When to resume one's exercise program after obstetric or gynecologic surgery is best depicted in the accompanying table.

EARLIEST TIME TO RESUME EXERCISE POSTOPERATIVELY

| | Aerobic Exercise | | | | | |
| | Nonwater Sports | | Water Sports | | Weight Training | |
Procedure	Light	Intense	Light	Intense	Light	Submaximal
D and C; first-trimester abortion	Same or next day	Same or next day	When bleeding has ceased	When bleeding has ceased	Same day	Same day
Vaginal delivery; second-trimester abortion	2 days	2 days	When bleeding has ceased	When bleeding has ceased	Same day	Same day
Diagnostic laparoscopy	1–2 days	1–2 days	1–2 days	1–2 days	1–2 days	1–2 days
Operative laparoscopy	21 days	21 days	21 days	21 days	21 days	21 days
Cesarean delivery; other laparotomy	7 days	21 days	21 days	21 days	7 days	21 days

III. Exercise Following Common Orthopedic Injuries and Operative Procedures

LETHA Y. GRIFFIN, M.D., Ph.D.

ANKLE SPRAIN

The proper time to return to activity following an ankle sprain depends on the severity of the injury. The level of severity is defined by a grading system: grade I refers to pain at the site of ligamentous injury but no laxity; grade II is pain at the site of ligamentous injury with mild laxity; and grade III describes pain at the site of ligamentous injury with significant laxity.

With grade I ankle sprains it may take from several days to several weeks for the patient to return to activity, whereas with grade III ankle sprains it will take a minimum of several weeks and may take up to several months. In grade I liga-mentous injuries about the ankle, initial protection, ice, compression, and ele-vation are followed by rapid rehabilitation, stressing increasing range of motion and strength, along with return of proprioceptive feedback from the ankle. Range of motion is achieved by having the athlete do figure-of-eights and circles with her foot. Rubber tubing can be used as a resistive device for gaining strength in dorsiflexion and plantarflexion and inversion-eversion.

Gains in proprioceptive feedback can often be maximized by having the ath-lete stand on the affected extremity with her eyes closed and relearn how to bal-ance. Also helpful in this regard is a tilt board, a flat board attached to a half circle of wood, on which the athlete tries to balance her weight with the good foot planted on the ground and only partial weight on the injured side, which is on the tilt board. She then gradually increases her weight on the injured side until she has good balance and can stand independently on it. When the athlete has full range of motion and 90% strength and can hop independently on her extrem-ity without pain, she can return to pivotal sports.

The rehabilitation programs for grade II and grade III sprains about the ankle are similar. However, the period of immobilization and protection is longer, to allow for initial healing.

ARTHROMENISCECTOMY

Following an arthromeniscectomy, the athlete is encouraged to ice and ele-vate her extremity for the first 48 hours. This initial period of rest, compression, elevation, and icing helps prevent swelling and, hence, minimizes the time off from sport following this procedure. If after 48 hours the athlete has minimal to no swelling and good range of motion, she can begin strengthening exercises, as well as functional strengthening activities such as biking and swimming (pro-vided sutures are removed), and within several weeks she can begin running. Pivotal activities are usually not allowed for 3 to 4 weeks, until the new meniscal rim has remodeled.

PATELLA-STABILIZATION PROCEDURES

Soft Tissue Releases

Following a soft tissue release for patella stabilization (typically a medial reefing or tightening of the medial muscles, as well as a release of the lateral mus-cles), the athlete's affected limb is initially protected, iced, and elevated for 5 to 7 days. This allows the initial inflammation to diminish. Isometric exercises for the quadriceps, especially the vastus medialis, are encouraged during this period of time. A muscle stimulation unit to maintain the oxidative enzyme con-tents of the involved muscle cells may be beneficial.

Quadriceps-setting exercises and short arc extension exercises are typically begun from 5 days to 2 weeks postoperatively. Biking, swimming, and walking can be begun as soon as the athlete has achieved control of her extremity and has a functional range of motion. Biking is often very useful in increasing range of motion, and therefore is to be encouraged. Return to pivotal sports may not be possible for up to 3 to 6 months, depending on the stability of the repair.

Bony Realignment Procedure for Patella Dislocation

Following a bony realignment of the patella, the timing for initiating range of motion and strengthening exercises is dependent upon the bony fixation device used (e.g., screws, staples, and so on). The period of immobilization varies and should be dictated by the orthopedist.

LUMBAR DISKECTOMY

Immediately following diskectomy, the athlete is encouraged to begin walking in her hospital room, progressing within 7 to 10 days to walking about the home and outside the home, going gradually from 10-minute walks to 30- to 45-minute walks, at an increasing pace. Sutures are removed in 10 to 14 days. If there is not marked swelling or spasm in the paravertebral muscles, the athlete is also encouraged to begin swimming at 2 to 3 weeks following surgery. Swimming, like running, develops abdominal and paravertebral muscle strength and is therefore to be encouraged.

Pivotal sports are generally permitted within 3 to 4 months, as soon as the athlete has good muscle strength and no pain with activities of daily living. General consensus is lacking on whether an athlete should be permitted to return to contact sports following diskectomy. Although many athletes have returned to long-distance running following diskectomy, one should encourage the athlete to choose a sport that does not require such impact loading on the lumbar spine.

BUNIONECTOMY

Bunionectomy is not a "simple" procedure. It frequently necessitates bony realignment of the first metatarsal. A special shoe with a nonflexible wooden sole may be needed to protect the osteotomy while walking. Ambulation can begin soon after the procedure, as long as protection is provided by such an appliance.

When early bony union is seen and pain and swelling have subsided, the hard-soled shoe may be replaced by a comfortable shoe with a nonelevated heel. Within 3 to 4 weeks, the athlete will probably be allowed to return to swimming and biking, as well as to weight-training routines, as long as they do not involve rising up on the toes or impact loading on the feet. Impact-loading activities such as running, soccer, tennis, and so forth should not be permitted until swelling is completely resolved, range of motion of the metatarsophalangeal joint of the great toe is restored, and good bony union is present at the osteotomy site, which may be any time from 3 to 6 months.

REMOVAL OF MORTON'S NEUROMA

The term "Morton's neuroma" refers to painful scarring about the intermetatarsal nerve in the foot. If the neuroma is unresponsive to nonoperative methods such as metatarsal pads, shoe modification, injection of steroids, and local anesthesia, then surgical excision can be accomplished.

Following this procedure, the athlete is instructed to keep the foot elevated for several days to diminish swelling. Within 3 to 4 days, she can be performing normal, routine activities. However, if foot swelling occurs when she attempts to do so, further elevation is necessary. Generally, swelling has resolved by the second or third week. If the athlete is pain-free, swimming and biking are then permitted. It may be 3 to 6 weeks before the athlete can resume running and pivotal activities without discomfort.

IV. Exercise Following an Infection

GABE MIRKIN, M.D.

It is probably all right to exercise during a systemic infection, provided that the athlete is afebrile and does not have myalgia before exercising. These same criteria should be used to determine when to return to exercising after recovering from an infection. However, each case should be decided on its own merits, rather than by general rules.

Exercising with a fever increases cardiac output far beyond exercising with a normal body temperature. The heart must pump extra blood to skin to prevent heat build-up, in addition to its usual tasks of supplying oxygen and nutrients to exercising muscle. Some viruses that infect the respiratory tract can also infect the myocardium.[1] The combination of increased workload and viral myocarditis can result in a fatal arrhythmia.[2]

When skeletal muscles are infected by respiratory viruses, they usually hurt during exercise. Exercising when muscles hurt markedly increases susceptibility to injury. Infected muscles have reduced strength[3] and endurance[4] and decreased levels of necessary enzymes such as glyceraldehyde 3-phosphate dehydrogenase.[5]

REFERENCES

1. Burch JA: Viral diseases of the heart. Acta Cardiol 1:5, 1979.
2. Roberts JA: Viral illnesses and sports performance. Sports Med 3:296, 1986.
3. Friman G: Effect of acute infectious disease on isometric muscle strength. Scand J Clin Lab Invest 37:303, 1977.
4. Arnold DL: Excessive intracellular acidosis of skeletal muscle on exercise in a patient with post-viral exhaustion syndrome. Lancet 1:1367, 1984.
5. Astrom E: Effect of viral and mycoplasma infections on ultrastructure and enzyme activities in human skeletal muscle. Acta Pathol Microbiol Immunol Scand 84:113, 1976.

Index

Page numbers followed by F indicate figures; page numbers followed by T indicate tables

Printed in the United Kingdom
by Lightning Source UK Ltd.
122446UK00001BA/2/A